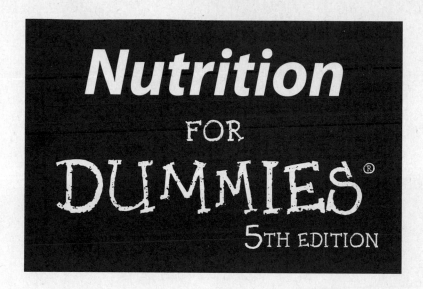

Nutrition

FOR

DUMMIES®

5TH EDITION

by Carol Ann Rinzler

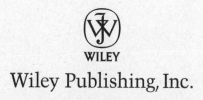

WILEY

Wiley Publishing, Inc.

Nutrition For Dummies®, 5th Edition

Published by
Wiley Publishing, Inc.
111 River St.
Hoboken, NJ 07030-5774
www.wiley.com

Copyright © 2011 by Wiley Publishing, Inc., Indianapolis, Indiana

Published by Wiley Publishing, Inc., Indianapolis, Indiana

Published simultaneously in Canada

For general information on our other products and services, please contact our Customer Care Department within the U.S. at 877-762-2974, outside the U.S. at 317-572-3993, or fax 317-572-4002.

For technical support, please visit www.wiley.com/techsupport.

Wiley also publishes its books in a variety of electronic formats. Some content that appears in print may not be available in electronic books.

Library of Congress Control Number: 2011927298

ISBN: 978-0-470-93231-5

ISBN 978-0-470-93231-5 (pbk); ISBN 978-1-118-09303-0 (ebk); ISBN 978-1-118-09304-7 (ebk); ISBN 978-1-118-09305-4 (ebk)

Manufactured in the United States of America

10 9 8 7 6 5 4 3 2

WILEY

About the Author

Carol Ann Rinzler is the author of more than 20 books on health and nutrition as well as columns for several newspapers and national magazines.

Dedication

For my husband, Perry Luntz. Always.

Author's Acknowledgments

In writing this book, I am indebted to those who took time to share with me their knowledge and expertise. Akiva Cohen of the University of Pennsylvania, School of Medicine and the Children's Hospital, Philadelphia; Roger Hartl of Weill Cornell Medical College; and Alex Bekker, Kalman Rubinson, and Donald Wilson of NYU Langone Medical Center–NYU School of Medicine, were each kind enough to read and comment on portions of this manuscript. Mel Rosenfeld, also of NYU Langone, generously opened for me the door to the extraordinary world of neuroscience

USDA FSIS Consumer Safety Officer Peter Duryea provided clarity on consumer safety issues. John S. Webster, Director, Public and Governmental Affairs, USDA Center for Nutrition Policy and Promotion was an invaluable guide to the Dietary Guidelines for Americans. Barbara Kloberdanz, Minna Elias, and Jeffrey Kolodny offered their welcome support.

As with previous editions of *Nutrition For Dummies,* once again, I am grateful to my technical editor Alfred Bushway of the University of Maine's Department of Food Science and Human Nutrition for his graceful, thorough and thoughtful editing. The same is true of the skilled and pleasant professionals at Wiley Publishing. Acquisitions Editor Michael Lewis shepherded the project from idea to completion; Project Editor Kelly Ewing kept things moving smoothly even through the inevitable crises; and Project Coordinator Sheree Montgomery handled the Composition side of things.

To each of these people, my thanks.

Publisher's Acknowledgments

We're proud of this book; please send us your comments at http://dummies.custhelp.com. For other comments, please contact our Customer Care Department within the U.S. at 877-762-2974, outside the U.S. at 317-572-3993, or fax 317-572-4002.

Some of the people who helped bring this book to market include the following:

Acquisitions, Editorial, and Media Development

Project Editor: Kelly Ewing

Acquisitions Editor: Michael Lewis

Copy Editor: Kelly Ewing

Assistant Editor: David Lutton

General Reviewer: Alfred Bushway

Senior Editorial Manager: Jennifer Ehrlich

Editorial Supervisor and Reprint Editor: Carmen Krikorian

Editorial Assistant: Jennette ElNaggar

Art Coordinator: Alicia B. South

Cover Photos: © istockphoto.com/ Elena Schweitzer

Cartoons: Rich Tennant (www.the5thwave.com)

Composition Services

Project Coordinator: Sheree Montgomery

Layout and Graphics: Claudia Bell, Andrea Hornberger, Corrie Socolovitch

Proofreaders: Laura Albert, Laura Bowman

Indexer: Becky Hornyak

Illustrator: Liz Kurtzman

Publishing and Editorial for Consumer Dummies

Kathleen Nebenhaus, Vice President and Executive Publisher

Kristin Ferguson-Wagstaffe, Product Development Director

Ensley Eikenburg, Associate Publisher, Travel

Kelly Regan, Editorial Director, Travel

Publishing for Technology Dummies

Andy Cummings, Vice President and Publisher

Composition Services

Debbie Stailey, Director of Composition Services

Table of Contents

Contents at a Glance

Part II: What You Get from Food........................ 73

Introduction

The first edition of *Nutrition For Dummies* in 1997 began by noting that once upon a time, people simply sat down to dinner, eating to fill up an empty stomach or just for the pleasure of it. Nobody said, "Wow, that cream soup is loaded with calories," or asked whether the bread was a high-fiber loaf or fretted about the chicken being served with the skin still on. No longer. Today, the dinner table can be a battleground between health and pleasure. You plan your meals with the precision of a major general moving his troops into the front lines, and for most people, the fight to eat what's good for you rather than what tastes good has become a lifelong struggle.

The four editions since then have added new information designed to end the war between your need for good nutrition and your equally compelling need for tasty meals, with the facts and figures from nutrition researchers who continue to make it ever more clear that what's good for you can also be good to eat — and vice versa.

About This Book

Nutrition For Dummies, 5th Edition, doesn't aim to send you back to the class-room, sit you down, and make you take notes about what to put on the table every day from now until you're 104 years old. You're reading a reference book, so you don't have to memorize anything — when you want more info, just jump in anywhere to look it up.

Instead, this book means to give you the information you need to make wise food choices — which always means choices that please the palate and soul, as well as the body. Some of what you'll read here is really, *really* basic: definitions of vitamins, minerals, proteins, fats, carbohydrates, and, yes, plain (and not so plain) water. You'll also read tips about how to put together a nutritious shopping list and how to use food to make meals so good you can't wait to eat them.

For those who know absolutely nothing about nutrition except that it deals with food, this book is a starting point. For those who know more than a little about nutrition, this book is a refresher course to bring you up to speed on what has happened since the last time you checked out a calorie chart.

For those who want to know *absolutely everything,* this 5th edition of *Nutrition For Dummies* is up to date, with hot new info from the 2010 revisions of the *Dietary Guidelines for Americans,* new recommended daily allowances for all the nutrients a healthy body needs, plus all the twisty "this is good for you" and "this is not" bits and pieces of food info that nutrition scientists have come up with since, well, the last edition.

Conventions Used in This Book

The following conventions are used throughout the text to make things consistent and easy to understand:

- All Web addresses appear in `monofont`.
- New terms appear in *italic* and are closely followed by an easy-to-understand definition.
- **Bold** is used to highlight the action parts of numbered steps, as well as key words in bulleted lists.
- Nutrition experts commonly use metric terms such as gram (g), milligram (mg), and microgram (mcg) to describe quantities of protein, fat, carbohydrates, vitamins, minerals, and other nutrients.

What You Don't Have to Read

What? Not read something printed in a book? Well, yeah. Some small parts of this book are fun or informative but not necessarily vital to your understanding of nutrition. For example:

- **Text in sidebars:** The sidebars are the shaded boxes that appear here and there. They share personal stories and observations but aren't necessary reading.
- **Anything with a Technical Stuff icon attached:** This information is interesting but not critical to your understanding of nutrition.
- **The stuff on the copyright page:** No kidding. You'll find nothing here of interest unless you're inexplicably enamored by legal language and Library of Congress numbers.

Foolish Assumptions

Every book is written with a particular reader in mind, and this one is no different. As I wrote this book, I made the following basic assumptions about who you are and why you plunked down your hard-earned cash for an entire volume about nutrition:

  ✔ You didn't study nutrition in high school or college and now you've discovered that you have a better shot at staying healthy if you know how to put together well-balanced, nutritious meals.

  ✔ You're confused by conflicting advice on vitamins and minerals, protein, fats, and carbs. In other words, you need a reliable road map through the nutrient maze.

  ✔ You want basic information, but you don't want to become an expert in nutrition or spend hours digging your way through medical textbooks and journals.

How This Book Is Organized

The following is a brief summary of each part in *Nutrition For Dummies,* 5th Edition. You can use this guide as a fast way to check out what you want to read first. One really nice thing about this book is that you don't have to start with Chapter 1 and read straight through to the end. *Au contraire,* as the French like to say when they mean "on the contrary," you can dive in absolutely anywhere and still come up with tons of tasty information about how food helps your body work.

Part 1: The Basic Facts about Nutrition

Chapter 1 defines nutrition and its effects on your body. This chapter also tells you how to read a nutrition study and how to judge the value of nutrition information in newspapers, magazines, and on TV. Chapter 2 is a really clear guide to how your digestive system works to transform food and beverages into the nutrients you need to sustain a healthy body. Chapter 3 concentrates on calories, the energy factor in food and beverages. Chapter 4 covers the present state of the average American body which is larger than it should be. Chapter 5 tells you how much of each nutrient you need to stay in tiptop form. Chapter 6 details some of the rules on dietary supplements — the pills, powders, and potions that add nutritional punch to your regular diet.

Part II: What You Get from Food

Chapter 7 gives you the facts about protein: where you get it and what it does in your body. Chapter 8 does the same job for dietary fat, while Chapter 9 explains carbohydrates: sugars, starches, and dietary fiber, the indigestible but totally vital substance in carbohydrate foods. Chapter 10 outlines the risks and — surprise! — some newly proven benefits of alcohol beverages.

Chapter 11 is about vitamins, the substances in food that trigger so many vital chemical reactions in your body. Chapter 12 is about minerals, substances that often work in tandem with vitamins. Chapter 13 is about water, the essential liquid that comprises as much as 70 percent of your body weight. This chapter also describes the functions of electrolytes, special minerals that maintain your fluid balance (the correct amount of water inside and outside your body cells).

Part III: Healthy Eating

Chapter 14 is about *hunger* (the need for food) and *appetite* (the desire for food). Balancing these two eating factors makes maintaining a healthful weight possible for you. Chapter 15 on the other hand, is about food preference: why you like some foods and really, really hate others. (Broccoli, anyone?) Chapter 16 tells you how to assemble a healthful diet. It's based on the *Dietary Guidelines for Americans* created by the U.S. Departments of Agriculture and Health and Human Services, plus some recent updates from the National Academy of Sciences' Institute of Medicine, so you know it's good for you. Chapter 17 explains how to use nutritional guidelines to plan nutritious, appetizing meals at home. Chapter 18 shows you how to take the guidelines out to dinner so that you can judge the value of foods in all kinds of restaurants, from the posh white-tablecloth ones to fast-food havens.

Part IV: Food Processing

Chapter 19 asks and answers this simple question: What is food processing? Chapter 20 shows you how cooking affects the way food looks and tastes, as well as its nutritional value. Chapter 21 does the same for freezing, canning, drying, and irradiating techniques. Chapter 22 gives you the lowdown on chemicals used to keep food fresh, safe, and appetizing.

Part V: Food and Medicine

Chapter 23 explains why some food gives some people hives and presents strategies for identifying and avoiding the food to which you may be allergic. Chapter 24 focuses on how what you eat affects your brain at every stage of life. Chapter 25 tells you how foods may interact with medical drugs — an important subject for anyone who ever has taken, now takes, or ever plans to take medicine. Chapter 26 tells you how some foods may actually act as preventive medicine or relieve the symptoms of certain illnesses ranging from the horrible-but-not-really-serious common cold to the Big Two: heart disease and cancer.

Part VI: The Part of Tens

Could there even be a *For Dummies* book without The Part of Tens? Not a chance. This part (Chapters 27, 28, 29, and 30) provides ten great nutritional Web site addresses, lists ten common foods with near-magical status and ten healthful foods beginning with the letter "P," and last — but definitely not least — lays out ten easy ways to cut calories from food.

Icons Used in This Book

Icons are a handy *For Dummies* way to catch your attention as you slide your eyes down the page. The icons come in several varieties, each with its own special meaning:

Nutrition is full of stuff that "everybody knows." This masked marvel clues you in to the real facts when (as often happens) everybody's wrong!

This time, the same smart fella is pointing to clear, concise explanations of technical terms and processes — details that are interesting but not necessarily critical to your understanding of a topic. In other words, skip them if you want, but try a few first.

Bull's-eye! This is time- and stress-saving information that you can use to improve your diet and health.

This is a watch-out-for-the-curves icon, alerting you to nutrition pitfalls such as (oops!) leaving the skin on the chicken — turning a lowfat food into one that is high in fat and cholesterol. This icon also warns you about physical dangers such as supplements to avoid because they may do more damage than good to your health.

Where to Go from Here

For Dummies books are not linear (proceeding from Chapter 1 to 2 to 3 and so on). In fact, you can dive right in anywhere, say at L, M, or N, and still make sense of what you're reading because each chapter delivers a complete message.

For example, if proteins are your passion, go right to Chapter 7. If you want to know why you absolutely cannot resist chocolate-covered pretzels, go to Chapter 15. If you're fascinated by food processing, your choice is Chapter 19. Use the table of contents to find broad categories of information or the index to look up more specific things.

On the other hand, if you're not sure where you want to go, why not just begin at the beginning, Part I, Chapter 1? It gives you all the basic info you need to understand nutrition and points to places where you can find more detailed information.

Part I
The Basic Facts about Nutrition

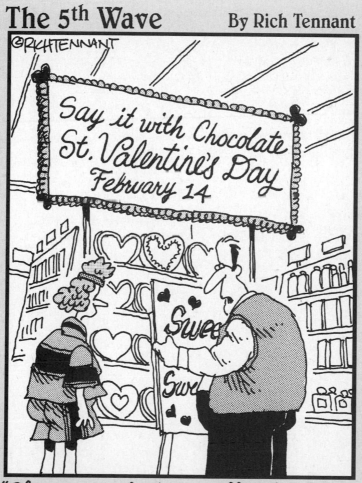

"Of course you're better off eating grains and vegetables, but for St. Valentine's Day, we've never been very successful with 'Say it with Legumes.'"

In this part . . .

To use food wisely, you need a firm grasp of the basics. This part defines nutrition and offers a detailed explanation of digestion (how your body turns food into nutrients). It also documents the expansion of the average American body, explains why calories are useful, and sets forth a no-nonsense starter guide to your daily requirements of vitamins, minerals, and other good stuff.

Chapter 1

What's Nutrition, Anyway?

You are *what* you eat. You are also *how* you eat. And *when* you eat.

Choosing a varied diet of healthful foods supports any healthy mind and body, but *which* healthful foods you choose says much about your personal tastes as well as the culture from which you come.

How you eat may do the same: Do you use a knife and fork? A pair of sticks? Your hands and a round of bread? Each is a cultural statement. As for *when* you eat (and when you stop), that is a purely personal physiological response to signals from your digestive organs and your brain: "Get food now!" or "Thank you, that's enough."

If you read chapter by chapter through this book, you can follow what you eat and drink as it moves from your plate to your mouth to your digestive tract and into every tissue and cell. Along the way, you discover how your organs and systems work. You observe firsthand why some foods and beverages are essential to your health. And you find out how to manage your diet so that you can get the biggest bang (nutrients) for your buck (calories).

Nutrition Equals Life

Technically speaking, *nutrition* is the science of how the body uses food. In fact, nutrition is life. All living things, including you, need food and water to live. Beyond that, you need good food, meaning food with the proper nutrients, to live well. If you don't eat and drink, you'll die. Period. If you don't eat and drink nutritious food and beverages:

- ✔ Your bones may bend or break (not enough calcium).
- ✔ Your gums may bleed (not enough vitamin C).
- ✔ Your blood may not carry oxygen to every cell (not enough iron).

And on, and on, and on. Understanding how good nutrition protects you against these dire consequences requires a familiarity with the language and concepts of nutrition. Knowing some basic chemistry is helpful. (Don't panic: Chemistry can be a cinch when you read about it in plain English.) A smattering of sociology and psychology is also useful because although nutrition is mostly about how food revs up and sustains your body, it's also about the cultural traditions and individual differences that explain how you choose your favorite foods (see Chapter 15).

To sum it up: Nutrition is about why you eat what you eat and how the food you get affects your body and your health.

First principles: Energy and nutrients

Nutrition's primary task is figuring out which foods and beverages (in what quantities) provide the energy and building material you need to construct and maintain every organ and system. To do this, nutrition concentrates on food's two basic attributes: energy and nutrients.

Energy from food

Energy is the ability to do work. Virtually every bite of food gives you energy, even when it doesn't give you nutrients. The amount of energy in food is measured in *calories,* the amount of heat produced when food is burned (metabolized) in your body cells. You can read all about calories in Chapter 3. But right now, all you need to know is that food is the fuel on which your body runs. Without enough food, you don't have enough energy.

Nutrients in food

Nutrients are chemical substances your body uses to build, maintain, and repair tissues. They also empower cells to send messages back and forth to conduct essential chemical reactions, such as the ones that make it possible for you to

- ✔ Breathe
- ✔ Move
- ✔ Eliminate waste
- ✔ Think

- ✔ See
- ✔ Hear
- ✔ Smell
- ✔ Taste

. . . and do everything else natural to a living body.

Food provides two distinct groups of nutrients:

- ✔ **Macronutrients (macro = big):** Protein, fat, carbohydrates, and water
- ✔ **Micronutrients (micro = small):** Vitamins and minerals

What's the difference between these two groups? The amount you need each day. Your daily requirements for macronutrients generally exceed 1 gram. (For comparison's sake, 28 grams equal 1 ounce.) For example, the average man needs about 63 grams of protein a day (slightly more than 2 ounces), and the average woman needs about 50 grams (slightly less than 2 ounces).

Your daily requirements for micronutrients are much smaller. For example, the Recommended Dietary Allowance (RDA) for vitamin C is measured in milligrams ($\frac{1}{1,000}$ of a gram), while the RDAs for vitamin D, vitamin B12, and folate are even smaller and are measured in micrograms ($\frac{1}{1,000,000}$ of a gram). You can find out much more about the RDAs, including how they vary for people of different ages, in Chapter 4.

What's an essential nutrient?

A reasonable person may assume that an essential nutrient is one you need to sustain a healthy body. But who says a reasonable person thinks like a nutritionist? In nutritionspeak, an *essential nutrient* is a very special thing:

✔ **An essential nutrient cannot be manufactured in the body.** You have to get essential nutrients from food or from a nutritional supplement.

✔ **An essential nutrient is linked to a specific deficiency disease.** For example, people who go without protein for extended periods of time develop the protein-deficiency disease *kwashiorkor*. People who don't get enough vitamin C develop the vitamin C–deficiency disease *scurvy*. A diet rich in the essential nutrient cures the deficiency disease, but you need the proper nutrient. In other words, you can't cure a protein deficiency with extra amounts of vitamin C.

Not all nutrients are essential for all species of animals. For example, vitamin C is an essential nutrient for human beings but not for dogs. A dog's body makes the vitamin C it needs. Check out the list of nutrients on a can or bag of dog food. See? No C. The dog already has the C it — sorry, he or she — requires.

Essential nutrients for human beings include many well-known vitamins and minerals, several *amino acids* (the so-called building blocks of proteins), and at least two fatty acids. For more about these essential nutrients, see Chapters 6, 7, 11, and 12.

Protecting the nutrients in your food

Identifying nutrients is one thing. Making sure you get them into your body is another. Here, the essential idea is to keep nutritious food nutritious by preserving and protecting its components.

Some people see the term *food processing* as a nutritional dirty word. Or words. They're wrong. Without food processing and preservatives, you and I would still be forced to gather (or kill) our food each morning and down it fast before it spoiled. For more about which processing and preservative techniques produce the safest, most nutritious — and yes, delicious — dinners, check out Part IV.

Considering how vital food preservation can be, you may want to think about when you last heard a rousing cheer for the anonymous cook who first noticed that salting or pickling food could extend food's shelf life. Or for the guys who invented the refrigeration and freezing techniques that slow food's natural tendency to degrade (translation: spoil). Or for Louis Pasteur, the man who made it ab-so-lute-ly clear that heating food to boiling kills bugs (translation: microorganisms) that might otherwise cause food poisoning. Hardly ever, that's when. So give them a hand, right here. Cool.

Essential nutrients for Fido, Fluffy, and your pet petunia

Vitamin C isn't the only nutrient that's essential for one species but not for others. Many organic compounds (substances similar to vitamins) and elements (minerals) are essential for your green or furry friends but not for you because you can synthesize them from the food you eat.

One good example is the organic compound myoinositol. *Myoinositol* is an essential nutrient for gerbils and rats who cannot make it in their own bodies and thus must get what they need from food. Human beings, on the other hand, synthesize myoinositol naturally and then use it in many body processes, such as transmitting signals between cells.

Here's a handy list of nutrients that are essential for (some) animals and/or plants but not for you:

Organic Compounds	*Elements*
Carnitine	Arsenic
Myoinositol	Cadmium
Taurine	Lead
	Nickel
	Silicon
	Tin
	Vanadium

Other interesting substances in food

The latest flash in the nutrition sky is caused by phytochemicals. *Phyto* is the Greek word for plants, so *phytochemicals* are simply — yes, you've got it — chemicals from plants. Although the 13-letter group name may be new to you, you're already familiar with some phytochemicals. Pigments such as beta carotene, the deep yellow coloring in fruits and vegetables that your body can convert to a form of vitamin A, are phytochemicals.

And then there are *phytoestrogens,* hormone-like chemicals that grabbed the spotlight when it was suggested that a diet high in phytoestrogens, such as the isoflavones found in soybeans, may lower the risk of heart disease and reduce the incidence of reproductive cancers (cancers of the breast, ovary, uterus, and prostate). More recent studies suggest that phytoestrogens may have some problems of their own, so to find out more about phytochemicals, including phytoestrogens, check out Chapter 22.

You are what you eat

Oh boy, I bet you've heard this one before. But it bears repeating, because the human body really is built from the nutrients it gets from food: water, protein, fat, carbohydrates, vitamins, and minerals. On average, when you step on the scale

- About 60 percent of your weight is water.
- About 20 percent of your weight is fat.
- About 20 percent of your weight is a combination of mostly protein (especially in your muscles) plus carbohydrates, minerals, and vitamins.

An easy way to remember your body's percentage of water, fat, and protein and other nutrients is to think of it as the "60-20-20 Rule."

What's a body made of?

Sugar and spice and everything nice . . . Oops. What I meant to say was the human body is made of water and fat and protein and carbohydrates and vitamins and minerals.

On average, when you step on the scale, approximately 60 percent of your weight is water, 20 percent is body fat (slightly less for a man), and 20 percent is a combination of mostly protein, plus carbohydrates, minerals, vitamins, and other naturally occurring biochemicals.

Based on these percentages, you can reasonably expect that an average 140-pound person's body weight consists of about

- 84 pounds of water
- 28 pounds of body fat
- 28 pounds of a combination of protein (up to 25 pounds), minerals (up to 7 pounds), carbohydrates (up to 1.4 pounds), and vitamins (a trace).

Yep, you're right: Those last figures do total more than 28 pounds. That's because "up to" (as in "up to 25 pounds of protein") means that the amounts may vary from person to person. Ditto for minerals and carbohydrates.

For example, a young person's body has proportionately more muscle and less fat than an older person's, while a woman's body has proportionately less muscle and more fat than a man's. As a result, more of a man's weight comes from protein and muscle and bone mass, while more of a woman's weight comes from fat. Protein-packed muscles and mineral-packed bones are denser tissue than fat.

Weigh a man and a woman of roughly the same height and size, and his greater bone and muscle mass means he's likely to tip the scale higher every time.

The National Research Council, Recommended Dietary Allowances (Washington D.C.: National Academy Press, 1989); Sharon Rady Rolfes, Kathryn Pinna, Ellie Whitney, Understanding Normal and Clinical Nutrition, 7th edition (Belmont CA: Thomson Wadsworth, 2006)

Your nutritional status

Nutritional status is a phrase that describes the state of your health as related to your diet. For example, people who are starving do not get the nutrients or calories they need for optimum health. These people are said to be *malnourished* (mal = bad), which means their nutritional status is, to put it gently, definitely not good. Malnutrition may arise from

- ✔ **A diet that doesn't provide enough food.** This situation can occur in times of famine or through voluntary starvation because of an eating disorder or because something in your life disturbs your appetite. For example, older people may be at risk of malnutrition because of tooth loss or age-related loss of appetite or because they live alone and sometimes just forget to eat.

- ✔ **A diet that, while otherwise adequate, is deficient in a specific nutrient.** This kind of nutritional inadequacy can lead to — surprise! — a deficiency disease, such as beriberi, the disease caused by a lack of vitamin B1 (thiamine).

- ✔ **A metabolic disorder or medical condition that prevents your body from absorbing specific nutrients, such as carbohydrates or protein.** One common example is diabetes, the inability to produce enough insulin, the hormone your body uses to metabolize (digest) carbohydrates. Another is celiac disease, a condition that makes it impossible for the body to digest gluten, a protein in wheat. Need more info on either diabetes or celiac disease? Check out *Diabetes For Dummies,* 2nd Edition, by Alan L. Rubin, MD, and *Living Gluten-Free For Dummies,* by Danna Korn (both published by Wiley — of course).

Doctors and registered dieticians have many tools with which to rate your nutritional status. For example, they can

- ✔ Review your medical history to see whether you have any conditions (such as dentures) that may make eating certain foods difficult or that interfere with your ability to absorb nutrients.

- ✔ Perform a physical examination to look for obvious signs of nutritional deficiency, such as dull hair and eyes (a lack of vitamins?), poor posture (not enough calcium to protect the spinal bones?), or extreme thinness (not enough food? An underlying disease?).

- ✔ Order laboratory blood and urine tests that may identify early signs of malnutrition, such as the lack of red blood cells that characterizes anemia caused by an iron deficiency.

At every stage of life, the aim of a good diet is to maintain a healthy nutritional status.

Fitting food into the medicine chest

Food is medicine for the body and the soul. Good meals make good friends, and modern research validates the virtues of not only Granny's chicken soup but also heart-healthy sulfur compounds in garlic and onions, anticholesterol dietary fiber in grains and beans, bone-building calcium in milk and greens, and mood elevators in coffee, tea, and chocolate.

Of course, foods pose some risks as well: food allergies, food intolerances, food and drug interactions, and the occasional harmful substances such as the dreaded *saturated fats* and *trans fats* (quick — Chapter 8!). In other words, constructing a healthful diet can mean tailoring food choices to your own special body. Not to worry: You can do it. Especially after reading through Part V. Would a *For Dummies* book leave you unarmed? Not a chance!

Finding Nutrition Facts

Getting reliable information about nutrition can be a daunting challenge. For the most part, your nutrition information is likely to come from TV and radio talk shows or news, your daily newspaper, your favorite magazine, a variety of nutrition-oriented books, and the Internet. How can you tell whether what you hear or read is really right?

Nutritional people

The people who make nutrition news may be scientists, reporters, or simply someone who wandered in with a new theory (Artichokes prevent cancer! Never eat cherries and cheese at the same meal! Vitamin C gives you hives!), the more bizarre the better. But several groups of people are most likely to give you news you can use with confidence. For example:

- **Nutrition scientists:** These are people with graduate degrees (usually in chemistry, biology, biochemistry, or physics) engaged in research dealing primarily with the effects of food on animals and human beings.

- **Nutrition researchers:** Researchers may be either nutrition scientists or professionals in another field, such as medicine or sociology, whose research (study or studies) concentrates on the effects of food.

- ✔ **Nutritionists:** These are people who concentrate on the study of nutrition. In some states, a person who uses the title "nutritionist" must have a graduate degree in basic science courses related to nutrition.

- ✔ **Dietitians:** These people have undergraduate degrees in food and nutrition science or the management of food programs. A person with the letters R.D. after his or her name has completed a dietetic internship and passed an American Dietetic Association licensing exam.

- ✔ **Nutrition reporters and writers:** These are people who specialize in giving you information about the medical and/or scientific aspects of food. Like reporters who concentrate on politics or sports, nutrition reporters gain their expertise through years of covering their beat. Most have the science background required to translate technical information into language nonscientists can understand; some have been trained as dietitians, nutritionists, or nutrition scientists.

Consumer alert: Regardless of the source, nutrition news should always pass what you may call *The Reasonableness Test*. In other words, if a story or report or study sounds ridiculous, it probably is.

The next section offers some guidelines for evaluating nutrition studies.

Can you trust this study?

You open your morning newspaper or turn on the evening news and read or hear that a group of researchers at an impeccably prestigious scientific organization has published a study showing that yet another thing you've always taken for granted is hazardous to your health. For example, the study says drinking coffee stresses your heart, adding salt to food raises blood pressure, or fatty foods increase your risk of cancer or heart disease.

So you throw out the offending food or drink or rearrange your daily routine to avoid the once-acceptable, now-dangerous food, beverage, or additive. And then what happens? Two weeks, two months, or two years down the road, a second, equally prestigious group of scientists publishes a study conclusively proving that the first group got it wrong: In fact, this study shows coffee has no effect on the risk of heart disease — and may even improve athletic performance; salt does not cause hypertension except in certain sensitive individuals; only *some* fatty foods are risky.

Who's right? Nobody seems to know. That leaves you, a layperson, on your own to come up with the answer. Never fear — you may not be a nutritionist, but that doesn't mean you can't apply a few common-sense rules to any study you read about, rules that say, "Yes, this may be true," or "No, this may not be."

Does this study include human beings?

True, animal studies can alert researchers to potential problems, but working with animals alone cannot give you conclusive proof.

Different species react differently to various chemicals and diseases. For example, although cows and horses can digest grass and hay, human beings can't. And while outright poisons such as cyanide clearly traumatize any living body, many foods or drugs that harm a laboratory rat won't harm you. And vice versa. For example, mouse and rat embryos suffer no ill effects when their mothers are given thalidomide, the sedative that's known to cause deformed fetal limbs when given to pregnant monkeys — and human beings — at the point in pregnancy when limbs are developing. (And here's an astounding turn: Modern research shows that thalidomide is beneficial for treating or preventing *human* skin problems related to Hansen's disease [leprosy], cancer, and/or autoimmune conditions, such as rheumatoid arthritis, in which the body mistakenly attacks its own tissues.)

Are enough people in this study?

Hey, researchers' saying, "Well, I did give this to a couple of people," is simply not enough. The study must include sufficient numbers and a variety of individuals, too. If you don't have enough people in the study — several hundred to many thousand — to establish a pattern, there's always the possibility that an effect occurred by chance.

If you don't include different types of people, which generally means young and old men and women of different racial and ethnic groups, your results may not apply across the board. For example, the original studies linking high blood cholesterol levels to an increased risk of heart disease and linking small doses of aspirin to a reduced risk of a second heart attack involved only men. It wasn't until follow-up studies were conducted with women that researchers were able to say with any certainty that high cholesterol is dangerous and aspirin is protective for women as well — but not in quite the same way: In January 2006, the *Journal of the American Medical Association* reported that men taking low dose aspirin tend to lower their risk of heart attack. For women, the aspirin reduces the risk of stroke. Vive la difference!

Is there anything in the design or method of this study that may affect the accuracy of its conclusions?

Some testing methods are more likely to lead to biased or inaccurate conclusions. For example, a retrospective study (which asks people to tell what they did in the past) is always considered less accurate than a prospective study (one that follows people while they're actually doing what the researchers are studying), because memory isn't always accurate. People tend to forget details or, without meaning to, alter them to fit the researchers' questions.

Was this study reviewed by the author's peers?

Serious researchers subject their studies to review by others working in the same field, a process called *peer review*. All reliable scientific journals have studies reviewed before they're published.

Are the study's conclusions reasonable?

When a study comes up with a conclusion that seems illogical to you, chances are the researchers feel the same way. For example, in 1990, the long-running Nurses' Study at the Harvard School of Public Health reported that a high-fat diet raised the risk of colon cancer. But the data showed a link only to diets high in beef. No link was found to diets high in dairy fat. In short, this study was begging for a second study to confirm (or deny) its results, and in 2005, a large study of more than 60,000 Swedish women, reported in the *American Journal of Clinical Nutrition,* showed that eating lots of high-fat dairy foods actually reduced the risk of colorectal cancer.

Finally, the nature of life is a continuing surprise. Even in nutrition. Consider dioxin, a toxic contaminant found in some fish. Consider Olestra, the calorie-free fat substitute that makes some tummies rumble. As you read this page, dioxin's still a bad actor, but in 2005, researchers at the University of Cincinnati and the University of Western Australia announced that eating foods containing Olestra may speed your body's elimination of — you guessed it — dioxin.

Chapter 2

Digestion: The 24/7 Food Factory

*W*hen you see (or smell) something appetizing, your digestive organs leap into action. Your mouth waters. Your stomach contracts. Intestinal glands begin to secrete the chemicals that turn food into the nutrients that build new tissues and provide the energy you need to keep zipping through the days, months, and years.

This chapter provides a basic primer on the digestive system and explains exactly how your body digests the many different kinds of foods you eat, all the while extracting the nutrients you need to keep on truckin'.

Introducing the Digestive System

Your *digestive system* is a collection of organs specifically designed to turn complex substances (food) into basic components (nutrients) during the two-part process known as *digestion*.

The digestive organs

Although exceedingly well organized, your digestive system is basically one long tube that starts at your mouth, continues down through your throat to your stomach, and then goes on to your small and large intestines and past the rectum to end at your anus.

In between, with the help of the liver, pancreas, and gallbladder, the usable (digestible) parts of everything that you eat are converted to simple compounds that your body can easily absorb to burn for energy or to build new tissue. The indigestible residue is bundled off and eliminated as waste.

Figure 2-1 shows the body parts and organs that comprise your digestive system.

Digestion: A two-part process

Digestion is a two-part process — half mechanical, half chemical:

✔ *Mechanical digestion* takes place in your mouth and your stomach. Your teeth break food into small pieces that you can swallow without choking. In your stomach and small intestine, a churning action called *peristalsis* continues to break food into smaller particles.

✔ *Chemical digestion* occurs at every point in the digestive tract where enzymes and other substances, such as *hydrochloric acid* (from stomach glands) and *bile* (from the liver), dissolve food, releasing the nutrients inside.

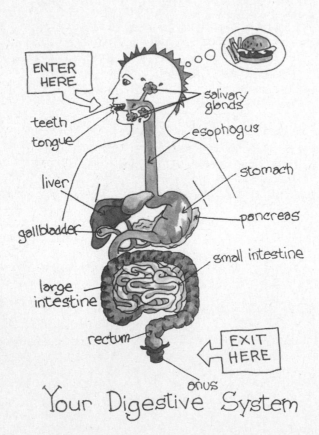

Figure 2-1:
Your digestive system in all its glory.

Understanding How Your Body Digests Food

Each organ in the digestive system plays a specific role in the digestive drama. But the first act occurs in two places that are never listed as part of the digestive tract: your brain, your eyes, and your nose.

The brain, eyes, and nose

When you see appetizing food, you experience a conditioned response. (For the lowdown on how your digestive system can be conditioned to respond to food, see Chapter 14; for information on your food preferences, see Chapter 15.) In other words, your thoughts — "Wow! That looks good!" — stimulate your brain to tell your digestive organs to get ready for action.

What happens in your nose is purely physical. The tantalizing aroma of good food is transmitted by molecules that fly from the surface of the food to settle on the membrane lining of your nostrils; these molecules stimulate the receptor cells on the olfactory nerve fibers that stretch from your nose back to your brain. When the receptor cells communicate with your brain — your brain sends encouraging messages to your mouth and digestive tract.

In both cases — eyes and nose — the results are the same: In other words, the sight and scent of food has made your mouth water and your stomach contract in anticipatory hunger pangs.

But wait! Suppose that you hate what you see or smell? For some people, even the thought of liver is enough to make them want to barf — or simply leave the room. At that point, your body takes up arms to protect you: You experience a *rejection reaction* — a reaction similar to that exhibited by babies given something that tastes bitter or sour. Your mouth purses, and your nose wrinkles as if to keep the food (and its odor) as far away as possible. Your throat tightens, and your stomach *turns* — muscles contracting not in anticipatory pangs but in movements preparatory for vomiting up the unwanted food. Not a pleasant moment.

But assume that you like what's on your plate. Go ahead. Take a bite.

The mouth

Lift your fork to your mouth, and your teeth and salivary glands swing into action. Your teeth chew, grinding the food, breaking it into small, manageable pieces. As a result:

✔ You can swallow without choking.

✔ You break down the indigestible wrapper of fibers surrounding the edible parts of some foods (fruits, vegetables, whole grains) so that your digestive enzymes can get to the nutrients inside.

At the same time, salivary glands under your tongue and in the back of your mouth secrete the watery liquid called *saliva,* which performs two important functions:

✔ Moistening and compacting food so that your tongue can push it to the back of your mouth and you can swallow, sending the food down the slide of your *gullet* (esophagus) into your stomach.

✔ Providing *amylases,* enzymes that start the digestion of complex carbo-hydrates (starches), breaking the starch molecules into simple sugars (Check out Chapter 9 for more on carbs.)

No protein digestion occurs in your mouth, though saliva does contain very small amounts of lingual lipases, fat-busting enzymes secreted by cells at the base of the tongue; however, the amount is so small that the fat digestion that occurs in the mouth is insignificant.

Turning starches into sugars

Salivary enzymes (like amylases) don't lay a finger on proteins and leave fats pretty much alone, but they do begin to digest complex carbohydrates, breaking the long, chainlike molecules of starches into individual units of sugars. This simple experiment enables you to taste firsthand the effects of amylases on carbohydrates.

1. **Put a small piece of plain, unsalted cracker on your tongue.**

   No cheese, no chopped liver — just the cracker, please.

2. **Close your mouth and let the cracker sit on your tongue for a few minutes.**

   Do you taste a sudden, slight sweetness? That's the salivary enzymes breaking a long, complex starch molecule into its component parts (sugars).

3. **Now swallow.**

   The rest of the digestion of the starch takes place farther down, in your small intestine.

The stomach

If you were to lay your digestive tract out on a table, most of it would look like a simple, rather narrow, tube. The exception is your stomach, a pouchy part just below your *gullet* (esophagus).

Like most of the digestive tube, your stomach is circled with strong muscles whose rhythmic contractions — called *peristalsis* — move food smartly along and turn your stomach into a sort of food processor that mechanically breaks pieces of food into ever smaller particles. While this is going on, glands in the stomach wall are secreting *stomach juices* — a potent blend of enzymes, hydrochloric acid, and mucus.

One stomach enzyme — *gastric alcohol dehydrogenase* — digests small amounts of alcohol, an unusual nutrient that can be absorbed directly into your bloodstream even before it's been digested. For more about alcohol digestion, including why men can drink more than women without becoming tipsy, see Chapter 10.

Other enzymes, plus stomach juices, begin the digestion of proteins and fats, separating them into their basic components — amino acids and fatty acids.

Stop! If the words amino acids and fatty acids are completely new to you and if you're suddenly consumed by the desire to know more about them this instant, stick a pencil in the book to hold your place and flip to Chapters 7 and 8, where I discuss them in detail.

Stop again!! For the most part, digestion of carbohydrates comes to a temporary halt in the stomach because the stomach juices are so acidic that they deactivate *amylases,* the enzymes that break complex carbohydrates apart into simple sugars. However, stomach acid can break some carbohydrate bonds, so a bit of carb digestion does take place.

Back to the action. Eventually, your churning stomach blends its contents into a thick soupy mass called *chyme* (from *cheymos,* the Greek word for juice). When a small amount of chyme spills past the stomach into the small intestine, the digestion of carbohydrates resumes in earnest, and your body begins to extract nutrients from food.

The small intestine

Open your hand and put it flat against your belly button, with your thumb pointing up to your waist and your pinkie pointing down.

Your hand is now covering most of the relatively small space into which your 20-foot-long small intestine is neatly coiled. When the soupy, partially digested chyme spills from your stomach into this part of the digestive tube, a whole new set of gastric juices are released:

- *Pancreatic and intestinal enzymes* that finish the digestion of proteins into amino acids

- *Bile,* a greenish liquid (made in the liver and stored in the gallbladder) that enables fats to mix with water

- *Alkaline pancreatic juices* that make the chyme less acidic so that amylases (the enzymes that break down carbohydrates) can go back to work separating complex carbohydrates into simple sugars

- *Intestinal alcohol dehydrogenase,* which digests alcohol not previously absorbed into your bloodstream

While these chemicals are working, contractions of the small intestine continue to move the food mass down through the tube so that your body can absorb sugars, amino acids, fatty acids, vitamins, and minerals into cells in the intestinal wall.

The lining of the small intestine is a series of folds covered with projections that have been described as "finger-like" or "small nipples." The technical name for these small structures is *villi.* Each villus is covered with smaller projections called *microvilli,* and every villus and microvillus is programmed to accept a specific nutrient — and no other.

Nutrients are absorbed not in their order of arrival in the intestine but according to how fast they're broken down into their basic parts:

- Carbohydrates — which separate quickly into single sugar units — are absorbed first.

- Proteins (as amino acids) go next.

- Fats — which take longest to break apart into their constituent fatty acids — are last. That's why a high-fat meal keeps you feeling fuller longer than a meal such as chow mein or plain tossed salad, which are mostly lowfat carbohydrates.

- Vitamins that dissolve in water are absorbed earlier than vitamins that dissolve in fat.

Peephole: The first man to watch a living human gut at work

William Beaumont, MD, was a surgeon in the United States Army in the early 19th century. His name survives in the annals of medicine because of an excellent adventure that began on June 6, 1822. Alexis St. Martin, an 18-year-old French Canadian fur trader, was wounded by a musket ball that discharged accidentally, tearing through his back and out his stomach, leaving a wound that healed but didn't close.

St. Martin's injury seems not to have affected what must have been a truly sunny disposition: Two years later, when all efforts to close the hole in his gut had failed, he granted Beaumont permission to use the wound as the world's first window on a working human digestive system. (To keep food and liquid from spilling out of the small opening, Beaumont kept it covered with a cotton bandage.)

Beaumont's method was simplicity itself. At noon on August 1, 1825, he tied small pieces of food (cooked meat, raw meat, cabbage, bread) to a silk string, removed the bandage, and inserted the food into the hole in St. Martin's stomach.

An hour later, he pulled the food out. The cabbage and bread were half digested; the meat, untouched. He reinserted the food into the hole. After another hour, he pulled the string out again. This time, only the raw meat remained untouched, and St. Martin, who now had a headache and a queasy stomach, called it quits for the day. But in more than 230 later trials, Beaumont — with the help of his remarkably compliant patient — discovered that although carbohydrates (cabbage and bread) were digested rather quickly, it took up to eight hours for the stomach juices to break down proteins and fats (the beef). Beaumont attributed this to the fact that the cabbage had been cut into small pieces and the bread was porous. Modern nutritionists know that carbohydrates are simply digested faster than proteins and that digesting fats (including those in beef) takes longest of all.

By withdrawing gastric fluid from St. Martin's stomach, keeping it at 100°F (the temperature recorded on a thermometer stuck into the stomach), and adding a piece of meat, Beaumont was able to clock exactly how long the meat took to fall apart: 10 hours.

Beaumont and St. Martin separated in 1833 when the patient, who was then a sergeant in the United States Army, was posted elsewhere, leaving the doctor to write "Experiments and Observations on the Gastric Juice and the Physiology of Digestion." The treatise is now considered a landmark in the understanding of the human digestive system.

After you've digested your food and absorbed its nutrients through your small intestine:

- ✔ Amino acids, sugars, vitamin C, the B vitamins, iron, calcium, and magnesium are carried through the bloodstream to your liver, where they are processed and sent out to the rest of the body.

- ✔ Fatty acids, cholesterol, and vitamins A, D, E, and K go into the lymphatic system and then into the blood. They, too, end up in the liver, are processed, and are shipped out to other body cells.

Inside the cells, nutrients are *metabolized,* or burned for heat and energy or used to build new tissues. The metabolic process that gives you energy is called *catabolism* (from *katabole,* the Greek word for casting down). The metabolic process that uses nutrients to build new tissues is called *anabolism* (from *anabole,* the Greek word for raising up).

How the body uses nutrients for energy and new tissues is, alas, a subject for another chapter. In fact, this subject is enough to fill seven different chapters, each devoted to a specific kind of nutrient. For information about metabolizing proteins, turn to Chapter 7. I discuss fats in Chapter 8, carbohydrates in Chapter 9, alcohol in Chapter 10, vitamins in Chapter 11, minerals in Chapter 12, and water in Chapter 13.

The large intestine

After every useful, digestible ingredient other than water has been wrung out of your food, the rest — indigestible waste such as fiber — moves into the top of your large intestine, the area known as your *colon.* The colon's primary job is to absorb water from this mixture and then to squeeze the remaining matter into the compact bundle known as feces.

Feces (whose brown color comes from leftover bile pigments) are made of indigestible material from food, plus cells that have sloughed off the intestinal lining and bacteria — quite a lot of bacteria. In fact, about 30 percent of the entire weight of the feces is bacteria, microorganisms that live in permanent colonies in your colon, where they

  ✔ Manufacture vitamin B12, which is absorbed through the colon wall

  ✔ Produce vitamin K, also absorbed through the colon wall

  ✔ Break down amino acids and produce nitrogen (which gives feces a characteristic odor)

  ✔ Feast on indigestible complex carbohydrates (fiber), excreting the gas that sometimes makes you physically uncomfortable — or a social pariah

When the bacteria have finished, the feces — perhaps the small remains of yesterday's copious feast — pass down through your rectum and out through your anus. But not necessarily right away: Digestion of any one meal may take longer than a day to complete.

After that, digestion's done!

Chapter 3

Calories: The Energizers

Automobiles burn gasoline to get the energy they need to move. Your body burns *(metabolizes)* food to produce energy in the form of heat. This heat warms your body and (as energy) powers every move you make.

The amount of heat produced by metabolizing food is measured in units called kilocalories. A *kilocalorie* is the amount of energy it takes to raise the temperature of 1 kilogram of water 1 degree on a Centigrade (Celsius) thermometer at sea level.

In common use, nutritionists substitute the word *calorie* for *kilocalorie*. Strictly speaking, a calorie is really $\frac{1}{1000}$ of a kilocalorie. But the word calorie is easier to say and easier to remember, so that's the term you see whenever you read about the energy in food. Read on to find out what calories mean to you and your nutrition.

Counting the Calories in Food

When you read that a serving of food — say, one banana — has 105 calories, that means your metabolizing the banana produces 105 calories of heat that your body can use for work.

TECHNICAL STUFF

Measuring the number of calories

Nutrition scientists measure the number of calories in food by actually burning the food in a *bomb calorimeter,* which is a box with two chambers, one inside the other. The researchers weigh a sample of the food, put the sample in a dish, and put the dish into the inner chamber of the calorimeter. They fill the inner chamber with oxygen and then seal it so the oxygen can't escape. The outer chamber is filled with a measured amount of cold water, and the oxygen in the first chamber (inside the chamber with the water) is ignited with an electric spark. When the food burns, an observer records the rise in the temperature of the water in the outer chamber. If the temperature of the water goes up 1 degree per kilogram, the food has 1 calorie; 2 degrees, 2 calories; 235 degrees, 235 calories — or one 8-ounce chocolate malted made with powder mix and whole milk.

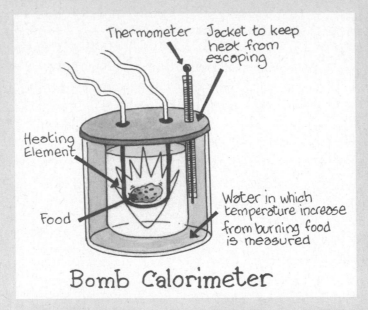

Bomb Calorimeter

You may wonder which kinds of food have the most calories. Here's how the calories measure up in 1 gram of the four basic food types:

- **Protein:** 4 calories
- **Carbohydrates:** 4 calories
- **Alcohol:** 7 calories
- **Fat:** 9 calories

In other words, ounce for ounce, proteins and carbohydrates give you fewer than half as many calories as fat. That's why — again, ounce for ounce — high-fat foods, such as cream cheese, are high in calories, while lowfat foods, such as bagels (minus the cream cheese, of course) are not.

Sometimes foods that seem to be equally low-calorie really aren't. You have to watch all the angles, paying attention to fat in addition to protein and carbo-hydrates. Here's a good example: A chicken breast and a hamburger are both high-protein foods. Both should have the same number of calories per ounce. But if you serve the chicken without its skin, it contains very little fat, while the hamburger is chock-full of it. A 3-ounce serving of skinless chicken pro-vides 140 calories, while a 3-ounce burger yields 230 to 245 calories, depend-ing on the cut of the meat and its fat content.

Empty calories

All food provides calories. All calories provide energy. But some foods are said to give you *empty calories.* This term has nothing to do with the calorie's energy potential; it simply describes a calorie with no extra benefits, such as amino acids, fatty acids, fiber, vitamins, and minerals.

The best-known empty-calorie foods are table sugar and *ethanol* (the kind of alcohol found in beer, wine, and spirits). On their own, sugar and ethanol give you energy — but no nutrients. (See Chapter 9 for more about sugar and Chapter 10 for more about alcohol.)

Of course, sugar and alcohol are ingredients often found in foods that do provide other nutrients. For example, sugar is found in bread, and alcohol is found in beer — two very different foods that both have calcium, phospho-rus, iron, potassium, sodium, and B vitamins.

In the United States, some people are malnourished because they can't afford enough food to get the nutrients they need. The school lunch program started by President Franklin Delano Roosevelt in 1935 and expanded by almost every president, Republican and Democrat, since then has been a largely successful attempt to prevent malnutrition among poor schoolchildren.

But many Americans who can afford enough food nevertheless are malnourished because they simply don't know how to choose a diet that gives them nutrients as well as calories. For these people, eating too many foods with empty calories can cause significant health problems, such as weak bones, bleeding gums, skin rashes, mental depression, and preventable birth defects as well as being over-weight or underweight (yes, being too thin can be a problem).

Every calorie counts

People who say that "calories don't count" or that "some calories count less than others" are usually trying to convince you to follow a diet that concentrates on one kind of food to the exclusion of most others. One common example that seems to arise like a phoenix in every generation of dieters is the *high-protein diet.*

The high-protein diet tells you to cut back or even entirely eliminate carbohydrate foods on the assumption that because your muscle tissue is mostly protein, the protein foods you eat will go straight from your stomach to your muscles, while everything else turns to fat. In other words, this diet says that you can stuff yourself with protein foods because no matter how many calories you get, they'll all be protein calories, and they'll all end up in your muscles, not on your hips. Wouldn't it be nice if that were true? The problem is, it isn't. All calories, regardless of where they come from, give you energy. If you take in more energy (calories) than you spend each day, you'll gain weight. If you take in fewer calories than you use up, you'll lose weight. This nutrition rule is an equal opportunity, one-size-fits-all proposition that applies to everyone. No exceptions.

How Many Calories Do You Need?

Think of your energy requirements as a bank account. You make deposits when you consume calories. You make withdrawals when your body spends energy on work. Nutritionists divide the amount of energy you withdraw each day into two parts:

✔ The energy you need when your body is at rest

✔ The energy you need to do your daily "work"

To keep your energy account in balance, you need to take in enough each day to cover your withdrawals. As a general rule, infants and adolescents burn more energy per pound than adults do, because they're continually making large amounts of new tissue. Similarly, an average man burns more energy than an average woman because his body is larger and has more muscle (see the upcoming section "Sex, glands, and chocolate cake"), thus leading to the totally unfair but totally true proposition that a man who weighs, say, 150 pounds can consume about 10 percent more calories than a woman who weighs 150 pounds and still not gain weight. For the numbers, check out the next section and Table 3-1.

Resting energy expenditure (REE)

Even when you're at rest, your body is busy. Your heart beats. Your lungs expand and contract. Your intestines digest food. Your liver processes nutrients. Your glands secrete hormones. Your muscles flex, usually gently. Cells send electrical impulses back and forth among themselves, and your brain continually signals to every part of your body.

The energy that your resting body uses to do all this stuff is called (surprise! surprise!) *resting energy expenditure,* abbreviated REE. The REE, also known as the *basal metabolism,* accounts for a whopping 60 to 70 percent of all the energy you need each day.

To find your resting energy expenditure (REE), you must first figure out your weight in kilograms (kg). One kilogram equals 2.2 pounds. So to get your weight in kilograms, divide the number in pounds by 2.2. For example, if you weigh 150 pounds, that's equal to 68.2 kg (150 ÷ 2.2). Plug that into the appropriate equation in Table 3-1 — and bingo! You have your REE.

What do you do with this information? First, simply appreciate its scientific value in describing the most basic fact about how many calories you need to survive. Second, and more pragmatically, regard it as a base on which to build a nutritional, real-life, daily menu.

Table 3-1   How Many Calories Do You Need When You're Resting?

Sex and Age	Equation to Figure Out Your REE
Males	
18–30 years	$(15.3 \times \text{weight in kg}) + 679$
31–60 years	$(11.6 \times \text{weight in kg}) + 879$
Older than 60 years	$(13.5 \times \text{weight in kg}) + 487$
Females	
18–30 years	$(14.7 \times \text{weight in kg}) + 496$
31–60 years	$(8.7 \times \text{weight in kg}) + 829$
Older than 60 years	$(10.5 \times \text{weight in kg}) + 596$

The National Research Council, Recommended Dietary Allowances (Washington, D.C.: National Academy Press, 1989)

Sex, glands, and chocolate cake

A *gland* is an organ that secretes *hormones,* which are chemical substances that can change the function — and sometimes the structure — of other body parts.

Hormones secreted by three glands — the pituitary, the thyroid, and the adrenals — influence how much energy you use when your body's at rest.

Your pituitary gland, a small structure in the center of your brain, stimulates your thyroid gland (which sits at the front of your throat) to secrete hormones that impact the rate at which your tissues burn nutrients to produce energy.

Muscle versus fat versus weight loss

Muscle weighs more than fat. This is why many people who take up exercise to lose weight discover, one month or so into the barbells and step-up-step-down routine, their clothes fit better, but the scale points slightly higher. They've traded lightweight fat for heavier muscle, proving that sometimes you can't win for losing.

When your thyroid gland doesn't secrete enough hormones (a condition known as *hypothyroidism*), you burn food more slowly, and your REE drops. When your thyroid secretes excess amounts of hormones (a condition known as *hyperthyroidism*), you burn food faster, and your REE is higher.

When you're frightened or excited, your adrenal glands (two small glands, one on top of each kidney) release *adrenaline,* the hormone that serves as your body's call to battle stations. Your heartbeat increases. You breathe faster. Your muscles clench. And you burn food faster, converting it as fast as possible to the energy you need for the reaction commonly known as *fight or flight.* But these effects are temporary. The effects of your sex glands, on the other hand, last as long as you live.

If you're a woman, you know that your appetite may rise and fall in tune with your menstrual cycle. In fact, this fluctuation parallels what's happening to your REE, which goes up just before or at the time of ovulation. Your appetite is highest when menstrual bleeding starts and then falls sharply. Yes, you really are hungrier (and need more energy) just before you get your period.

Being a man (and making lots of testosterone) makes satisfying your nutritional needs on a normal American diet easier. Your male bones are naturally denser, so you're less dependent on dietary or supplemental calcium to prevent *osteoporosis* (severe loss of bone tissue) late in life. You don't lose blood through menstruation, so you need only less than half as much iron (8 mg for an adult male; 18 mg for a premenopausal woman who is neither pregnant nor nursing). Best of all, you can consume about 10 percent more calories than a woman of the same weight without adding pounds.

It is no accident that while teenage boys' are developing wide shoulders and biceps, teenage girls are getting hips. Testosterone, the male hormone, promotes the growth of muscle and bone. Estrogen gives you fatty tissue. As a result, the average male body has proportionally more muscle; the average female body, proportionally more fat.

Muscle is active tissue. It expands and contracts. It works. And when a muscle works, it uses more energy than fat (which insulates the body and provides a source of stored energy but does not move an inch on its own). What this muscle versus fat battle means is that the average man's REE is about 10 percent higher than the average woman's. In practical terms, that means a 140-pound man can hold his weight steady while eating about 10 percent more than a 140-pound woman who is the same age and performs the same amount of physical work.

No amount of dieting changes this unfair situation. A woman who exercises strenuously may reduce her body fat so dramatically that she no longer menstruates — an occupational hazard for some professional athletes. But she'll still have proportionately more body fat than an adult man of the same weight. If she eats what he does, and they perform the same amount of physical work, she still requires fewer calories than he to hold her weight steady.

Energy for work

Your second largest chunk of energy after the REE is the energy you withdraw to spend on physical work, everything from brushing your teeth in the morning to planting a row of petunias in the garden or working out in the gym.

Your total energy requirement (the number of calories you need each day) is your REE plus enough calories to cover the amount of work you do.

Does thinking about this use up energy? Yes, but not as much as you'd like to imagine. To solve a crossword puzzle — or write a chapter of this book — the average brain uses about 1 calorie every four minutes. That's only one-third the amount needed to keep a 60-watt bulb burning for the same length of time.

Table 3-2 defines the energy level of various activities ranging from the least energetic (sleep) to the most (playing football, digging ditches). Table 3-3 shows how many calories you use in an hour's worth of different kinds of work.

Table 3-2	How Active Are You When You're Active?
Activity Level	*Activity*
Resting	Sleeping, reclining
Very light	Seated and standing activities, painting, driving, laboratory work, typing, sewing, ironing, cooking, playing cards, and playing a musical instrument

(continued)

Table 3-2 *(continued)*

Activity Level	Activity
Light	Walking on a level surface at 2.5 to 3 mph, garage work, electrical trades, carpentry, restaurant trades, house-cleaning, child care, golfing, sailing, and table tennis
Moderate	Walking 3.5 to 4 mph, weeding and hoeing, carrying a load, cycling, skiing, tennis, and dancing
Heavy	Walking with a load uphill, tree felling, heavy manual digging, basketball, climbing, football, and soccer
Exceptionally heavy	Professional athletic training

The National Research Council, Recommended Dietary Allowances (Washington, D.C.: National Academy Press, 1989)

Table 3-3	How Many Calories Do You Need to Do the Work You Do?
Activity Level	**Calories Needed for This Work for One Hour**
Very light	80–100
Light	110–160
Moderate	170–240
Heavy	250–350
Exceptionally heavy	350+

"Food and Your Weight," House and Garden Bulletin, No. 74 (Washington, D.C.: U.S. Department of Agriculture)

How Many Calories Do You Really Need?

Figuring out exactly how many calories to consume each day can be a consuming task. Luckily, the Institute of Medicine, the group whose Food and Nutrition Board determines the RDAs for vitamins, minerals and other nutrients, has created a list of the average daily calorie allowance for healthy people from infants to senior citizens who maintain a healthful weight (see Chapter 4) based on the amount of activity a person performs each day.

Table 3-4 shows the calorie recommendations. Note that in this context, *sedentary* means a lifestyle with only the light physical activity associated with daily living; *moderately active* means a lifestyle that adds physical activity equal to a daily 1.5–3 mile walk at a speed of 3–4 miles per hour; *active* means adding physical activity equal to walking 3 miles a day at the 3–4 mph clip.

Table 3-4		**Estimated Daily Calorie Requirements for Healthy Adults* Based on Activity Level**		
	Age (Years)	*Sedentary*	*Moderate*	*Active*
Women	19–30	2000	2000–2200	2300
	31–50	1800	2000	2200
	51+	1600	1800	2000–2200
Men	19–30	2400	2600–2800	3000
	31–50	2200	2400–2600	2800–3000
	51+	2000	2200–2400	2400–2800

* These calorie recommendations assume a person of healthful weight, that is women with a Body Mass Index (BMI) of 21.5 and men with a BMI of 22.5 (for more on BMI, see Chapter 4).

Source: Institute of Medicine, "Estimated Energy Requirements (EER), IOM Dietary Reference Intakes macronutrients report," 2002.

The Last Word on Calories

Calories are not your enemy. On the contrary, they give you the energy you need to live a healthy life.

The trick is to manage your calories and not let them manage you. After you know that fats are more fattening than proteins and carbohydrates and that your body burns food to make energy, you can strategize your energy intake to match your energy expenditure, and vice versa. Chapter 16 covers the details of a healthful diet. Chapter 17 shows how to plan nutritious meals.

Chapter 4

Big, Bigger, Biggest: The Growing American Body

A mericans are fat. And getting fatter.

According to the Dietary Guidelines 2010 (see Chapter 16), in 1970, about 15 percent of all Americans were obese. By 2008, that figure had more than doubled to 34 percent, and in 32 of the 50 states, more than one in every four people were obese.

And the kids are *not* all right. Overall, the National Survey of Children's Health (2007) says that more than 12 million American children and adolescents are obese, and the National Center for Health Statistics says that the number of obese 6- to 11-year-olds has quadrupled since 1970.

This excess poundage isn't pretty, and it comes at a cost. The Centers for Disease Control and Prevention (CDC) puts the price of treating obesity-related illnesses at nearly $150 billion each year, an amount equal to about 10 percent of all medical spending in the United States, including your health insurance premiums.

And if these trends continue, researchers at the Johns Hopkins Bloomberg School of Public Health, the Agency for Healthcare Research and Quality, and the University of Pennsylvania School of Medicine predict that by the year 2030, nearly 90 percent of American adults will be overweight, and the cost of treating their obesity-related health problems will approach $1 trillion a year.

No wonder the American Heart Association says we're in the grip of an obesity epidemic.

The Obesity Epidemic

The word *epidemic* conjures up images of polio, plague, flu, measles — a host of contagious illnesses that pass more or less easily from one person to another.

But does obesity qualify? Maybe.

In 2007, Nicholas Christakis, who teaches sociology at Harvard, and James Fowler, a political scientist at the University of California, San Diego, suggested in *The New England Journal of Medicine* that gaining weight may be a "socially contagious" event. In other words, people in groups tend to adopt similar behavior, and gaining or losing weight in tandem with friends and relatives may be one of those activities.

To reach this conclusion, Christakis and Fowler had analyzed more than 30 years' worth of information for more than 12,000 volunteers in the famed Framingham Heart Study, the project that has tracked the incidence and causes of heart disease in a Massachusetts city since 1948.

The Framingham people were weighed during checkups every two to four years. When Christakis and Fowler toted up the results, they discovered that the risk of becoming obese rose nearly 60 percent for someone with an obese friend, 40 percent for someone with an obese brother or sister, and 37 percent for someone whose husband or wife is obese. And these people didn't even have to live close to each other for the risk to rise: The co-incidence of obesity existed even when the subjects lived in different cities.

And here's a fascinating factoid: Other studies show that you can actually pinpoint the places where Americans are most likely to be overweight on a map of the United States.

The Obesity Map

For several years, *Men's Health* magazine has rated the top fattest and fittest (leanest) cities in the United States. To do these rankings, *Men's Health* looks at

- The percentage of the city's population that is overweight
- The percentage of people in the city who have been diagnosed with Type 2 diabetes

- ✔ The percentage of residents who haven't left the couch in a month (the figures comes from the CDC Behavioral Risk Factor Surveillance System, an ongoing telephone survey)
- ✔ The amount of money these people spend on junk food as reported by the Bureau of Labor Statistics)
- ✔ The number of people who ate fast food nine or more times in a month

Then the editors crunch the numbers to come up with the list of the fattest and fittest cities. The 2010 version is in Table 4-1.

Table 4-1	The Ten Fattest and Leanest U.S. Cities
Fattest Cities (Fattest First)	*Leanest Cities (Leanest First)*
Corpus Christi	San Francisco
Charleston (WV)	Burlington
El Paso	Washington, D.C.
Dallas	Seattle
Memphis	Austin
Kansas City (MO)	Albuquerque
San Antonio	Portland (OR)
Baltimore	Cincinnati
Houston	Denver
Birmingham	Aurora (CO)

Source: " America's Fattest Cities," Men's Health, May 2010. www.menshealth.com/ fattestcities2010

You may want a more global picture of who's fat and who's not, in which case you will be pleased to hear that The Trust for America's Health and the Robert Woods Johnson Foundation have collected data from the CDC to produce that list (see Table 4-2).

What do the fattest cities and states have in common? According to Michael Wimberly of the Geographic Information Science Center of Excellence at South Dakota State University, the people living there are less likely to engage in physical activity, less likely to eat five servings of fruits and veggies a day, more likely to eat the "wrong" foods, and likely to be living somewhere pretty far away from a really good supermarket. Wimberly calls this an *obesogenic environment,* a situation that encourages weight gain.

Do you live in one of the 30 states not included in Table 4-2? Not to worry. Type this address into your search bar to access an interactive map of the United States with the appropriate stats per state: `http://healthy americans.org/reports/obesity2010`.

Table 4-2	The Fattest and Leanest U.S. States		
Fattest State	**% of Adults Who Are Obese**	**Leanest State**	**% of Adults Who Are Obese**
Mississippi	33.8	Colorado	19.1
Alabama	31.6	Connecticut	21.4
Tennessee	31.6	Washington, D.C.	21.5
West Virginia	31.3	Massachusetts	31.7
Louisiana	31.2	Hawaii	22.6
Oklahoma	30.6	Vermont	22.8
Kentucky	30.5	Rhode Island	22.0
Arkansas	30.1	Utah	23.2
South Carolina	29.9	Montana	23.5
North Carolina	29.4	New Jersey	23.9
Michigan	29.4		

Source: Trust for America's Health & Robert Woods Johnson Foundation, "F as in Fat: How Obesity Threatens America's Future," June 2010. `http://healthyamericans.org/reports/obesity2010`

How Much Should You Really Weigh?

Through the years, many health organizations ranging from insurance companies to the U.S. federal government have created charts and tables purporting to establish *healthy weight* standards for adult Americans.

Some of these efforts set the figures so low that you can hardly get there without severely restricting your diet — or being born again with a different body, preferably with light bones and no curves.

Others are more reasonable.

Weight charts and tables

In 1959, the Metropolitan Life Insurance Company published the first set of standard weight charts. The weights were drawn from insurance statistics showing what the healthiest, longest-living people weighed — with clothes on and (for the women) wearing shoes with one-inch heels. The problem? At the time, the class of people with insurance was so small and so narrow that it was hard to say with certainty that their weight could predict healthy poundage for the rest of the population.

Thirty-one years later, the government published the weight chart shown in Table 4-3. This moderate, eminently usable set appeared in the 1990 edition of *Dietary Guidelines for Americans* produced by the U.S. Department of Agriculture and the U.S. Department of Health and Human Services. The weights are listed in ranges for both men and women of specific heights. Here, height is measured without shoes, and weight is measured without clothes. (For more on the latest Dietary Guidelines, see Chapter 16.)

Because most people gain some weight as they grow older, the people who compiled these recommendations did a really sensible thing, dividing the ranges into two broad categories, one for people age 19 to 34, the other for those age 35 and older.

Obviously, individuals with a small frame and proportionately more fat tissue than muscle tissue (muscle is heavier than fat) are likely to weigh in at the low end. People with a large frame and proportionately more muscle than fat are likely to weigh in at the high end. As a general (but by no means invariable) rule, that means that women — who have smaller frames and less muscle — weigh less than men of the same height and age.

Later editions of the Dietary Guidelines omitted the higher weight allowances for older people, so that the "healthy" weights for everyone, young or old, became the ones listed in 1990 in the column for 19- to 34-year-olds. I'm going to go out on a limb here to say that I prefer the 1990 recommendations because they are

✔ Achievable without constant dieting

✔ Realistic about how your body changes as you get older

✔ Less likely to make you totally crazy about your weight

Which is a pretty good description of how nutritional guidelines need to work, don't you think?

Table 4-3	How Much Should You Weigh?	
Height	*Weight (Pounds) for 19- to 34-Year-Olds*	*Weight (Pounds) for 35-Year-Olds and Older*
5'	97–128	108–138
5'1"	101–132	111–143
5'2"	104–137	115–148
5'3"	107–141	119–152
5'4"	111–146	122–157
5'5"	114–150	126–162
5'6"	118–155	130–167
5'7"	121–160	134–172
5'8"	125–164	138–178
5'9"	129–169	142–183
5'10"	132–174	146–188
5'11"	136–179	151–194
6'	140–184	155–199
6'1"	144–189	159–205
6'2"	148–195	164–210
6'3"	152–200	168–216
6'4"	156–205	173–222
6'5"	160–211	177–228
6'6"	164–216	182–234

Nutrition and Your Health: Dietary Guidelines for Americans, 3rd ed. (Washington D.C.: U.S. Department of Agriculture, U.S. Department of Health and Human Services, 1990)

The BMI: Another way to rate your weight

The *Body Mass Index* (BMI) is a number that measures the relationship between your weight and your height.

In the United States, a BMI below 18.5 is currently considered underweight, 18.5–24.9 is normal, 25.0–29.9 is overweight, 30.0 to 39.9 is obese, and 40.00 or greater is severely obese. Previously, other countries were slightly more lenient in their estimate of normal and overweight (for example, in Australia, a BMI of less than 20 was considered underweight). Today, the American standards are generally accepted around the world.

The equation used to calculate your BMI is called the *Quetelet Index,* named after the 19th century Belgian mathematician and astronomer who invented the concept of "the average man" (see the sidebar in this section). The equation is W/H^2, which originally meant weight (in kilograms) divided by height (in meters, squared).

To figure your BMI, divide your weight (in pounds) by your height (in inches, squared). The new equation looks like this:

W/H^2 x 705

For example, if you are 5'3" tall and weigh 138 pounds, the equation for your BMI looks like this:

$BMI = W/H^2$ x 705

= (138 pounds/63 x 63 inches) x 705

= (138/3,969) x 705

= 24.5 BMI

Or you could just run your finger down the table in Figure 4-1, which does the math for men and women from 4'10" to 6'4" tall, weighing 91 to 443 pounds.

The man who invented the average man

Lambert Adolphe Jacques Quetelet (1795–1874) was a Belgian mathematician, astronomer, statistician, and sociologist who invented the concept of the *homme moyen* (middle man), the average Joe who stands at the center of any bell curve.

Quetelet's main concern was predicting criminal behavior. To this end, he hoped to develop statistical patterns based on a person's deviation from average (read: normal) social behavior that could be used to predict his actions including moral (good) and criminal (bad) behavior. While this idea provoked many lively discussions among 19th-century social scientists, it never really worked as a crime-fighting tool. But it is extremely useful in estimating health risks.

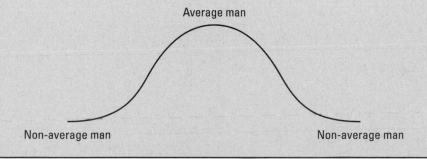

Figure 4-1:
Calculating your BMI the easy way.

Body Mass Index Table

	Normal						Overweight					Obese										Extreme Obesity														
BMI	19	20	21	22	23	24	25	26	27	28	29	30	31	32	33	34	35	36	37	38	39	40	41	42	43	44	45	46	47	48	49	50	51	52	53	54
Height (inches)												Body Weight (pounds)																								
58	91	96	100	105	110	115	119	124	129	134	138	143	148	153	158	162	167	172	177	181	186	191	196	201	205	210	215	220	224	229	234	239	244	248	253	258
59	94	99	104	109	114	119	124	128	133	138	143	148	153	158	163	168	173	178	183	188	193	198	203	208	212	217	222	227	232	237	242	247	252	257	262	267
60	97	102	107	112	118	123	128	133	138	143	148	153	158	163	168	174	179	184	189	194	199	204	209	215	220	225	230	235	240	245	250	255	261	266	271	276
61	100	106	111	116	122	127	132	137	143	148	153	158	164	169	174	180	185	190	195	201	206	211	217	222	227	232	238	243	248	254	259	264	269	275	280	285
62	104	109	115	120	126	131	136	142	147	153	158	164	169	175	180	186	191	196	202	207	213	218	224	229	235	240	246	251	256	262	267	273	278	284	289	295
63	107	113	118	124	130	135	141	146	152	158	163	169	175	180	186	191	197	203	208	214	220	225	231	237	242	248	254	259	265	270	278	282	287	293	299	304
64	110	116	122	128	134	140	145	151	157	163	169	174	180	186	192	197	204	209	215	221	227	232	238	244	250	256	262	267	273	279	285	291	296	302	308	314
65	114	120	126	132	138	144	150	156	162	168	174	180	186	192	198	204	210	216	222	228	234	240	246	252	258	264	270	276	282	288	294	300	306	312	318	324
66	118	124	130	136	142	148	155	161	167	173	179	186	192	198	204	210	216	223	229	235	241	247	253	260	266	272	278	284	291	297	303	309	315	322	328	334
67	121	127	134	140	146	153	159	166	172	178	185	191	198	204	211	217	223	230	236	242	249	255	261	268	274	280	287	293	299	306	312	319	325	331	338	344
68	125	131	138	144	151	158	164	171	177	184	190	197	203	210	216	223	230	236	243	249	256	262	269	276	282	289	295	302	308	315	322	328	335	341	348	354
69	128	135	142	149	155	162	169	176	182	189	196	203	209	216	223	230	236	243	250	257	263	270	277	284	291	297	304	311	318	324	331	338	345	351	358	365
70	132	139	146	153	160	167	174	181	188	195	202	209	216	222	229	236	243	250	257	264	271	278	285	292	299	306	313	320	327	334	341	348	355	362	369	376
71	136	143	150	157	165	172	179	186	193	200	208	215	222	229	236	243	250	257	265	272	279	286	293	301	308	315	322	329	338	343	351	358	365	372	379	386
72	140	147	154	162	169	177	184	191	199	206	213	221	228	235	242	250	258	265	272	279	287	294	302	309	316	324	331	338	346	353	361	368	375	383	390	397
73	144	151	159	166	174	182	189	197	204	212	219	227	235	242	250	257	265	272	280	288	295	302	310	318	325	333	340	348	355	363	371	378	386	393	401	408
74	148	155	163	171	179	186	194	202	210	218	225	233	241	249	256	264	272	280	287	295	303	311	319	326	334	342	350	358	365	373	381	389	396	404	412	420
75	152	160	168	176	184	192	200	208	216	224	232	240	248	256	264	272	279	287	295	303	311	319	327	335	343	351	359	367	375	383	391	399	407	415	423	431
76	156	164	172	180	189	197	205	213	221	230	238	246	254	263	271	279	287	295	304	312	320	328	336	344	353	361	369	377	385	394	402	410	418	426	435	443

Source: Adapted from Clinical Guidelines on the Identification, Evaluation, and Treatment of Overweight and Obesity in Adults: The Evidence Report.

Adapted from Clinical Guidelines on the Identification, Evaluation, and Treatment of Overweight and Obesity in Adults: The Evidence Report.

High-tech fat figuring

A tape measure or a weight chart is a low-tech tool anyone can handle. But science loves complexity, so weight experts have several complicated ways to figure out if you're fat. Here are three of the most interesting. *Caveat:* These are not your handy home tests — they're performed in some doctor's office, but more likely in a research hospital or bariatric clinic.

Bioelectric impedance. Your body is full of fluids packed with *electrolytes,* such as sodium and potassium, ions that conduct the electrical impulses that send messages back and forth among your cells. Muscle tissue contains more fluid than fat tissue, so a body with more muscle than fat is less resistant to an outside electrical current. To measure your body's resistance to electrical current (a phenomenon known as *impedance*), the technician conducting the test places electrodes at your wrists and ankles and

zaps a harmless low-intensity electrical current through. Then, she calculates how resistant your tissues were to the current. The final number indicates how much body fat you have.

The Bod Pod. This egg-shape chamber measures how much air you displace when you step in. Because muscle is more dense than body fat and displaces more air, the tech running the test can calculate the amount of fat in your body by looking at your weight and then at the amount of air you push aside when you enter the chamber.

Dual Energy X-Ray Absorptiometry (DEXA). This test uses X-rays to measure muscle, bone, and body fat. The test — which takes about 10 minutes — produces an image of the tissues that allows the tech to estimate the amount of body fat.

Surprise: The "normal" weights on this chart are within a pound or two of the healthful weights proposed for people younger than 35 in the 1990 *Dietary Guidelines for Americans.*

How Reliable Are the Numbers?

Weight charts and tables and numbers and stats are so plentiful that you may think they're totally reliable in predicting who's healthy and who's not. They aren't. Real people and their real differences keep sneaking into the equation.

For example, BMI is not a reliable guide for

- ✔ Women who are pregnant or nursing
- ✔ People who are very tall or very short
- ✔ Professional athletes or weight trainers with very well-developed muscle tissue. ***Remember:*** Muscle weighs more than fat, so a person with lots of muscle tissue may have a higher BMI and still be really healthy.

In addition, the value of the Body Mass Index in predicting your risk of illness appears to be tied to your age. If you're in your 30s, a lower BMI is clearly linked to better health. If you're in your 70s or older, no convincing evidence points to your weight playing a significant role in determining how healthy you are or how much longer you'll live. In between, from age 30 to age 74, the relationship between your BMI and your health is, well, in between — more important early on, less important later in life.

Increasing the odds of accuracy

To make the BMI a more accurate tool for predicting the health risks of carrying extra weight, the National Institutes of Health suggests adding a second measurement, the waist circumference — in other words, the apple/pear test.

If you look like an apple, with a lot of fat around your waist rather than around your hips (the pear shape), your risk of diabetes, high blood pressure, and heart disease go up. (And, yes, some people are neither apples nor pears, simply humans with relatively flat tummies and hips.)

To figure out which one you are, wrap a measuring tape around your middle, just above your hip bones. Take a deep breath. Let it out. Measure. That's your waist. Table 4-4 shows the relative risks associated with different waist measurements.

Table 4-4	Estimated Risk of Type 2 Diabetes, Hypertension, and Heart Disease Linked to BMI and Waist Size		
	BMI	Risk at Waist size <40 Inches (Men), <35 Inches (Women)	Risk at Waist Size >40 Inches (Men), >35 Inches (Women)
Underweight	<18.5	—	—
Normal	19–24.9	—	—
Overweight	25–29.9	Increased	High
Obese	30–34.9	High	Very high
	35–39.9	Very high	Very high
	>40	Extremely high	Extremely high

Source: National Heart, Lung and Blood Institute, National Institutes of Health, `www.nhlbi.nih.gov/health/public/heart/obesity/lose_wt/bmi_dis.htm`.

Confounding the predictions

Although an increasing number of Americans should work at losing weight, the fact is that many larger people, even people who are clearly obese, do live long, happy, and healthy lives.

To figure out why some overweight people's health status does not follow the "rules," many nutrition scientists now focus on the importance of *confounding variables,* sciencespeak for "something else is going on here."

Here are three potential confounding variables in the obesity/health equation:

- Maybe people who are overweight are more prone to illness because they exercise less, in which case stepping up the workouts may reduce the perceived risk of being overweight.

- People who are overweight may be more likely to be sick because they eat lots of foods containing high-calorie ingredients, such as saturated fat, that can trigger adverse health effects; in this case, the remedy may simply be a change in diet.

- Maybe people who are overweight have a genetic predisposition to a serious disease. If that's true, you'd have to ask whether losing 20 pounds really reduces their risk of disease to the level of a person who is naturally 20 pounds lighter. Perhaps not: In a few studies, people who successfully lost weight actually had a higher rate of death.

Seeing red flags on weight and health

Regardless of your BMI, the risk of health problems rises if you have

- High blood pressure
- High levels of LDL ("bad") cholesterol
- Low levels of HDL ("good") cholesterol
- High levels of triglycerides (a kind of fat found in blood)
- A family history of premature heart disease, meaning one or more close relatives who suffered a heart attack before age 50 for a man or age 60 for a woman
- Not being physically active or being a smoker

If the profile fits, check with your doctor about a sensible weight loss plan.

Facing the Numbers When They Don't Fit Your Body

Right about here, you probably feel the strong need for a really big chocolate bar — not such a bad idea now that nutritionists have discovered that dark chocolate is rich in disease-fighting antioxidants that benefit your various organs (so long as you stick to a 1-ounce daily "dose").

But it makes sense to consider the alternative — realistic rules that enable you to control your weight safely and effectively.

- ✔ **Rule No. 1: Not everybody starts out with the same set of genes — or fits into the same pair of jeans.** Some people are naturally larger and heavier than others. If that's you, and all your vital stats satisfy your doctor, don't waste time trying to fit someone else's idea of perfection. Relax and enjoy your own body.

- ✔ **Rule No. 2: If you're overweight and your doctor agrees with your decision to diet, you don't have to set world records to improve your health.** Even a moderate drop in poundage can be highly beneficial. According to *The New England Journal of Medicine* (www.nejm.org on the Net), losing just 10 to 15 percent of your body weight can lower high blood sugar, high cholesterol, and high blood pressure, reducing your risks of diabetes, heart disease, and stroke.

- ✔ **Rule No. 3: The number you really need to remember is 3,500, the number of calories it takes to gain or lose one pound of body fat.** In other words, 3,500 food calories equal one pound of body weight. So if you simply

  - Cut your calorie consumption from 2,000 calories a day to 1,700 and continue to do the same amount of physical work, you'll lose one pound of fat in just 12 days.

  - Go the other way, increasing calories from 1,700 to 2,000 a day without increasing the amount of work you do, 12 days later you'll be one pound heavier.

✔ **Rule No.4: Moderation is the best path to weight control.** Moderate calorie deprivation on a sensible diet produces healthful, moderate weight loss; this diet includes a wide variety of different foods containing sufficient amounts of essential nutrients. Abusing this rule and cutting calories to the bone can turn you literally into skin and bones, depriving you of the nutrients you need to live a normal healthy life. For more on the potentially devastating effects of starvation, voluntary and otherwise, check out Chapter 14.

✔ **Rule No. 5: Be more active.** Exercise allows you to take in more calories and still lose weight. In addition, exercise reduces the risk of many health problems, such as heart disease. Sounds like a recipe for success.

Snooze to lose

Two 2010 studies, one at the University of Chicago Medical Center and the other at the Division of Sleep Medicine at Brigham and Women's Hospital and Beth Israel Deaconess Medical Center in Boston, link sleep deprivation to weight gain. In the first study, dieters who had a full 7 to 8 hours of sleep each night lost fat when they lost weight. In the second study, teenagers who slept fewer than eight hours a night ate more fatty foods than did those who caught a full night's sleep.

Why? Some believe the answer may lie in the sleep-satisfied body's ability to regulate hormones that control appetite, but conclusive evidence must wait for another study.

In the meantime, here's a motto for the weight conscious: 40 winks or 40 pounds.

Chapter 5

How Much Nutrition Do You Need?

A healthful diet provides sufficient amounts of all the nutrients that your body needs. The question is, how much is enough?

Today, three sets of recommendations provide the answers, and each comes with its own virtues and deficiencies. The first, and most familiar, is the *RDA* (short for *Recommended Dietary Allowance*). The second, originally known as the *Estimated Safe and Adequate Daily Dietary Intakes (ESADDI),* now shortened to *Adequate Intake* or simply *AI,* describes recommended amounts of nutrients for which no RDAs exist. The third is the *DRI (Dietary Reference Intake),* an umbrella term that includes RDAs plus several innovative categories of nutrient recommendations.

Confused? Not to worry. This chapter spells it all out.

RDAs: Guidelines for Good Nutrition

The Recommended Dietary Allowances (RDAs) were created in 1941 by the Food and Nutrition Board, a subsidiary of the National Research Council, which is part of the National Academy of Sciences in Washington, D.C.

RDAs originally were designed to make planning several days' meals in advance easy for you. The *D* in RDA stands for dietary, not daily, because the RDAs are an average. You may get more of a nutrient one day and less the next, but the idea is to hit an average over several days.

For example, the current RDA for vitamin C is 75 mg for a woman and 90 mg for a man (age 18 and older). One 8-ounce glass of fresh orange juice has 120 mg vitamin C, so a woman can have an 8-ounce glass of orange juice on Monday and Tuesday, skip Wednesday, and still meet the RDA for the three days. A man may have to toss in something else — maybe a stalk of broccoli — to be able to do the same thing. No big deal.

The amounts recommended by the RDAs provide a margin of safety for healthy people, but they're not therapeutic. In other words, RDA servings won't cure a nutrient deficiency, but they can prevent one from occurring.

The essentials

RDAs offer recommendations for protein and 18 essential vitamins and minerals, a list that includes

Vitamin A	Folate	Vitamin B12
Vitamin E	Phosphorus	Vitamin K
Magnesium	Vitamin C	Iron
Thiamin (vitamin B1)	Zinc	Riboflavin (vitamin B2)
Copper	Niacin	Iodine
Vitamin B6	Selenium	

The newest essential nutrient, choline, won its wings in 2002, but no RDAs have yet been established. Calcium also has an Adequate Intake (AI) rather than an RDA.

Recommendations for carbohydrates, fats, dietary fiber, and alcohol

What nutrients are missing from the RDA list of essentials? Carbohydrates, fiber, fat, and alcohol. The reason is simple: If your diet provides enough protein, vitamins, and minerals, it's almost certain to provide enough carbohydrates and probably more than enough fat. Although no specific RDAs exist for carbohydrates and fat, guidelines definitely exist for them and for dietary fiber and alcohol.

In 1980, the U.S. Public Health Service and the U.S. Department of Agriculture joined forces to produce the first edition of *Dietary Guidelines for Americans* (see Chapter 16). A new edition of the Dietary Guidelines has been issued every five years since then to set parameters for what you can consider reasonable amounts of calories, carbohydrates, dietary fiber, fats, protein, and alcohol. According to these guidelines, several general rules advise you to

✔ **Balance your calorie intake with energy output in the form of regular exercise.** Check out Chapter 3 for specifics on how many calories a person of your weight, height, and level of activity (couch potato? marathon runner?) needs to consume each day.

✔ **Eat enough carbohydrates (primarily the complex ones from fruits, vegetables, and whole grains) to account for 45 to 65 percent of your total daily calories.** That's 900 to 1,300 calories on a 2,000-calorie diet (25 grams dietary fiber on a 2,000 calorie/day diet).

✔ **Keep your saturated fat intake to no more than 7 percent of your daily calories.** But to be realistic, you can consider starting with no more than 10 percent and then moving on to the more healthful lower amount. Your daily diet should have less than 300 mg cholesterol; people at risk of heart disease should lower their intake to 200 mg per day. Read the Nutrition Facts label on your food to avoid trans fats created in producing foods such as margarines. (For the skinny on saturated, unsaturated, and trans fats, plus cholesterol, check out Chapter 8.)

✔ **Drink alcohol only in moderation.** That means one drink a day for a woman and two for a man.

Different people, different needs

Because different bodies require different amounts of nutrients, RDAs currently address as many as 22 specific categories of human beings: boys and girls, men and women, from infancy through middle age. The RDAs recently were expanded to include recommendations for groups of people ages 50 to 70 and 70 and older. Eventually, recommendations will be made for people older than 85. These expanded groupings are a *really* good idea. In 1990, the U.S. Census counted 31.1 million Americans older than 65. By 2050, the U.S. government expects more than 60 million mostly active older citizens.

If age is important, so is gender. For example, because women of childbearing age lose iron when they menstruate, their RDA for iron is higher than the RDA for men. On the other hand, because men who are sexually active lose zinc through their ejaculations, the zinc RDA for men is higher than the zinc RDA for women. And gender affects body composition, which influences other RDAs, such as protein: The RDA for protein is set in terms of grams of protein per kilogram (2.2 pounds) of body weight. Because the average man weighs more than the average woman, his RDA for protein is higher than hers. The RDA for an adult male, age 19 or older, is 56 grams; for a woman, it's 46 grams.

AIs: The Nutritional Numbers Formerly Known as ESADDIs

In addition to the RDAs, the Food and Nutrition Board has created an *Adequate Intake* (AI) for eight nutrients considered necessary for good health, even though nobody really knows exactly how much your body needs. Not to worry: Sooner or later some smart nutrition researcher will come up with a hard number and move the nutrient to the RDA list.

You can find the AIs for biotin, choline, pantothenic acid, and vitamin D in Chapter 11, along with the requirements for other vitamins. The AIs for the minerals calcium, chromium, molybdenum, and manganese are in Chapter 12 with the other dietary minerals.

DRI: The Totally Complete Nutrition Guide

In 1993, the Food and Nutrition Board's Dietary Reference Intakes committee set up several panels of experts to review the RDAs and other recommendations for major nutrients (vitamins, minerals, and other food components) in light of new research and nutrition information.

The first order of business was to establish a new standard for nutrient recommendations called the *Dietary Reference Intake* (DRI). DRI is an umbrella term that embraces several categories of nutritional measurements for vitamins, minerals, and other nutrients. It includes

- **Estimated Average Requirement (EAR):** The amount that meets the nutritional needs of half the people in any one group (such as teenage girls or people older than 70). Nutritionists use the EAR to figure out whether an entire population's normal diet provides adequate amounts of nutrients.

- **Recommended Dietary Allowance (RDA):** The RDA, now based on information provided by the EAR, is still a daily average that meets the needs of 97 percent of a specific population, such as women age 18 to 50 or men aged 70 and older.

- **Adequate Intake (AI):** The AI is a new measurement, providing recommendations for nutrients for which no RDA is set. (**Note:** AI replaces ESADDI.)

- **Tolerable Upper Intake Level (UL):** The UL is the highest amount of a nutrient you can consume each day without risking an adverse effect.

Reviewing terms used to describe nutrient recommendations

Nutrient listings use the metric system. RDAs for protein are listed in grams. The RDA and AIs for vitamins and minerals are shown in milligrams (mg) and micrograms (mcg). A milligram is $\frac{1}{100}$ of a gram; a microgram is $\frac{1}{100}$ of a milligram.

Vitamin A, vitamin D, and vitamin E are special cases. For instance, one form of vitamin A is *preformed vitamin A,* a form of the nutrient that your body can use right away. Preformed vitamin A, known as *retinol,* is found in food from animals — liver, milk, and eggs. Carotenoids (red or yellow pigments in plants) also provide vitamin A. But to get vitamin A from carotenoids, your body has to convert the pigments to chemicals similar to retinol. Because retinol is a ready-made nutrient, the RDA for vitamin A is listed in units called retinol equivalents (RE). One mcg (microgram) RE is approximately equal to 3.33 international units (IU, the former unit of measurement for vitamin A).

Vitamin D consists of three compounds: vitamin D1, vitamin D2, and vitamin D3. Cholecalciferol, the chemical name for vitamin D3, is the most active of the three, so the RDA for vitamin D is measured in equivalents of cholecalciferol.

Your body gets vitamin E from two classes of chemicals in food: tocopherols and tocotrienols. The compound with the greatest vitamin E activity is a tocopherol: *alpha*-tocopherol. The RDA for vitamin E is measured in milligrams of *alpha*-tocopherol equivalents (a-TE).

The DRI panel's first report, listing new recommendations for calcium, phosphorus, magnesium, and fluoride, appeared in 1997. Its most notable change was upping the recommended amount of calcium from 800 mg to 1,000 mg for adults ages 31 to 50 as well as post-menopausal women taking estrogen supplements; for post menopausal women not taking estrogen, the recommendation is 1,500 mg.

The DRI panel's second report appeared in 1998. The report included new recommendations for thiamin, riboflavin, niacin, vitamin B6, folate, vitamin B12, pantothenic acid, biotin, and choline. The most important revision was increasing the folate recommendation to 400 mcg a day based on evidence showing that folate reduces a woman's risk of giving birth to a baby with spinal cord defects and lowers the risk of heart disease for men and women. (See the sidebar "Reviewing terms used to describe nutrient recommendations" in this chapter to brush up on your metric abbreviations.)

As a result of the 1989 DRI panel's report, the FDA ordered food manufacturers to add folate to flour, rice, and other grain products. (Multivitamin products already contain 400 mcg of folate.) In May 1999, data released by the Framingham Heart Study, which has followed heart health among residents of a Boston suburb for nearly half a century, showed a dramatic increase in blood levels of folate. Before the fortification of foods, 22 percent of the study participants had folate deficiencies; after the fortification, the number fell to 2 percent.

A DRI report with revised recommendations for vitamin C, vitamin E, the mineral selenium, beta-carotene, and other antioxidant vitamins was published in 2000. In 2001, new DRIs were released for vitamin A, vitamin K, arsenic, boron, chromium, copper, iodine, iron, manganese, molybdenum, nickel, silicon, vanadium, and zinc. In 2004, the Institute of Medicine (IOM) released new recommendations for sodium, potassium, chloride, and water, plus a special report on recommendations for two groups of older adults (ages 50 to 70 and 71 and over). By 2005, the Food and Nutrition Board had established an AI of 600 IU vitamin D for men and women older than 71. Put all these findings together, and they spell out the recommendations you find in this chapter.

Table 5-1 shows the most recent RDAs for vitamins for healthy adults; Table 5-2 shows RDAs for minerals for healthy adults. Where no RDA is given, an AI is indicated by an asterisk (*) by the column heading. The complete reports on which these tables are based are available online at www.iom.edu/ Object.File/Master/21/372/0.pdf. (If you want an idea of what kinds of foods provide these vitamins and minerals, check out Chapters 11 and 12.)

Hankering for more details? Notice something missing? Right — no recommended allowances for protein, fat, carbohydrates, and, of course, water. You can find those (respectively) in Chapters 7, 8, 9, and 13.

Table 5-1	Vitamin RDAs for Healthy Adults				
Age (Years)	Vitamin A (RE/IU)†	Vitamin D (mcg/IU)‡*	Vitamin E (a-TE)	Vitamin K (mcg)*	Vitamin C (mg)
Males					
19–30	900/2,970	15/600	15	120	90
31–50	900/2,970	15/600	15	120	90
51–70	900/2,970	15/600	15	120	90
Older than 70	900/2,970	20/800	15	120	90
Females					
19–30	700/2,310	15/600	15	90	75
31–50	700/2,310	15/600	15	90	75
51–70	700/2,310	15/600	15	90	75
Older than 70	700/2,310	20/900	15	90	75

Adequate Intake (AI)
† The "official" RDA for vitamin A is still 1,000 RE/5,000 IU for a male, 800 RE/4,000 IU for a female who isn't pregnant or nursing; the lower numbers listed on this chart are the currently recommended levels for adults.
‡ The current recommendations are the amounts required to prevent vitamin D deficiency disease; recent studies suggest that the optimal levels for overall health may actually be higher, in the range of 800–1,000 IU a day.

Age (years)	Thiamin (Vitamin B1) (mg)	Riboflavin (Vitamin B2) (mg)	Niacin (NE)	Pantothenic acid (mg)*	Vitamin B6 (mg)	Folate (mcg)	Vitamin B12 (mcg)	Biotin (mcg)*
Males								
19–30	1.2	1.3	16	5	1.3	400	2.4	30
31–50	1.2	1.3	16	5	1.3	400	2.4	30
50–70	1.2	1.3	16	5	1.7	400	2.4	30
Older than 70	1.2	1.1	16	5	1.7	400	2.4	30
Females								
19–30	1.1	1.1	14	5	1.3	400	2.4	30
31–50	1.1	1.1	14	5	1.3	400	2.4	30
51–70	1.1	1.1	14	5	1.5	400	2.4	30
Older than 70	1.1	1.1	14	5	1.5	400	2.4	30
Pregnant	1.4	1.1	18	6	1.9	600	2.6	30
Nursing	1.4	1.1	17	7	2.0	500	2.8	35

* Adequate Intake (AI)

How much is that?

Nutrient amounts are measured in various units:

✔ g = gram

✔ mg = milligram = ¹⁄₁₀₀₀th of a gram

✔ mcg = microgram = ¹⁄₁,₀₀₀,₀₀₀th of a gram

✔ IU = international unit

✔ RE = retinol equivalent = the amount of "true" vitamin A in an IU

✔ a-TE = alpha-tocopherol equivalent = the amount of alpha-tocopherol in a unit of vitamin E

Table 5-2		Mineral RDAs for Healthy Adults				
Age (years)	Calcium (mg)*	Phosphorus (mg)	Magnesium (mg)	Iron (mg)	Zinc (mg)	Copper (mcg)
Males						
19–30	1,000	700	400	8	11	900
31–50	1,000	700	420	8	11	900
51–70	1,200	700	420	8	11	900
Older than 70	1,200	700	420	8	11	900
Females						
19–30	1,000	700	310	18	8	900
31–50	1,000	700	320	18	8	900
51–70	1,000/1,500**	700	320	8	8	900
Older than 70	1,000/1,500**	700	320	8	8	900
Pregnant	1,000–1,300	700–1,250	350–400	27	11–12	1,000
Nursing	1,000–1,300	700–1,250	310–350	9–10	12–13	1,300

* Adequate Intake (AI)
** The lower recommendation is for postmenopausal women taking estrogen supplements; the higher figure is for postmenopausal women not taking estrogen supplements.

Age (years)	Iodine (mcg)	Selenium (mcg)	Molybdenum (mcg)	Manganese (mg)*	Fluoride (mg)*	Chromium (mcg)*	Choline (mg)*
Males							
19–30	150	55	45	2.3	4	36	550
31–50	150	55	45	2.3	4	36	550
51–70	150	55	45	2.3	4	30	550
Older than 70	150	55	45	2.3	4	30	550
Females							
19–30	150	55	45	1.8	3	25	425
31–50	150	55	45	1.8	3	25	425
51–70	150	55	45	1.8	3	20	425
Older than 70	150	55	45	1.8	3	20	425
Pregnant	220	60	50	2.0	1.5–4.0	29–30	450
Nursing	290	70	50	2.6	1.5–4.0	44–45	550

*Adequate Intake (AI)
Adapted with permission from Recommended Dietary Allowances (Washington D.C.: National Academy Press, 1989), and DRI panel reports, 1997–2004

No Sale Ever Is Final

The slogan "No Sale Ever Is Final," printed on the sales slips at one of my favorite clothing stores, definitely applies to nutritional numbers. RDAs, AIs, and DRIs should always be regarded as works in progress, subject to revision at the first sign of a new study. In other words, in an ever-changing world, here's one thing of which you can be *absolutely* certain: The numbers in this chapter will change. Sorry about that.

Chapter 6

A Supplemental Story

In This Chapter

▶ Assessing the value of dietary supplements

▶ Finding out who regulates dietary supplements

▶ Getting your nutrients from food

The Food and Drug Administration (FDA) estimates that Americans spend nearly $25 billion each year on dietary supplements. You can stir up a good food fight in any group of nutrition experts simply by asking whether all these products are (a) necessary, (b) economical, or (c) safe. But when the argument's over, you still may not have a satisfactory *official* answer, so this brief chapter aims to provide the information you need to make your own sensible choices.

Introducing Dietary Supplements

The vitamin pill you may pop each morning is a dietary supplement. So are the calcium antacids many American women consider standard nutrition and the vanilla, chocolate, or strawberry liquid your granny chug-a-lugs each afternoon before setting out on her power walk. In fact, according to the Food and Drug Administration, any pill, tablet, capsule, powder, or liquid you take by mouth that contains a dietary ingredient is a dietary supplement. That includes

✔ Vitamins

✔ Minerals

✔ Herbs

✔ Amino acids (the "building blocks of protein" described in Chapter 7)

✔ Enzymes

✔ Organ tissue, such as that dried liver

✔ Some hormones, such as melatonin, the purported sleep aid

   ✔ Metabolites (substances produced when nutrients are digested)

   ✔ Extracts

Dietary supplements may be single-ingredient products, such as vitamin E capsules, or they may be combination products, such as multivitamin and mineral pills, or the newly popular "energy drinks." In a country where food is plentiful and affordable, you have to wonder why so many people opt to rely on these products instead of just plain food.

Examining Why People Use Dietary Supplements

Many people consider supplements a quick an easy way to get nutrients without much shopping and kitchen time and without all the pesky fats and sugars in food. Others take supplements as nutritional insurance. (For more on recommended dietary allowances of vitamins and minerals, see Chapter 5.) And some use supplements as substitutes for medical drugs.

In general, nutrition experts, including the American Dietetic Association, the National Academy of Sciences, and the National Research Council, prefer that you invest your time and money whipping up meals and snacks that supply the nutrients you need in a balanced diet of real food.

Nonetheless, every expert worth his or her vitamin D admits that in certain circumstances, supplements can be a definite plus.

When food isn't enough

Certain metabolic disorders and diseases of the digestive organs (liver, gallbladder, pancreas, and intestines) interfere with the normal digestion of food and the absorption of nutrients. Some medicines may also interfere with normal digestion, meaning you need supplements to make up the difference. People who suffer from certain chronic diseases or who have experienced a major injury (such as a serious burn), or who have just been through surgery may need more nutrients than they can get from food.

To be safe, check with your doctor before opting for a supplement you hope will have medical effects (make you stronger, smooth your skin, ease your anxiety). The bad old days when doctors were total ignoramuses about nutrition may not be gone forever, but they're fading fast. Besides, your doctor is the person most familiar with your health, knows what medications you're taking, and can caution you about potential side effects.

Supplementing aging appetites

As you grow older, your appetite may decline and your sense of taste and smell may falter. If food no longer tastes as good as it once did, if you have to eat alone all the time and don't enjoy cooking for one, or if dentures make chewing difficult, you may not be taking in all the foods that you need to get the nutrients you require. Dietary supplements may be the answer.

Meeting a woman's special needs

At various stages of their reproductive lives, women benefit from supplements. For example:

- **Before menopause:** Women, who lose iron each month through menstrual bleeding, rarely get sufficient amounts of iron from a typical American diet providing fewer than 2,000 calories a day. For them, and for women who are often on a diet to lose weight, iron supplements may be the only practical answer. Deciding which iron pill to choose? Check out Chapter 12.

- **During pregnancy and lactation:** Women who are pregnant or nursing often need supplements to provide the nutrients they need to build new maternal and fetal tissue or to produce nutritious breast milk. In addition, supplements of the B vitamin folate are known to decrease a woman's risk of giving birth to a child with a neural tube defect (a defect of the spinal cord and column).

  Never self-prescribe supplements while you're pregnant. Large amounts of some nutrients may actually be hazardous for your baby. For example, taking megadoses of vitamin A while pregnant may increase the risk of birth defects.

- **Through adulthood:** True, women older than 19 can get the calcium they require (1,000 milligrams/day) from four 8-ounce glasses of nonfat skim milk a day, three 8-ounce or four 6-ounce containers of yogurt made with nonfat milk, 22 ounces of canned salmon (with the soft edible bones; definitely not the hard bones in fresh salmon!), or any combination of the above. However, expecting women to do this nutritional balancing act every single day may be unrealistic. The simple alternative is calcium supplements.

Boosting a special diet

Vitamin B12 is found only in food from animals, such as meat, milk, and eggs. (Some seaweed does have B12, but the suspicion is that the vitamin comes from microorganisms living in the plant.) Once upon a time, *vegans* (people who eat only plant foods — no dairy foods or eggs allowed) would almost certainly have had to get their B12 from supplements. Today, fortified grains may do the trick, but some vegans still add B12 supplements to be sure.

Using supplements as insurance

Healthy people who eat a nutritious diet still choose supplements to make sure they're getting adequate nutrition.

At first glance, it seemed they might be right. In 2002, the American Medical Association (AMA), which for decades had turned thumbs down on vitamin supplements, changed its collective mind after a review of 26 years' worth of scientific studies relating vitamin levels to the risk of chronic illness. Robert H. Fletcher and Kathleen M. Fairfield, the Harvard-based authors of the study, which was published in the *Journal of the American Medical Association (JAMA)*, noted that while true vitamin-deficiency diseases such as scurvy and beriberi are rare in Western countries, *suboptimal vitamin levels* — sciencespeak for slightly less than you need — are a real problem. If "slightly less than you need" sounds slightly less than important, consider this:

- ✔ Suboptimal intake of folate and two other B vitamins (B6 and B12) may raise your risk of heart disease, colon cancer, breast cancer, and birth defects.

- ✔ Suboptimal vitamin D intake means a higher risk of rickets and osteoporosis.

Of course, as Isaac Newton so nicely put it in 1686 in his Third Law of Motion, "For every action, there is an equal and opposite reaction." Thus, in 2007, when the National Cancer Institute toted up the data from nearly 300,000 men enrolled in the National Institutes of Health's AARP Diet and Health Study, the numbers showed no link between taking a multivitamin and the risk of developing prostate cancer. But — and it's a big one — men who took a daily supplement were nearly one-third more likely to develop advanced prostate cancers and nearly (98 percent) 100 percent more likely to die from their disease.

And two years later, in 2009, a report in *The Archives of Internal Medicine* summarizing data from an analysis of more than 150,000 women showed that taking multivitamins every day had no effect on the risk for breast cancer, colorectal cancer, endometrial cancer, lung cancer, ovarian cancer, heart attack, stroke, blood clots, or mortality. The study's author, Marian L. Neuhouser, a nutritional epidemiologist with the Fred Hutchinson Cancer Research Center in Seattle, was quoted as concluding that "buying more fruits and vegetables might be a better choice." Tastes better, too.

Supplement Safety: An Iffy Proposition

As its name implies, the Food and Drug Administration (FDA) regulates drugs *and* food. Before the agency allows a new food or a new drug on the market, the manufacturer must submit proof that the product is safe. Drug manufacturers must also meet a second test, showing that their new medi-cine is *efficacious,* meaning that it works and that the drug and the dosage in which it's sold will cure or relieve the condition for which it's prescribed.

Nobody says the drug-regulation system's perfect. Reality dictates that manu-facturers test a drug only on a limited number of people for a limited period of time. So you can bet that some new drugs will trigger unexpected, serious, maybe even life-threatening side effects when used by thousands of people or taken for longer than the testing period. For proof, look no further than Avandia, the diabetes drug that appeared safe when approved but turned out to be a heart hazard after it reached pharmacy shelves.

But at least the FDA can require that premarket safety and/or effectiveness info be displayed on foods and drugs. Unfortunately, the agency has no such power when it comes to dietary supplements.

In 1994, Congress passed and President Clinton signed into law the Dietary Supplement Health and Education Act, which limits the FDA's control over dietary supplements. Under this law, the FDA can't

✔ Require premarket tests to prove that supplements are safe and effective

✔ Limit the dosage in any dietary supplement

✔ Halt or restrict sales of a dietary supplement unless evidence shows that the product has caused illness or injury *when used according to the direc-tions on the package;* in other words, if you experience a problem after taking slightly more or less of a supplement than directed on the label, the FDA can't help you

If the dietary supplement contains a "new dietary ingredient(s)," the law says the manufacturer or distributor must tell the FDA about the/these new ingredient(s) and "the notification must include information that is the basis on which the manufacturers/distributors have concluded that a dietary supplement contain-ing a new dietary ingredient will reasonably be expected to be safe under the conditions of use recommended or suggested in the labeling." Whew!

Sweet trouble

Experience dictates that making pills — even vitamin pills — taste good can be hazardous to a child's health. Some nutrients are seriously troublesome in high doses (see Chapters 11 and 12), especially for kids. The best example: iron pills. The Food and Drug Administration warns that the lethal dose for young children may be as low as 3 grams (3,000 milligrams) elemental iron, the amount in 49 tablets with 65 milligrams iron apiece. If you have youngsters in your house, protect them by buying neutral-tasting supplements and keeping all pills, nutrient and otherwise, in a safe cabinet, preferably high off the floor, locked tightly to resist prying fingers.

As a result, the FDA has found it virtually impossible to take products off drugstore shelves even after reports of illness and injury. For example, supplements containing the herb *ephedra* are reputed to enhance weight loss and sports performance. More than 600 reports of illness and at least 100 deaths have been linked to the use of ephedra supplements. The herb is banned by professional football and college athletics in the United States and by the Olympics. However, the FDA didn't act until February 2003, following the death of Baltimore Orioles pitcher Steve Bechler, who reportedly had been using ephedra products to control his weight. Bechler's untimely death rang warning bells across the country, including in Washington, D.C., where the FDA ruled that henceforth every bottle of ephedra must carry strong warnings that the popular herb can cause potentially lethal heart attacks or strokes. In the sports world, ephedra was immediately forbidden in minor-league but not major-league baseball. The FDA then banned all ephedra products, and despite a challenge from an ephedra manufacturer, the ban was upheld by the U.S. Court of Appeals for the Tenth Circuit in 2006.

By the way, ephedra isn't the only herbal supplement that can make you *really* uncomfortable. In 2010, *Consumer Reports* issued a list of 12 hazardous ingredients they named The Dirty Dozen (see Table 6-1).

Table 6-1	Some Potentially Hazardous Herbals
Herb	*Known Side Effects and Reactions*
Aconite, aka Monkshood	Dizziness, gastric upset, muscle spasms, irregular heart beat
Bitter orange	Fast heart beat and high blood pressure
Chaparral	Liver damage
Colloidal silver	Seizures, liver damage
Coltsfoot	Liver damage, cancer
Comfrey	Liver damage, liver cancer
Country mallow	Headache, gastric upset, insomnia, irregular heartbeat, irritability, dizziness, insomnia
Germanium	Toxic to kidney, liver, and nerves
Greater celandine	Potential liver disease, bile duct obstruction
Kava	Liver damage
Lobelia	Rapid heartbeat, falling blood pressure, coma
Yohimbe	Rapid heartbeat, changes in blood pressure

Sources: Memorial Sloan-Kettering Cancer Center, "About Herbs, Botanicals and Other Products, `www.mskcc.org/mskcc/html/11570.cfm`; *WebMD, "Find a vitamin or supplement"* `www.webmd.com/vitamins-supplements/default.aspx`

Choosing the Most Effective Supplements

Okay, you've read about the virtues and drawbacks of supplements. You've decided which supplements you think may do you some good. Now it's crunch time, and all you really want to know is how to choose the safest, most effective, products. The following guidelines can help:

- **Pick a well-known brand.** Even though the FDA can't require manufacturers to submit safety and effectiveness data, a respected name on the label offers some assurance of a quality product. It also promises a fresh product; well-known brands generally sell out more quickly. The initials *USP* (U.S. Pharmacopoeia, a reputable testing organization) are another quality statement, and so are the words "release assured" or "proven release," which mean the supplement is easily absorbed by your body.

- **Look for the expiration date.** Over time, all dietary supplements become less potent. Always choose the product with the longest useful shelf life. Pass on the ones that will expire before you can use all the pills, such as the 100-pill bottle with an expiration date 30 days from now.

- **Read the storage requirements.** Even when you buy a product with the correct expiration date, it may be less effective if you don't keep it in the right place. Some supplements must be refrigerated; the rest you need to store, like any food product, in a cool, dry place. Avoid putting dietary supplements in a cabinet above the stove or refrigerator — true, the fridge is cold inside, but the motor pulsing away outside emits heat.

- **Stick with a safe dose.** Unless your doctor prescribes a dietary supplement as medicine, you don't need products marked "therapeutic," "extra-strength," or any variation thereof. Pick one that gives you no more than the RDA for any ingredient.

- **Avoid hype.** When the label promises something that's too good to be true, you know it's too good to be true. The FDA doesn't permit supplement marketers to claim that their products cure or prevent disease (that would make them medicines that require premarket testing). But the agency does allow claims that affect function, such as "maintains your cholesterol" (the medical claim would be "lowers your cholesterol").

Another potential hype zone is the one labeled "natural," as in "natural vitamins are better." If you took Chem 101 in college, you know that the ascorbic acid (vitamin C) in oranges has exactly the same chemical composition as the ascorbic acid some nutritional chemist cooks up in her lab. But the ascorbic acid in a "natural" vitamin pill may come without additives, such as coloring agents or fillers used in "regular" vitamin pills. In other words, if you aren't sensitive to the coloring agents or fillers in plain old pills, don't spend the extra dollars for "natural." If you are sensitive, do. What could be simpler? (For more on "natural" versus "synthetic" food ingredients, see Chapter 22.)

✔ **Check the ingredient list.** In the early 1990s, the FDA introduced the consumer-friendly nutrition food label with its mini-nutrition guide to nutrient content, complete ingredient listings, and dependable information about how eating certain foods may affect your risk of chronic illnesses, such as heart disease and cancer. (For more about the nutrition labels, see Chapter 17.)

TIP

The FDA's new supplement labels must list all ingredients. The label for vitamin and mineral products must give you the quantity per nutrient per serving plus the *%DV* (percentage daily value), the percentage of the RDA (Recommended Dietary Allowance). The listings for other dietary supplements, such as botanicals (herbs) and phytochemicals (see Chapter 12), must show the quantity per serving plus the part of the plant from which the ingredient is drawn (root, leaves, and so on). A manufacturer's own proprietary blend of two or more botanicals must list the weight of the total blend.

The boost in a bottle

It all started with Gatorade. In the summer of 1965, a football coach at the University of Florida asked a team of university physicians to explain why so many players wilted in the heat. The answer: Loss of fluid and electrolytes (see Chapter 13) when sweating. The result: A thirst-quenching hydrating fluid replacement beverage called, yes, Gatorade that soon had the Florida Gators walking over their opponents to end up with a winning season and a win at the Orange Bowl in 1966. (In 2010, Gatorade introduced a new generation of sugarfree products.)

Nothing succeeds like success, of course. Fairly soon, other universities began ordering up some Gatorade for their teams, pro teams bought in, and, by 1983, Gatorade was the official sports drink of the NFL — a title it holds to this day. Eventually, the hydrating liquid for serious athletes morphed into an "energy drink" for amateur athletes with nutrient-packed beverages promising to increase performance and, sometimes, just keep a person awake and alert. Not surprising, one of the most common ingredients in these beverages is the original awake-and-alert substance, caffeine, as in coffee or guarana, a caffeinated berry native to Brazil and Venezuela. Other prominent ingredients are taurine, an amino acid whose name comes from the Latin word for *bull,* a clear hint of strength, and ginseng, the reputed healing herb. And often, vitamins — primarily the Bs — are also in the mix. And sometimes there is sugar to sweeten an otherwise bland cocktail. The value of the herbs in these products is questionable, as is the value of vitamins for healthy people who eat a varied diet.

However, I have three cautions. First, sugar is fattening. Second, adding vitamins to a daily diet via energy drinks might trip a person who is taking other supplements into overdose territory (see Chapter 11). Third, watch the caffeine level. Yes, caffeine keeps you awake and has been proven to improve endurance for athletes such as distance runners. But too much caffeine, whether from coffee, tea, or energy drinks, leads to the inevitable results: A nervous, irritable insomniac with a rapid heartbeat and maybe even high blood pressure. And this is not a minor matter: According to a 2003 report from the *Journal of the American Pharmaceutical Association,* there have been at least four case reports of caffeine-associated deaths and four documented cases of seizures associated with energy drinks.

Anyone here want a glass of water?

Figure 6-1 shows an example of the supplement labels.

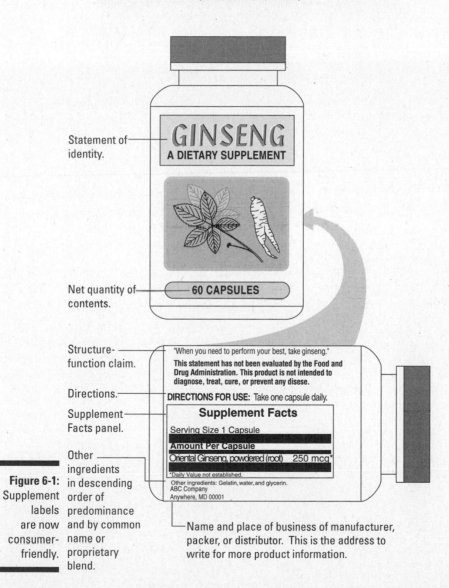

Nutrition Labeling for Dietary Supplements

(Effective March 1999)

Statement of identity.

GINSENG
A DIETARY SUPPLEMENT

Net quantity of contents.

60 CAPSULES

Structure-function claim.

"When you need to perform your best, take ginseng."

This statement has not been evaluated by the Food and Drug Administration. This product is not intended to diagnose, treat, cure, or prevent any disese.

Directions.

DIRECTIONS FOR USE: Take one capsule daily.

Supplement Facts panel.

Supplement Facts

Serving Size 1 Capsule

Amount Per Capsule

Oriental Ginseng, powdered (root)   250 mcg*

*Daily Value not established.

Other ingredients: Gelatin, water, and glycerin.
ABC Company
Anywhere, MD 00001

Other ingredients in descending order of predominance and by common name or proprietary blend.

Name and place of business of manufacturer, packer, or distributor. This is the address to write for more product information.

Figure 6-1: Supplement labels are now consumer-friendly.

Good Reasons for Getting Nutrients from Food Rather Than Supplements

Despite this chapter's focus on the wonders of supplements, I feel obligated to play devil's advocate and report to you the arguments in favor of healthy people getting all or most of their nutrients from food rather than supplements.

- ✔ **Cost:** If you're willing to plan and prepare nutritious meals, you can almost always get your nutrients less expensively from fresh fruits, vegetables, whole grains, dairy products, meat, fish, and poultry. Besides, food usually tastes better than supplements.

- ✔ **Unexpected bonuses:** Food is a package deal containing vitamins, minerals, protein, fat, carbohydrates, and dietary fiber, plus a cornucopia of phytochemicals (phyto = plant) that may be vital to your continuing good health.

- ✔ **Safety:** Several common nutrients may be toxic in *megadose servings* (amounts several times larger than the RDAs). Not only are large doses of vitamin A linked to birth defects, but they may also cause symptoms similar to a brain tumor. Niacin megadoses may cause liver damage. Megadoses of vitamin B6 may cause (temporary) damage to nerves in arms, legs, fingers, and toes. All these effects are more likely to occur with supplements. Pills slip down easily, but regardless of how hungry you are, you probably won't eat enough food to reach toxic levels of nutrients. (To read more about the hazards of megadoses, see Chapters 11 and 12.)

The best statement about the role of supplements in good nutrition may be a paraphrase of Abraham Lincoln's famous remark about politicians and voters: "You may fool all the people some of the time; you can even fool some of the people all the time; but you can't fool all of the people all the time." If Honest Abe were with us now and were a sensible nutritionist rather than a president, he might amend his words: "Supplements are valuable for all people some of the time and for some people all the time, but they're probably not necessary for all people all the time."

Part II
What You Get from Food

The 5th Wave By Rich Tennant

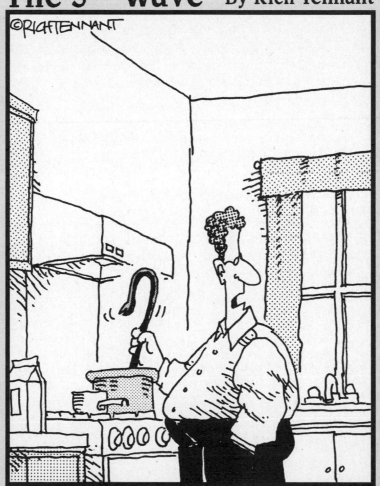

©RICHTENNANT

"I'm not sure we're getting enough iron in our diet, so I'm stirring the soup with a crowbar."

In this part . . .

This part is an up-to-the-minute guide to nutrients you've heard about practically forever: protein, fat, carbohydrates, alcohol, vitamins, minerals, and water. This part provides the newest numbers available on how each works and how much of each one you need to keep your body humming happily.

Because this is a *For Dummies* book, you don't have to read straight through from protein to water to see how things work. You can skip from chapter to chapter, back and forth, side to side. Any way you take it, this part is bound to clue you in to the value of the nutrients in food.

Chapter 7

Powerful Protein

*P*rotein is an essential nutrient whose name comes from the Greek word *protos,* which means "first." To visualize a molecule of protein, close your eyes and see a very long chain, rather like a chain of sausage links. The links in the chains are *amino acids,* commonly known as the building blocks of protein. In addition to carbon, hydrogen, and oxygen atoms, amino acids contain a nitrogen (amino) group. The *amino group* is essential for synthesizing (assembling) specialized proteins in your body.

In this chapter, you can find out more — maybe even more than you ever wanted to know — about this molecule, how your body uses the proteins you take in as food, and how the body makes some special proteins you need for a healthy life.

How Your Body Uses Proteins

Your body uses proteins to build new cells, maintain tissues, and synthesize new proteins that make it possible for you to perform basic bodily functions.

The human body is chock-full of proteins. Proteins are present in the outer and inner membranes of every living cell. Here's where else protein makes an appearance:

➤ Your hair, your nails, and the outer layers of your skin are made of keratin, a *scleroprotein,* or a protein resistant to digestive enzymes. If you bite your nails, you can't digest them.

➤ Muscle tissue contains *myosin, actin, myoglobin,* and a number of other proteins.

✔ Bone's outer layer is hardened with minerals such as calcium, but the basic, rubbery inner structure is protein; and bone marrow, the soft material inside the bone, is also protein-rich.

✔ Red blood cells contain *hemoglobin,* a protein compound that carries oxygen throughout the body. *Plasma,* the clear fluid in blood, contains fat and protein particles known as *lipoproteins,* which ferry cholesterol around and out of the body.

About half the dietary protein that you consume each day goes into making *enzymes,* the specialized worker proteins that do specific jobs such as digesting food and assembling or dividing molecules to make new cells and chemical substances. To perform these functions, enzymes often need specific vitamins and minerals.

Your ability to see, think, hear, and move — in fact, to do just about everything that you consider part of a healthy life — requires your nerve cells to send messages back and forth to each other and to other specialized kinds of cells, such as muscle cells. Sending these messages requires chemicals called *neurotransmitters.* Making neurotransmitters requires proteins.

Finally, proteins play an important part in the creation of every new cell and every new individual. Your chromosomes consist of *nucleoproteins,* which are substances made of amino acids and nucleic acids. (See the "DNA/RNA" sidebar in this chapter for more information about nucleoproteins.)

DNA/RNA

Nucleoproteins are chemicals in the nucleus of every living cell. They're made of proteins linked to *nucleic acids* — complex compounds that contain phosphoric acid, a sugar molecule, and nitrogen-containing molecules made from amino acids.

Nucleic acids (molecules found in the chromosomes and other structures in the center of your cells) carry the genetic codes, the genes that help determine what you look like, your general intelligence, and who you are. They also contain one of two sugars, either *ribose* or *deoxyribose.* The nucleic acid containing ribose is called *ribonucleic acid* (RNA). The nucleic acid containing deoxyribose is called *deoxyribonucleic acid* (DNA).

DNA is a very long molecule with two strands twisting about each other (the *double helix*); it carries and transmits the genetic inheritance in your chromosomes. DNA's job is to provide instructions that determine how your body cells are formed and how they behave. RNA, a single-strand molecule, is created in the cell nucleus according to the pattern determined by the DNA. Then RNA carries the DNA's instructions to the rest of the cell,

DNA is the most distinctly "you" thing about your body. Chances that another person on Earth has exactly the same DNA as you are really small. That's why DNA analysis is so valuable in identifying individuals in various situations. Most commonly, this means criminal behavior, but some now propose that parents store a sample of their children's DNA to have a conclusive way of identifying a missing child, even years later.

How the Proteins You Eat Move Into Your Cells

The cells in your digestive tract can absorb only single amino acids or very small chains of two or three amino acids called *peptides.* So proteins from food are broken into their component amino acids by digestive enzymes — which are, of course, specialized proteins. Then other enzymes in your body cells build new proteins by reassembling the amino acids into specific compounds that your body needs to function. This process is called *protein synthesis.* During protein synthesis

- Amino acids hook up with fats to form *lipoproteins,* the molecules that ferry cholesterol around and out of the body. Or amino acids may join up with carbohydrates to form the *glycoproteins* found in the mucus secreted by the digestive tract.

- Proteins combine with phosphoric acid to produce *phosphoproteins,* such as casein, a protein in milk.

- Nucleic acids combine with proteins to create *nucleoproteins,* which are essential components of the cell nucleus and of cytoplasm, the living material inside each cell.

The carbon, hydrogen, and oxygen that are left over after protein synthesis is complete are converted to glucose and used for energy. The nitrogen residue (ammonia) isn't used for energy. It's processed by the liver, which converts the ammonia to urea. Most of the urea produced in the liver is excreted through the kidneys in urine; very small amounts are sloughed off in skin, hair, and nails.

Every day, you *turn over* (reuse) more proteins than you get from the food you eat, so you need a continuous supply to maintain your protein status. If your diet does not contain sufficient amounts of proteins, you start digesting the proteins in your body, including the proteins in your muscles and — in extreme cases — your heart muscle.

Differentiating Dietary Proteins

All the proteins in your food are made of building blocks called amino acids, but not all proteins contain all the amino acids you require. This section helps you figure out how you can get the most useful proteins from your varied diet.

Essential and nonessential proteins

To make all the proteins that your body needs, you require 22 different amino acids. Ten are considered *essential,* which means you can't synthesize them in your body and must obtain them from food. (Two of these, arginine and histidine, are essential only for children.) Several more are *nonessential:* If you don't get them in food, you can manufacture them yourself from fats, carbohydrates, and other amino acids. Three — glutamine, ornithine, and taurine — are somewhere in between essential and nonessential for human beings: They're essential only under certain conditions, such as with injury or disease.

Essential Amino Acids	*Nonessential Amino Acids*
Arginine*	Alanine
Histidine*	Asparagine
Isoleucine	Aspartic acid
Leucine	Citrulline
Lysine	Cysteine
Methionine	Glutamic acid
Phenlyalanine	Glycine
Threoniwne	Hydroxyglutamic acid
Tryptophan	Norleucine
Valine	Proline
	Serine
	Tyrosine

* Essential for children; nonessential for adults

High-quality and low-quality proteins

Because an animal's body is similar to yours, its proteins contain similar combinations of amino acids. That's why nutritionists call proteins from foods of animal origin — meat, fish, poultry, eggs, and dairy products — *high-quality proteins.* Your body absorbs these proteins more efficiently; they can be used without much waste to synthesize other proteins. The proteins from plants — grains, fruit, vegetables, legumes (beans), nuts, and seeds — often have limited amounts of some essential amino acids, which means their nutritional content is not as high as animal proteins.

Super soy: The special protein food

Nutrition fact No. 1: Food from animals has complete proteins. **Nutrition fact No. 2:** Vegetables, fruits, and grains have incomplete proteins. **Nutrition fact No. 3:** Nobody told the soybean.

Unlike other vegetables, including other beans, soybeans have complete proteins with sufficient amounts of all the amino acids essential to human health. In fact, food experts rank soy proteins on par with egg whites and casein (the protein in milk), the two proteins easiest for your body to absorb and use (see Table 7-1).

Some nutritionists think soy proteins are even better than the proteins in eggs and milk, because the proteins in soy come with no cholesterol and very little of the saturated fat known to clog your arteries and raise your risk of heart attack. Better yet, more than 20 recent studies suggest that adding soy foods to your diet can actually lower your cholesterol levels.

One-half cup (4 ounces) of cooked soybeans has 14 grams of protein; 4 ounces of tofu has 13. Either serving gives you approximately twice the protein you get from one large egg or one 8-ounce glass of skim milk, or two-thirds the protein in 3 ounces of lean ground beef. Eight ounces of fat-free soy milk has 7 grams protein — a mere 1 gram less than a similar serving of skim milk — and no cholesterol. Soybeans are also jam-packed with dietary fiber, which helps move food through your digestive tract.

The basic standard against which you measure the value of proteins in food is the egg. Nutrition scientists have arbitrarily given the egg a *biological value* of 100 percent, meaning that, gram for gram, it's the food with the best supply of complete proteins. Other foods that have proportionately more protein may not be as valuable as the egg because they lack sufficient amounts of one or more essential amino acids.

For example, eggs are 11 percent protein, and dry beans are 22 percent protein. However, the proteins in beans don't provide sufficient amounts of *all* the essential amino acids, so they (the beans) are not as nutritionally complete as proteins from animal foods. The prime exception is the soybean, a legume that's packed with abundant amounts of all of the amino acids essential for adults. Soybeans are an excellent source of proteins for vegetarians, especially *vegans,* which are vegetarians who avoid all products of animal origin, including milk and eggs.

The term used to describe the value of the proteins in any one food is *amino acid score.* Because the egg contains all the essential amino acids, it scores 100. Table 7-1 shows the protein quality of representative foods relative to the egg.

Table 7-1	Scoring the Amino Acids in Food	
Food	*Protein Content (Grams)*	*Amino Acid Score (Compared to the Egg)*
Egg	33	100
Fish	61	100
Beef	29	100
Milk (cow's whole)	23	100
Soybeans	29	100
Dry beans	22	75
Rice	7	62–66
Corn	7	47
Wheat	13	50
Wheat (white flour)	12	36

Nutritive Value of Foods (Washington, D.C.: U.S. Department of Agriculture, 1991); George M. Briggs and Doris Howes Calloway, Nutrition and Physical Fitness, 11th ed. (New York: Holt, Rinehart and Winston, 1984)

Complete proteins and incomplete proteins

Another way to describe the quality of proteins is to say that they're either complete or incomplete. A *complete protein* is one that contains ample amounts of all essential amino acids; an *incomplete protein* does not. A protein low in one specific amino acid is called a *limiting protein* because it can build only as much tissue as the smallest amount of the necessary amino acid. You can improve the protein quality in a food containing incomplete/limiting proteins by eating it along with one that contains sufficient amounts of the limited amino acids.

Matching foods to create complete proteins is called *complementarity,* a concept first popularized by Frances Moore Lappe in her bestselling book, Diet for a Small Planet (1971). Moore's intent was to convince people to become vegetarians or at least to increase the amount of plant foods in their diets while decreasing the amount of foods from animals so as to conserve energy and reduce the overall cost of producing food.

The lowdown on gelatin and your fingernails

Everyone knows that gelatin is a protein that strengthens fingernails. Too bad *everyone's* half-wrong.

Yes, gelatin is protein, and yes, protein makes nails strong. But, not the incomplete protein in gelatin, a food made by treating animal bones with acid, thus destroying the essential amino acid tryptophan.

Luckily, you can improve the protein value of gelatin by slicing a banana onto the dish (bananas are tryptophan-rich) and pouring on some milk (also a good source of tryptophan).

One example of complementarity is rice and beans. The rice is low in the essential amino acid lysine, and beans are low in the essential amino acid methionine. By eating rice with beans, you improve (or complete) the proteins in both. Another example is pasta and cheese. Pasta is low in the essential amino acids lysine and isoleucine; milk products have abundant amounts of these two amino acids. Shaking Parmesan cheese onto pasta creates a higher-quality protein dish. In each case, the foods have complementary amino acids. Other examples of complementary protein dishes are peanut butter with bread, and milk with cereal. Many such combinations are a natural and customary part of the diet in parts of the world where animal proteins are scarce or very expensive.

Table 7-2 shows how to combine foods to improve the quality of their proteins. Once upon a time, nutritionists insisted that you had to consume these combinations in rigorous combination — that is, in the same dish or the same meal. But time moves on, and so does nutrition knowledge. Today, those same nutritionists accept the idea that when you eat a food with incomplete proteins, the proteins hang around in your body several hours, long enough to hook up with incomplete proteins in other foods in your next meal, which certainly makes meal planning ever so much easier.

Table 7-2	How to Combine Foods to Complement Proteins	
This Food	*Complements This Food*	*Examples*
Whole grains	Legumes (beans)	Rice and beans
Dairy products	Whole grains	Cheese sandwich, pasta with cheese, pancakes (wheat and milk/egg batter)
Legumes (beans)	Nuts and/or seeds	Chili soup (beans) with caraway seeds
Dairy products	Legumes (beans)	Chili beans with cheese
Dairy products	Nuts and seeds	Yogurt with chopped nut garnish

How Much Protein Do You Need?

The National Academy of Sciences Food and Nutrition Board, which sets the requirements (for example, RDAs) for vitamins and minerals, also sets goals for daily protein consumption. As with other nutrients, the board has different recommendations for different groups of people: young, older, male, and female.

Calculating the correct amount

In 2005, the Academy set a Dietary Reference Intake (DRI) of 46 grams protein per day for a healthy adult woman and 56 grams per day for a healthy adult man. (Check out Chapter 5 for a complete explanation of the DRI.)

These amounts are easily obtained from two to three 3-ounce servings of lean meat, fish, or poultry (21 grams each). Vegetarians can get their protein from 2 eggs (12–16 grams), 2 slices of packaged fat-free cheese (10 grams), 4 slices of bread (3 grams each), and one cup of yogurt (10 grams). Vegans (those who do not eat any foods from animals, including dairy products) get the protein they need from a cup of oatmeal (6 grams) with a cup of soymilk (7 grams), 2 tablespoons peanut butter (8 grams) sandwiched on one large pita (5–6 grams), 6 ounces soy milk yogurt (6 grams), 6 ounces tofu (13 grams) with 1 cup cooked brown rice (5 grams), and 1 cup steamed broccoli (5 grams).

Muscle into fat? No way

An older body synthesizes new proteins less efficiently than a younger one, so muscle mass (protein tissue) diminishes while fat content stays the same or rises. This change is often erroneously described as muscle "turning to fat." The aging body still uses protein to build new tissue, however, including hair, skin, and nails, which continue to grow until death. By the way, the idea that nails continue to grow after death — a staple of shock movies and horror comics — arises from the fact that after death, tissue around the nails shrinks, making a corpse's nails simply look longer.

For the protein values in literally thousands of servings of literally thousands of foods, check out the USDA National Nutrient Database for Standard Reference at `www.nal.usda.gov/fnic/foodcomp/search`.

Dodging protein deficiency

The first sign of protein deficiency is likely to be weak muscles — the body tissue most reliant on protein. For example, children who do not get enough protein have shrunken, weak muscles. They may also have thin hair, their skin may be covered with sores, and blood tests may show abnormally low blood levels of *albumin,* a protein that helps maintain the body's fluid balance, keeping a proper amount of liquid in and around body cells.

A protein deficiency may also affect red blood cells. The cells live for only 120 days, so the body needs a regular supply of protein to make new ones. People who do not get enough protein may become *anemic,* having fewer red blood cells than they need. Other signs of protein deficiency are fluid retention (the big belly on a starving child), hair loss, and muscle wasting caused by the body's attempt to protect itself by digesting the proteins in its own muscle tissue, a phenomenon that explains why victims of starvation are, literally, skin and bones.

Given the high protein content of a normal American diet (which generally provides far more protein than you actually require), protein deficiency is rare in the United States except as a consequence of eating disorders such as *anorexia nervosa* (refusal to eat) and *bulimia* (regurgitation after meals).

Boosting your protein intake: Special considerations

Anyone who's building new tissue quickly needs extra protein. For example, the Dietary Reference Intake (DRI) for protein for women who are pregnant or nursing is 71 grams per day. Injuries also raise your protein requirements. An injured body releases above-normal amounts of protein-destroying hormones from the pituitary and adrenal glands. You need extra protein to protect existing tissues, and after severe blood loss, you need extra protein to make new hemoglobin for red blood cells. Cuts, burns, or surgical procedures mean that you need extra protein to make new skin and muscle cells. Fractures mean extra protein is needed to make new bone. The need for protein is so important when you've been badly injured that if you can't take protein by mouth, you'll be given an intravenous solution of amino acids with glucose (sugar) or emulsified fat.

Do athletes need more proteins than the rest of us? Recent research suggests that the answer may be yes, but athletes easily meet their requirements simply by eating more food, not necessarily increasing the amount of any specific food.

Avoiding protein overload

Yes, you can get too much protein. Several medical conditions make it difficult for people to digest and process proteins properly. As a result, waste products build up in different parts of the body.

People with liver disease or kidney disease either don't process protein efficiently into urea or don't excrete it efficiently through urine. The result may be uric acid kidney stones or *uremic poisoning* (an excess amount of uric acid in the blood). The pain associated with *gout* (a form of arthritis that affects nine men for every one woman) is caused by uric acid crystals collecting in the spaces around joints. Doctors may recommend a low-protein diet as part of the treatment in these situations.

Chapter 8

Facing Facts on Fat and Cholesterol

....

In This Chapter

▶ Defining the different kinds of fat in food

▶ Listing the good and bad points of dietary fat

▶ Explaining cholesterol's good and bad points

▶ Balancing the fat (and cholesterol) in your diet

....

The chemical family name for fats and related compounds, such as cholesterol, is *lipids,* from *lipos,* the Greek word for fat. Liquid fats are called *oils;* solid fats are called, well, *fat,* and the fat in food is called *dietary fat.*

With the exception of *cholesterol* (a fatty substance that has no calories and provides no energy), dietary fats are high-energy nutrients. Gram for gram, fats have more than twice as much energy potential (calories) as protein and carbohydrates: 9 calories per fat gram versus 4 calories per gram for the other two. (For more calorie information, see Chapter 3.)

This chapter cuts the fat away from the subject of fats and zeroes in on what you need to put together a diet with just enough fat to control your cholesterol.

How Your Body Uses Fats

Dietary fats are sources of energy that add flavor to food — the characteristic sizzle on the steak, so to speak. Unfortunately, this tasty nutrient may also be hazardous to your health. The trick is to separate the good from the bad.

What fats do for you

A healthy body needs fats to build body tissues and manufacture biochemicals, such as hormones. Some of the *adipose* (fatty) tissue in your body is plain to see. For example, even though your skin covers it, you can *see* the fat deposits in female breasts, hips, thighs, buttocks, and belly or on the male abdomen and shoulders.

This relatively visible body fat

- ✔ Provides a source of stored energy
- ✔ Gives shape to your body
- ✔ Cushions your skin (imagine sitting in a chair without your buttocks to pillow your bones)
- ✔ Acts as an insulation blanket that reduces heat loss

Other body fat is tucked away in and around your internal organs. This hidden fat is

- ✔ Part of every cell membrane (the outer skin that holds each cell together)
- ✔ A component of *myelin,* the fatty material that sheathes nerve cells and makes it possible for them to send the electrical messages that enable you to think, see, speak, move, and perform the multitude of tasks natural to a living body (Your brain is about 60 percent fat, giving a whole new meaning to the term "fat head.")
- ✔ A constituent of hormones and other biochemicals, such as vitamin D and bile
- ✔ A shock absorber that protects your organs (as much as possible) if you fall or are injured

Pulling energy from fat

Although dietary fat has more energy (calories) per gram than protein and carbohydrates, your body has a more difficult time pulling the energy out of fatty foods than out of foods high in protein and carbs.

Imagine a chain of long balloons — the kind people twist into shapes that resemble dachshunds, flowers, and other amusing things. When you drop one of these balloons into water, it floats. That's exactly what happens when you swallow fat-rich foods. The fat floats on top of the watery food-and-liquid mixture in your stomach, which limits the effects of *lipases,* the enzymes that break fats apart so you can digest them. As a result, fat is digested more slowly than proteins and carbohydrates, so you feel fuller, a condition called *satiety* (pronounced *say-ty-eh-tee*) longer after eating high-fat food.

Into the intestines

When the fat moves down your digestive tract into your small intestine, an intestinal hormone called *cholecystokinin* alerts your gallbladder to release *bile.* Bile is an emulsifier, a substance that enables fat to mix with water so that lipases can start breaking the fat into *glycerol* and *fatty acids.* These smaller fragments may be stored in special cells (fat cells) in adipose tissue, or they may be absorbed into cells in the intestinal wall, where one of the following happens:

✔ They're combined with oxygen (or burned) to produce heat/energy, water, and the waste product carbon dioxide.

✔ They're used to make lipoproteins that haul fats, including cholesterol, through your bloodstream.

Into the body

Glucose, the molecule you produce by digesting carbohydrates, is the body's basic source of energy. Burning glucose is easier and more efficient than burning fat, so your body always goes for carbohydrates first. But if you've used up all your available glucose — maybe you're stranded in a cabin in the Arctic, you haven't eaten for a week, a blizzard's howling outside, and the corner deli 500 miles down the road doesn't deliver — then it's time to start in on your body fat.

The first step is for an enzyme in your fat cells to break up stored *triglycerides* (the form of fat in adipose tissue). The enzyme action releases glycerol and fatty acids, which travel through your blood to body cells, where they combine with oxygen to produce heat/energy, plus water — lots of water — and the waste product carbon dioxide.

As anyone who has used a high-protein/high-fat/low-carb weight-loss diet such as the Atkins regimen can tell you, in addition to all that water, burning fat without glucose produces a second waste product called *ketones.* In extreme cases, high concentrations of ketones (a condition known as ketosis) may alter the acid/alkaline balance (or pH) of your blood (a condition known as ketoacidosis) and may trip you into a coma. Left untreated, ketoacidosis can lead to death. Medically, ketoacidosis is most likely to occur among people with diabetes. For people on a low-carb diet, the most likely sign of ketoacidosis is stinky urine or breath that smells like acetone (nail polish remover).

Defining fatty acids and their relationship to dietary fat

Fatty acids are the building blocks of fats. Chemically speaking, a *fatty acid* is a chain of carbon atoms with hydrogen atoms attached and a *carbon-oxygen-oxygen-hydrogen group* (the unit that makes it an acid) at one end.

Exploring the chemical structure of fatty acids

Molecules are groups of atoms hooked together by chemical bonds. Different atoms form different numbers of bonds with other atoms. For example, a hydrogen atom can form one bond with one other atom; an oxygen atom can form two bonds with other atoms; and a carbon atom can form four bonds to other atoms.

To actually see how this bonding works, visualize a carbon atom as one of those round pieces in a child's Erector set or Tinkertoy kit. Your carbon atom (C) has — figuratively speaking, of course — four holes: one on top, one on the bottom, and one on each side. If you stick a peg into each hole and attach a small piece of wood representing a hydrogen atom (H) to the pegs on the top, the bottom, and the left, you have a structure that looks like this:

Methyl Group

This unit, called a *methyl group,* is the first piece in any fatty acid. To build the rest of the fatty acid, you add carbon atoms and hydrogen atoms to form a chain. At the end, you tack on a group with one carbon atom, two oxygen atoms, and a hydrogen atom. This group is called an *acid group,* the part that makes the chain of carbon and hydrogen atoms a fatty acid.

Saturated Fatty Acid

The preceding molecule is a *saturated fatty acid* because it has a hydrogen atom at every available carbon link in the chain. A *monounsaturated fatty acid* drops two hydrogen atoms and forms one double bond (two lines instead of one) between two carbon atoms. A *polyunsaturated fatty acid* drops more hydrogen atoms and forms several (poly) double bonds between several carbon atoms. Every hydrogen atom still forms one bond, and every carbon atom still forms four bonds, but they do so in a slightly different way. These sketches are not pictures of real fatty acids, which have many more carbons in the chain and have their double bonds in different places, but they can give you an idea of what fatty acids look like up close.

Instead of this: (a saturated fatty acid)

You get this: (a monosaturated fatty acid)

or

(a polyunsaturated fatty acid)

And that's the whole deal!

An *essential fatty acid* is one that your body needs but cannot assemble from other fats. You have to get it whole, from food. Linoleic acid, found in vegetable oils, is an essential fatty acid. Two others — linolenic acid and arachidonic acid — occupy a somewhat ambiguous position. You can't make them from scratch, but you can make them if you have enough linoleic acid on hand, so food scientists often argue about whether linolenic and arachidonic acids are actually "essential."

In practical terms, who cares? Linoleic acid is so widely available in food, you're unlikely to experience a deficiency of any of the three — linoleic, linolenic, or arachidonic acid — as long as a measly 2 percent of the calories you get each day come from fat.

Focusing on the fats in food

Food contains three kinds of fats: triglycerides, phospholipids, and sterols. Here's how they differ:

- **Triglycerides:** You use these fats to make adipose tissue to burn for energy.

- **Phospholipids:** Phospholipids are hybrids — part lipid, part phosphate (a molecule made with the mineral phosphorus) — that ferry hormones and the fat-soluble vitamins A, D, E, and K through your blood and back and forth in the watery fluid that flows across cell membranes.

- **Sterols (steroid alcohols):** These are fat and alcohol compounds with no calories. VItamin D is a sterol. So is the sex hormone testosterone. And so is cholesterol, the base on which your body builds hormones and vitamins.

The fatty acids in food

All the fats in food are combinations of fatty acids. Nutritionists characterize fatty acids as saturated fatty acids (SFA), monounsaturated fatty acids (MUFA), or polyunsaturated fatty acids (PUFA), depending on how many hydrogen atoms are attached to the carbon atoms in the chain. The more hydrogen atoms, the more saturated the fatty acid. Depending on which fatty acids predominate, a food fat is likewise characterized as saturated, monounsaturated, or polyunsaturated.

- A *saturated fat,* such as butter, has mostly saturated fatty acids. Saturated fats are solid at room temperature and get harder when chilled.

- A *monounsaturated fat,* such as olive oil, has mostly monounsaturated fatty acids. Monounsaturated fats are liquid at room temperature; they get thicker when chilled.

- A *polyunsaturated fat,* such as corn oil, has mostly polyunsaturated fatty acids. Polyunsaturated fats are liquid at room temperature; they stay liquid when chilled.

So why is margarine, which is made from unsaturated fats such as corn and soybean oil, a solid? Because it's been artificially saturated by food chemists who add hydrogen atoms to some of its unsaturated fatty acids. This process, known as *hydrogenation,* turns an oil, such as corn oil, into a solid fat that can be used in products such as margarines without leaking out all over the table. A fatty acid with extra hydrogen atoms is called a *hydrogenated fatty acid.* (*Trans fatty acids* are hydrogenated fatty acids.) Because of those extra hydrogen atoms, hydrogenated fatty acids behave like saturated fats, clogging arteries and raising the levels of cholesterol in your blood.

One answer to the problem of hydrogenated fatty acids is plant *sterols* and *stanols.* Plant sterols are natural compounds in the oils in grains, fruits, and vegetables, including soybeans. *Stanols* are compounds created by adding hydrogen atoms to sterols from wood pulp and other plant sources; the first commercial stanol food was Benecol (bene = good, col = cholesterol) spread.

Sterols and stanols work like little sponges, sopping up cholesterol in your intestines before it can make its way into your bloodstream. As a result, your total cholesterol levels and your levels of low-density lipoproteins (LDLs or "bad cholesterol") go down. In some studies, one to two 1-tablespoon servings a day of sterols and stanols can lower levels of bad cholesterol by 10 to 17 percent, with results showing up in as little as two weeks.

Table 8-1 shows the kinds of fatty acids found in some common dietary fats and oils. Fats are characterized according to their predominant fatty acids. For example, as you can plainly see in the table, nearly 25 percent of the fatty acids in corn oil are monounsaturated fatty acids. Nevertheless, because corn oil has more polyunsaturated fatty acid, corn oil is considered a polyunsaturated fatty acid. Note for math majors: Some totals in Table 8-1 don't add up to 100 percent because these fats and oils also contain other kinds of fatty acids in amounts so small that they don't affect the basic character of the fat.

Table 8-1	What Fatty Acids Are in That Fat or Oil?			
Fat or Oil	**Saturated Fatty Acid (%)**	**Monounsaturated Fatty Acid (%)**	**Polyunsaturated Fatty Acid (%)**	**Kind of Fat or Oil**
Canola oil	7	53	22	Mono-unsaturated
Corn oil	13	24	59	Poly-unsaturated
Olive oil	14	74	9	Mono-unsaturated
Palm oil	52	38	10	Saturated
Peanut oil	17	46	32	Mono-unsaturated
Safflower oil	9	12	74	Poly-unsaturated
Soybean oil	15	23	51	Poly-unsaturated

Fat or Oil	Saturated Fatty Acid (%)	Monounsaturated Fatty Acid (%)	Polyunsaturated Fatty Acid (%)	Kind of Fat or Oil
Soybean-cotton-seed oil	18	29	48	Poly-unsaturated
Butter	62	30	5	Saturated
Lard	39	45	11	Saturated*

Because more than one-third of its fats are saturated, nutritionists label lard a saturated fat. Nutritive Value of Foods (Washington, D.C.: U.S. Department of Agriculture); Food and Life (New York: American Council on Science and Health)

Identifying the foods with fats

As a general rule:

- Fruits and vegetables have only traces of fat, primarily unsaturated fatty acids.
- Grains have small amounts of fat, up to 3 percent of their total weight.
- Dairy products vary. Cream is a high-fat food. Regular milks and cheeses are moderately high in fat. Skim milk and skim milk products are lowfat foods. Most of the fat in any dairy product is saturated fatty acids.
- Meat is moderately high in fat, and most of its fats are saturated fatty acids.
- Poultry (chicken and turkey), without the skin, is relatively low in fat.
- Fish may be high or low in fat, primarily unsaturated fatty acids that — lucky for the fish — remain liquid even when the fish is swimming in cold water. (Remember, saturated fats harden when cooled.)
- Vegetable oils, butter, and lard are high-fat foods. Most of the fatty acids in vegetable oils are unsaturated; most of the fatty acids in lard and butter are saturated.
- Processed foods, such as cakes, breads, canned or frozen meat, and vegetable dishes, are generally higher in fat than plain grains, meats, fruits, and vegetables.

 Here's a simple guide to finding which foods are high (or low) in fat. Oils are virtually 100 percent fat. Butter and lard are close behind. After that, the fat level drops, from 70 percent for some nuts down to 2 percent for most bread. The rule to take away from these numbers? A diet high in grains and plants always is lower in fat than a diet high in meat and oils.

A nutritional fish story

When Sir William Gilbert, lyricist to songsmith Sir Arthur Sullivan, wrote, "Here's a pretty kettle of fish!" he may well have been talking about the latest skinny on seafood.

The good news from a 2002 Harvard survey of more than 43,000 male health professionals was that those who ate 3 to 5 ounces of fish just once a month have a 40 percent lower risk of *ischemic stroke,* a stroke caused by a blood clot in a cranial artery. The Harvard study did not include women, but a report on women and stroke published in the *Journal of the American Medical Association* in 2000 showed that women who consume about 4 ounces of fish — think one small can of tuna — two to four times a week appear to cut their risk of stroke by a similar 40 percent.

These benefits are, in large part, because of the presence of *omega-3 fatty acids,* unsaturated fatty acids found most commonly in fatty fish such as salmon and sardines. The primary omega-3 is *alpha*-linolenic acid, which your body converts to hormone-like substances called eicosanoids. The *eicosanoids* — eicosapentaenoic acid (EPA) and docosahexaenoic acid (DHA) — reduce inflammation, perhaps by inhibiting an enzyme called COX-2, which is linked to inflammatory diseases such as rheumatoid arthritis (RA).

Omega-3s also are heart-friendly. They make the tiny blood particles called platelets less sticky, reducing the possibility that they'll clump together to form blood clots that might obstruct a blood vessel and trigger a heart attack. Omega-3s also knock down levels of bad cholesterol so effectively that the American Heart Association recommends eating fish at least twice a week. Besides, fish also is a good source of *taurine,* an amino acid the journal *Circulation* notes helps maintain the elasticity of blood vessels.

Finally omega-3s are bone builders. Fish oils enable your body to create *calciferol,* a naturally occurring form of vitamin D, the nutrient that enables your body to absorb bone-building calcium — which may be why omega-3s appear to help hold minerals in bone — and increase the formation of new bone.

A pretty kettle of fish, indeed.

Consumer Alert No. 1

Not all omegas are equally beneficial. Omega-6 fatty acids — polyunsaturated fats found in beef, pork, and several vegetable oils, including corn, sunflower, cottonseed, soybean, peanut, and sesame oils — are chemical cousins of omega-3s, but the omega-6s lack the benefits of the omega-3s.

Consumer Alert No. 2

Despite all the benefits fish bring to a healthful diet, it is also true that some fish, particularly those caught in the wild (rather than raised on a fish farm), may be contaminated with metals such as methyl mercury, a hazardous metal that makes its way into the water as industrial pollution and may be hazardous for children as well as women who are or may be pregnant because mercury targets the developing fetus's and child's brain and spinal cord. To keep methyl mercury ingestion as low as possible, the 2010 Dietary Guidelines for Americans (see Chapter 16) say these people should avoid *all* King mackerel, shark, swordfish, and tile fish, species likely to be highly contaminated.

Getting the right amount of fat

Getting the right amount of fat in your diet is a delicate balancing act. Too much, and you increase your risk of obesity, diabetes, heart disease, and some forms of cancer. (The risk of colon cancer seems to be tied more clearly to a diet high in fat from meat rather than a diet high in fat from dairy products.) Too little fat, and infants don't thrive, children don't grow, and everyone, regardless of age, is unable to absorb and use fat-soluble vitamins that smooth the skin, protect vision, bolster the immune system, and keep reproductive organs functioning.

In 2002, the National Academies' Institute of Medicine (IOM) recommended that no more than 20 to 45 percent of daily calories should come from fat. On a 2,000-calorie daily diet, that's 400 to 900 calories from fats a day. The Dietary Guidelines for Americans 2010 (see Chapter 16) recommends that adults keep fat consumption at the lower end of the scale, say, 20 to 30 percent of total calories — 400 to 600 of the calories on a 2,000-calorie/day regimen.

This advice about fat intake is primarily for adults. Although many organizations, such as the American Academy of Pediatrics, the American Heart Association, and the National Heart, Lung, and Blood Institute, recommend restricting fat intake for older children, they stress that infants and toddlers require fatty acids for proper physical growth and mental development. Never limit the fat in your baby's diet without checking first with your pediatrician.

Considering Cholesterol and You

Every healthy body *needs* cholesterol. Look carefully, and you will find cholesterol in and around your cells, in your fatty tissue, in your organs, in your brain, and in your glands. What's it doing there? Plenty.

Cholesterol

- Protects the integrity of cell membranes

- Helps nerve cells to send messages back and forth

- Is a building block for vitamin D (a sterol), made when sunlight hits the fat just under your skin (for more about vitamin D, see Chapter 11)

- Enables your gallbladder to make *bile acids,* digestive chemicals that, in turn, enable you to absorb fats and fat-soluble nutrients such as vitamin A, vitamin D, vitamin E, and vitamin K

- Is a base on which you build steroid hormones such as estrogen and testosterone

Cholesterol and heart disease

Doctors measure your cholesterol level by taking a sample of blood and counting the milligrams of cholesterol in 1 deciliter (⅒ liter) of blood. When you get your annual report from the doctor, your total cholesterol level looks something like this: 225 mg/dL. In other words, you have 225 milligrams of cholesterol in every tenth of a liter of blood. The more cholesterol you have floating in your blood, the more cholesterol is likely to cross into your arteries, where it may stick to the walls, form deposits that eventually block the flow of blood, and thus increase your risk of heart attack or stroke.

As a general rule, the National Cholesterol Education Program (NCEP) defines total cholesterol levels this way:

✔ **<200 mg/dL:** Desirable with a low risk for coronary heart disease (CHD)

✔ **200 to 239 mg/dL:** Borderline high

✔ **>240 mg/dl:** High with double the risk of CHD as a person with <200 mg/dl

---

Cholesterol season

Even if you allow yourself to indulge in (a few) high-cholesterol ice cream cones and burgers every day of the year, your cholesterol level may still be naturally lower in the summer than in winter.

The basis for this intriguing culinary conclusion is the 2004 University of Massachusetts SEASONS (Seasonal Variation in Blood Lipids) Study of 517 healthy men and women ages 20 to 70. The volunteers started out with an average cholesterol level of 213 mg/dl (women) to 222 mg/dl (men). A series of five blood tests during the one-year study showed an average drop of 4 points in the summer for men and 5.4 points for women. People with high cholesterol (above 240 mg/dl) did better, dropping as much as 18 points in the summer.

U. Mass cardiologists say one explanation for the summer downswing may be the normal increase in human blood volume in hot weather. Cholesterol levels reflect the total amount of cholesterol in your bloodstream. With more blood in the stream, the amount of cholesterol per deciliter declines, producing a lower total cholesterol reading. A second possibility is that people tend to eat less and be more active in summer. They lose weight, and weight loss equals lower cholesterol.

The first bit of wisdom from this study is obvious: Being physically active reduces your cholesterol level. The second is that environment matters. In other words, if you're planning to start a new cholesterol-buster diet, you may just do better to start during the cool weather, when your efforts may lower your total cholesterol as much as 12 points over a reasonable period of time, say, six months. Then when your doctor runs a follow-up test the following summer, you'll get the added benefit of the seasonal slip to make you feel really, really good about how well you're doing. For more on controlling your cholesterol, check out *Controlling Cholesterol For Dummies,* 2nd Edition (Wiley), which I wrote with Martin W. Graf, MD.

But total cholesterol levels alone are not the entire story. Many people with high cholesterol levels live to a ripe old age, while others with low total cholesterol levels develop heart disease because cholesterol is only one of several risk factors for heart disease. Here are some more:

- An unfavorable ratio of lipoproteins (see the following section)
- Smoking
- Obesity
- Age (being older is riskier)
- Sex (being male is riskier)
- A family history of heart disease

Living with lipoproteins

A *lipoprotein* is a fat and protein particle that carries cholesterol through your blood. Your body makes four types of lipoproteins: chylomicrons, very low-density lipoproteins (VLDLs), low-density lipoproteins (LDLs), and high-density lipoproteins (HDLs). As a general rule, LDLs take cholesterol into blood vessels; HDLs carry it out of the body.

A lipoprotein is born as a *chylomicron,* made in your intestinal cells from protein and triglycerides (fats). After 12 hours of traveling through your blood and around your body, a chylomicron has lost virtually all of its fats. By the time the chylomicron makes its way to your liver, the only thing left is protein.

The liver, a veritable fat and cholesterol factory, collects fatty acid fragments from your blood and uses them to make cholesterol and new fatty acids. Time out! How much cholesterol you get from food may affect your liver's daily output: Eat more cholesterol, and your liver may make less. If you eat less cholesterol, your liver may make more. And so it goes.

Churning out harmful lipoproteins

Okay, after your liver has made cholesterol and fatty acids, it packages them with protein as very low-density lipoproteins (VLDLs), which have more protein and are denser than their precursors, the chylomicrons. As VLDLs travel through your bloodstream, they lose triglycerides, pick up cholesterol, and turn into low-density lipoproteins (LDLs). LDLs supply cholesterol to your body cells, which use it to make new cell membranes and manufacture sterol compounds such as hormones. That's the good news.

The bad news is that both VLDLs and LDLs are soft and squishy enough to pass through blood vessel walls. The larger and squishier they are, the more likely they are to slide into your arteries, which means that VLDLs are more hazardous to your health than LDLs although elevated levels of all LDLs are strongly linked to an increased risk of cardiovascular disease.

VLDLs and LDLs are sometimes called "bad cholesterol," but this characterization is a misnomer. They aren't cholesterol; they're just the rafts on which cholesterol sails into your arteries. Traveling through the body, LDLs continue to lose cholesterol. In the end, they lose so much fat that they become mostly protein — turning them into high-density lipoproteins, the particles sometimes called "good cholesterol." Once again, this label is inaccurate. HDLs aren't cholesterol: They're simply protein and fat particles too dense and compact to pass through blood vessel walls, so they carry cholesterol out of the body rather than into arteries.

That's why a high level of HDLs may reduce your risk of heart attack regardless of your total cholesterol levels. Conversely, a high level of LDLs may raise your risk of heart attack, even if your overall cholesterol level is low.

Setting limits on the bad guys

At one point, back in the Dawn of the Cholesterol Age, the "safe" upper limit for LDLs was assumed to be around 160 mg/dl. Now, the National Heart, Lung, and Blood Institute, American College of Cardiology, and the American Heart Association have all put their stamps of approval on the National Cholesterol Education Program's (NCEP) recommendations for new, lower levels of LDLs.

For healthy people with two or more risk factors, the *Optimal* level for LDLs is below 100 mg/dL; 100–129 mg/dL is considered *Near or above optimal.*

The "near" applies to healthy people; the "above," to those at high risk or with existing CHD. Very high-risk patients such as those who are hospitalized with heart disease or have heart disease plus several risk factors are often told to push their LDLs under 70 mg/dL, a level virtually impossible to reach without a cholesterol-busting drug, usually a statin, such as atorvastatin (Lipitor).

Diet and cholesterol

Most of the cholesterol that you need is made right in your own liver, which churns out about 1 gram (1,000 milligrams) a day from the raw materials in the proteins, fats, and carbohydrates that you consume. But you also get cholesterol from food of animal origin: meat, poultry, fish, eggs, and dairy products. Although some plant foods, such as coconuts and cocoa beans, are high in saturated fats, no plants produce cholesterol.

Table 8-2 lists the amount of cholesterol in normal servings of some representative foods.

Table 8-2	How Much Cholesterol Is on That Plate?	
Food	*Serving Size*	*Cholesterol (mg)*
Meat		
Beef (stewed) lean and fat	3 ounces	87
Beef (stewed) lean	2.2 ounces	66
Beef (ground) lean	3 ounces	74
Beef (ground) regular	3 ounces	76
Beef steak (sirloin)	3 ounces	77
Bacon	3 strips	16
Pork chop, lean	2.5 ounces	71
Poultry		
Chicken (roast) breast	3 ounces	73
Chicken (roast) leg	3 ounces	78
Turkey (roast) breast	3 ounces	59
Fish		
Clams	3 ounces	43
Flounder	3 ounces	59
Oysters (raw)	1 cup	120
Salmon (canned)	3 ounces	34
Salmon (baked)	3 ounces	60
Tuna (water canned)	3 ounces	48
Tuna (oil canned)	3 ounces	55
Cheese		
American	1 ounce	27
Cheddar	1 ounce	30
Cream	1 ounce	31
Mozzarella (whole milk)	1 ounce	22
Mozzarella (part skim)	1 ounce	15
Swiss	1 ounce	26
Milk		
Whole	8 ounces	33
2%	8 ounces	18
1%	8 ounces	18
Skim	8 ounces	10

(continued)

Table 8-2 *(continued)*

Food	Serving Size	Cholesterol (mg)
Other dairy products		
Butter	Pat	11
Other		
Eggs, large	1	213
Lard	1 tbsp.	12

Nutritive Value of Foods (Washington, D.C.: U.S. Department of Agriculture)

Chapter 9

Carbohydrates: A Complex Story

• •

In This Chapter

▶ Discovering the different kinds of carbohydrates

▶ Understanding how your body uses carbohydrates

▶ Choosing the foods with the best carbs

▶ Deciphering dietary fiber

• •

Carbohydrates — the name means carbon plus water — are sugar compounds that plants make when they're exposed to light. This process of making sugar compounds is called *photosynthesis,* from the Latin words for "light" and "putting together."

This chapter shines a bright light on the different kinds of carbohydrates, illuminating all the nutritional nooks and crannies to explain how each contributes to your vim and vigor — not to mention a tasty daily menu.

Checking Out Carbohydrates

Carbohydrates come in three varieties: simple carbohydrates, complex carbohydrates, and dietary fiber. All are composed of units of sugar. What makes one carbohydrate different from another is the number of sugar units it contains and how the units are linked together.

Simple carbohydrates

These carbohydrates have only one or two units of sugar.

> ✔ A carbohydrate with one unit of sugar is called a *simple sugar* or a *monosaccharide* (mono = one; saccharide = sugar). Fructose (fruit sugar) is a monosaccharide, and so are glucose (blood sugar), the sugar produced when you digest carbohydrates, and galactose, the sugar derived from digesting lactose (milk sugar).

✔ A carbohydrate with two units of sugar is called a *double sugar* or a *disaccharide* (di = two). Sucrose (table sugar), which is made of one unit of fructose and one unit of glucose, is a disaccharide.

Complex carbohydrates

These carbohydrates, which are also known as *polysaccharides* (poly = many), have more than two units of sugar linked together. Carbs with three to ten units of sugar are sometimes called *oligosaccharides* (oligo = few).

✔ Raffinose is a *trisaccharide* (tri = three) that's found in potatoes, beans, and beets. It has one unit each of galactose, glucose, and fructose.

✔ Stachyose is a *tetrasaccharide* (tetra = four) found in the same vegetables mentioned in the previous item. It has one fructose unit, one glucose unit, and two galactose units.

✔ Starch, a complex carbohydrate in potatoes, pasta, and rice, is a definite polysaccharide. In fact, it's an *oligosaccharide* built of many units of glucose.

Because complex carbohydrates may have anywhere from three to several thousand units of sugars, your body takes longer to digest them than it takes to digest simple carbohydrates. As a result, digesting complex carbohydrates releases glucose into your bloodstream more slowly and evenly than digesting simple carbs. (For more about digesting carbs, see the section "Carbohydrates and Energy: a Biochemical Love Story," later in this chapter.)

Dietary fiber

Dietary fiber is a term used to distinguish the fiber in food from the natural and synthetic fibers (silk, cotton, wool, nylon) used in fabrics. Dietary fiber is a third kind of carbohydrate.

Like the complex carbohydrates, dietary fiber (cellulose, hemicellulose, pectin, beta-glucans, gum) is a polysaccharide. Lignin, a different kind of chemical, is also called a dietary fiber.

Some kinds of dietary fiber also contain units of soluble or insoluble uronic acids, compounds derived from the sugars fructose, glucose, and galactose. For example, pectin — a soluble fiber in apples — contains soluble galacturonic acid.

Dietary fiber is not like other carbohydrates. The bonds that hold its sugar units together cannot be broken by human digestive enzymes. Although the bacteria living naturally in your intestines convert very small amounts of dietary fiber to fatty acids, dietary fiber is not considered a source of energy. (For more about fatty acids, see Chapter 8.)

Carbohydrates and Energy: a Biochemical Love Story

Your body runs on glucose, the molecules your cells burn for energy. (For more information on how you get energy from food, check out Chapter 3.)

Proteins, fats, and alcohol (as in beer, wine, and spirits) also provide energy in the form of calories. And protein does give you glucose, but it takes a long time, relatively speaking, for your body to get it.

When you eat carbohydrates, your pancreas secretes insulin, the hormone that enables you to digest starches and sugars. This release of insulin is sometimes called an *insulin spike,* also known as "insulin secretion."

Eating simple carbohydrates such as sucrose (table sugar) provokes higher insulin secretion than eating complex carbohydrates such as starch. If you have a metabolic disorder such as diabetes that keeps you from producing enough insulin, you must be careful not to take in more carbs than you can digest. (See "Some problems with carbohydrates," later in this chapter.)

Some perfectly healthful foods, such as carrots, potatoes, and white bread, have more simple carbs than others, such as apples, lentils, peanuts, and whole wheat bread. The Glycemic Index, a carbohydrate measurement scheme developed at the University of Toronto in 1981, gives you a handle on the amount of carbs by ranking foods according to how quickly they affect blood sugar levels when compared to glucose (the form of sugar your body uses as energy).

Most healthy people can metabolize even very large amounts of carbohydrate foods easily. Their insulin secretion rises to meet the demand and then quickly settles back to normal. In other words, although some popular weight loss programs, such as the South Beach Diet, rely on the Glycemic Index as a weight loss tool, the fact remains that for most people, a carb is a carb is a carb, regardless of how quickly the sugar enters the bloodstream. Check it out in *Diabetes For Dummies* (Wiley) by Dr. Alan L. Rubin, MD.

For info on why the difference between simple and complex carbs can matter for athletes, check out the section called "Who needs extra carbohydrates?"

How glucose becomes energy

Inside your cells, glucose is burned to produce heat and *adenosine triphosphate*, a molecule that stores and releases energy as required by the cell. By the way, nutrition scientists, who have as much trouble pronouncing polysyllabic words as you probably do, usually refer to adenosine triphosphate by its initials: ATP.

The transformation of glucose into energy occurs in one of two ways: with oxygen or without it. Glucose is converted to energy with oxygen in the *mitochondria* — tiny bodies in the jellylike substance inside every cell. This conversion yields energy (ATP, heat) plus water and carbon dioxide, a waste product.

Red blood cells do not have mitochondria, so they change glucose into energy without oxygen. This yields energy (ATP, heat) and lactic acid.

Glucose is also converted to energy in muscle cells. When it comes to producing energy from glucose, muscle cells are, well, double-jointed. They have mitochondria, so they can process glucose with oxygen. But if the level of oxygen in the muscle cell falls very low, the cells can just go ahead and change glucose into energy without it. This is most likely to happen when you've been exercising so strenuously that you (and your muscles) are, literally, out of breath.

Being able to turn glucose into energy without oxygen is a handy trick, but here's the downside: One byproduct is lactic acid. Why is that a big deal? Because too much lactic acid makes your muscles ache.

How pasta ends up on your hips when too many carbs pass your lips

Your cells budget energy very carefully. They do not store more than they need right now. Any glucose the cell does not need for its daily work is converted to glycogen (animal starch) and tucked away as stored energy in your liver and muscles.

Your body can pack about 400 grams (14 ounces) of glycogen into liver and muscle cells. A gram of carbohydrates — including glucose — has four calories. If you add up all the glucose stored in glycogen to the small amount of glucose in your cells and blood, it equals about 1,800 calories of energy.

If your diet provides more carbohydrates than you need to produce this amount of stored calories in the form of glucose and glycogen in your cells, blood, muscles, and liver, the excess will be converted to fat. And that's how your pasta ends up on your hips.

Other ways your body uses carbohydrates

Providing energy is an important job, but it isn't the only thing carbohydrates do for you. Carbohydrates also protect your muscles. When you need energy, your body looks for glucose from carbohydrates first. If none is available, because you're on a carbohydrate-restricted diet or have a medical condition that prevents you from using the carbohydrate foods you consume, your body begins to pull energy out of fatty tissue and then moves on to burning its own protein tissue (muscles). If this use of proteins for energy continues long enough, you run out of fuel and die.

A diet that provides sufficient amounts of carbohydrates keeps your body from eating its own muscles. That's why a carbohydrate-rich diet is sometimes described as *protein sparing*.

Carbohydrates also

- Regulate the amount of sugar circulating in your blood so that all your cells get the energy they need

- Provide nutrients for the friendly bacteria in your intestinal tract that help digest food

- Assist in your body's absorption of calcium

- May help lower cholesterol levels and regulate blood pressure (these effects are special benefits of dietary fiber (see "Dietary Fiber: The Non-Nutrient in Carbohydrate Foods," later in this chapter)

Finding the Carbohydrates You Need

The most important sources of carbohydrates are plant foods — fruits, vegetables, and grains. Milk and milk products contain the carbohydrate lactose (milk sugar), but meat, fish, and poultry have no carbohydrates at all.

The National Academy of Sciences Institute of Medicine (IOM) recommends that 45 to 65 percent of your daily calories come from carbohydrate foods such as grains (bread, cereals, pasta rice), fruit, and vegetables, foods that provide simple carbohydrates, complex carbohydrates, and the natural bonus of dietary fiber. Table sugar, honey, and sweets — which provide simple carbohydrates — are recommended only on a once-in-a-while basis.

One gram of carbohydrates has four calories. To find the number of calories from the carbohydrates in one food serving, multiply the number of grams of carbohydrates by four. For example, one whole bagel has about 38 grams of carbohydrates, equal to about 152 calories (38 × 4). (You have to say "about" because the dietary fiber in the bagel provides no calories, because the body can't metabolize it.) *Wait:* That number does not account for all the calories in the serving. Remember, the foods listed here may also contain at least some protein and fat, and these two nutrients add calories.

Some problems with carbohydrates

Some people have a hard time handling carbohydrates. For example, people with Type 1 ("insulin dependent") diabetes do not produce sufficient amounts of insulin, the hormones needed to carry all the glucose produced from carbohydrates into body cells. As a result, the glucose continues to circulate in the blood until it's excreted through the kidneys. That's why one way to tell whether someone has diabetes is to test the level of sugar in that person's urine.

Other people can't digest carbohydrates because their bodies lack the specific enzymes needed to break the bonds that hold a carbohydrate's sugar units together. For example, many (some say most) Asians, Africans, Middle Easterners, South Americans, and Eastern, Central, or Southern Europeans are deficient in lactase, the enzyme that splits lactose (milk sugar) into glucose and galactose. If these people drink milk or eat milk products, they end up with a lot of undigested lactose in their intestinal tracts. This undigested lactose makes the bacteria living there happy as clams — but not the person who owns the intestines: As bacteria feast on the undigested sugar, they excrete waste products that give their host gas and cramps.

To avoid this anomaly, many national cuisines purposely avoid milk as an ingredient. (Quick! Name one native Asian dish that's made with milk. No, coconut milk doesn't count.) To get the calcium their bodies need, these people simply substitute high-calcium foods such as greens or calcium-enriched soy products for milk.

Time out for the name game!

Here's an interesting bit of nutritional information. The names of all enzymes end in the letters *-ase*. An enzyme that digests a specific substance in food often has a name similar to the substance but with the letters *-ase* at the end. For example, *proteases* are enzymes that digest protein; *lipases* are enzymes that digest fats (lipids); and *galactase* is the enzyme that digests galactose.

A second solution for people who don't make enough lactase is to use a *predigested milk product,* such as yogurt or buttermilk or sour cream, all of which are created by adding friendly bacteria that digest the milk (that is, break the lactose apart) without spoiling it. Other solutions include lactose-free cheeses and enzyme-treated milk.

Who needs extra carbohydrates?

The small amount of glucose in your blood and cells provides the energy you need for your body's daily activities. The 400 grams of glycogen stored in your liver and muscles provides enough energy for ordinary bursts of extra activity.

But what happens when you have to work harder or longer than that? For example, what if you're a long-distance athlete, which means that you use up your available supply of glucose before you finish your competition? (That's why marathoners often run out of gas — a phenomenon called *hitting the wall* — at 20 miles, six miles short of the finish line.)

If you were stuck on an ice floe or lost in the woods for a month or so, after your body exhausts its supply of glucose, including the glucose stored in glycogen, it would start pulling energy first out of stored fat and then out of muscle. But extracting energy from body fat requires large amounts of oxygen — which is likely to be in short supply when your body has run, swum, or cycled 20 miles. So athletes have found another way to leap the wall: They load up on carbohydrates in advance.

Carbohydrate-loading is a dietary regimen designed to increase temporarily the amount of glycogen stored in your muscles in anticipation of an upcoming event. You start about a week before the event, says the University of Maine's Alfred A. Bushway, PhD, exercising to exhaustion so your body pulls as much glycogen as possible out of your muscles. Then, for three days, you eat foods high in fat and protein and low in carbohydrates to keep your glycogen level from rising again.

Three days before the big day, reverse the pattern. Now you want to build and conserve glycogen stores. What you need is a diet that's about 70 percent carbohydrates, providing 6 to 10 grams of carbohydrates for every kilogram (2.2 pounds) of body weight for men and women alike. And not just any carbohydrates, mind you. What you want are the complex carbohydrates in starchy foods like pasta and potatoes, rather than the simple ones more prominent in sugary foods like fruit. And of course, candy.

This carb-loading diet is not for everyday use, nor will it help people competing in events of short duration. It's strictly for events lasting longer than 90 minutes.

What about while you're running, swimming, or cycling? Will consuming simple sugars during the race give you extra short-term bursts of energy? Yes. Sugar is rapidly converted to glycogen and carried to the muscles. But you don't want plain table sugar (candy, honey) because it's *hydrophilic* (hydro = water; philic = loving), which means that it pulls water from body tissues into your intestinal tract. This can increase dehydration and trigger nausea. Getting the sugar you want from sweetened athletic drinks, which provide fluids along with the energy, is safer, especially since the athletic drink also contains salt (sodium chloride) to replace the salt that you lose when perspiring heavily. Turn to Chapter 13 to find out why this is important.

Dietary Fiber: The Non-Nutrient in Carbohydrate Foods

Dietary fiber is a group of complex carbohydrates that are not a source of energy for human beings. Because human digestive enzymes cannot break the bonds that hold fiber's sugar units together, fiber adds no calories to your diet and cannot be converted to glucose.

Ruminants (animals, such as cows, that chew the cud) have a combination of digestive enzymes and digestive microbes that enable them to extract the nutrients from insoluble dietary fiber (cellulose and some hemicelluloses). But not even these creatures can pull nutrients out of lignin, an insoluble fiber in plant stems and leaves and the predominant fiber in wood. As a result, the U.S. Department of Agriculture specifically prohibits the use of wood or sawdust in animal feed.

But just because you can't digest dietary fiber doesn't mean it isn't a valuable part of your diet. The opposite is true. Dietary fiber is valuable *because* you can't digest it!

The two kinds of dietary fiber

Nutritionists classify dietary fiber as either insoluble fiber or soluble fiber, depending on whether it dissolves in water.

✔ **Insoluble dietary fiber** includes cellulose, some hemicelluloses, and lignin found in whole grains and other plants. This kind of dietary fiber is a natural laxative. It absorbs water, helps you feel full after eating, and stimulates your intestinal walls to contract and relax. These natural contractions, called *peristalsis,* move solid materials through your digestive tract.

By moving food quickly through your intestines, insoluble fiber may help relieve or prevent digestive disorders such as constipation or diverticulitis (infection that occurs when food gets stuck in small pouches in the wall of the colon). Insoluble fiber also bulks up stool and makes it softer, reducing your risk of developing hemorrhoids and lessening the discomfort if you already have them.

✔ **Soluble dietary fiber** includes pectins (found in most fruit) and beta-glucans (found in oats and barley). Soluble dietary fiber seems to lower the amount of cholesterol circulating in your blood (your *cholesterol level*), which is why a diet rich in fiber appears to lower cholesterol levels and thus offer some protection against heart disease.

Here's a benefit for dieters: Soluble fiber forms gels in the presence of water, which is what happens when apples and oat bran reach your digestive tract. So, like insoluble fiber, soluble fiber can make you feel full without adding calories.

Ordinary soluble dietary fiber can't be digested, so your body doesn't absorb it. But in 2002, researchers at Detroit's Barbara Ann Karamonos Cancer Institute fed laboratory mice a form of soluble dietary fiber called *modified citrus pectin*. The fiber, which is made from citrus fruit peel, can be digested. When fed to laboratory rats, it appeared to reduce the size of tumors caused by implanted human breast and colon cancer cells. The researchers believe that the fiber prevents cancer cells from linking together to form tumors. Today, modified citrus pectin is being sold as a dietary supplement, but the American Cancer Society notes on its Web site that this fiber's effects on human bodies (and human cancers) remain unproven.

Getting dietary fiber from food

You will find absolutely no fiber in foods from animals: meat, fish, poultry, milk, milk products, and eggs. But you will find lots of dietary fiber in all plant foods — fruits, vegetables, and grains.

A balanced diet with plenty of foods from plants gives you both insoluble and soluble fiber. Most foods that contain fiber have both kinds, although the balance usually tilts toward one or the other. For example, the predominant fiber in an apple is pectin (a soluble fiber), but an apple peel also has some cellulose, hemicellulose, and lignin.

Table 9-1 shows you which foods are particularly good sources of specific kinds of fiber. A diet rich in plant foods (fruits, vegetables, grains) gives you adequate amounts of dietary fiber.

Table 9-1	Food Sources of Different Kinds of Fiber
Fiber	*Where Found*
Soluble fiber	
Pectin	Fruits (apples, strawberries, citrus fruits)
Beta-glucans	Oats, barley
Gums	Beans, cereals (oats, rice, barley), seeds, seaweed
Insoluble fiber	
Cellulose	Leaves (cabbage), roots (carrots, beets), bran, whole wheat, beans
Hemicellulose	Seed coverings (bran, whole grains)
Lignin	Plant stems, leaves, and skin

How much fiber do you need?

According to the U.S. Department of Agriculture, the average American woman gets about 12 grams of fiber a day from food; the average American man, 17 grams. Those figures are well below the new IOM (Institute of Medicine) recommendations that I conveniently list here:

- 25 grams a day for women age 19 to 50
- 38 grams a day for men age 19 to 50
- 21 grams a day for women older than 50
- 30 grams a day for men older than 50

The amounts of dietary fiber recommended by IOM are believed to give you the benefits you want without causing fiber-related unpleasantries.

Unpleasantries? Like what? And how will you know if you've got them?

Trust me: If you eat more than enough fiber, your body will tell you right away. All that roughage may irritate your intestinal tract, which will issue an unmistakable protest in the form of intestinal gas or diarrhea. In extreme cases, if you don't drink enough liquids to moisten and soften the fiber you eat so that it easily slides through your digestive tract, the dietary fiber may form a mass that can end up as an intestinal obstruction. (For more about water, see Chapter 13.)

If you decide to up the amount of fiber in your diet, follow this advice:

Fiber factoid

The amount of fiber in a serving of food may depend on whether the food is raw or cooked. For example, as you can see from Table 9-2, a 3.5-ounce serving of plain dried prunes has 7.2 grams of fiber while a 3.5-ounce serving of stewed prunes has 6.6 grams of fiber.

Why? When you stew prunes, they plump up — which means they absorb water. The water adds weight but (obviously) no fiber. So a serving of prunes-plus-water has slightly less fiber per ounce than a same-weight serving of plain dried prunes.

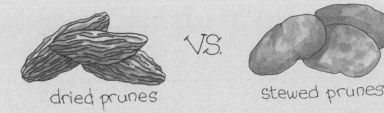

dried prunes   VS.   stewed prunes

✔ **Do it *very* gradually, a little bit more every day.** That way, you're less likely to experience intestinal distress. In other words, if your current diet is heavy on no-fiber foods such as meat, fish, poultry, eggs, milk, and cheese, and low-fiber foods such as white bread and white rice, don't load up on bran cereal (35 grams dietary fiber per 3.5-ounce serving) or dried figs (9.3 grams per serving) all at once. Start by adding a serving of cornflakes (2.0 grams dietary fiber) at breakfast, maybe an apple (2.8 grams) at lunch, a pear (2.6 grams) at mid-afternoon, and a half cup of baked beans (7.7 grams) at dinner. Four simple additions, and already you're up to 15 grams dietary fiber.

✔ **Always check the nutrition label whenever you shop.** (For more about the wonderfully informative guides, see Chapter 17.) When choosing between similar products, just take the one with the higher fiber content per serving. For example, white pita bread generally has about 1.6 grams dietary fiber per serving. Whole wheat pita bread may have as much as 7.4 grams.

✔ **Get enough liquids.** Dietary fiber is like a sponge. It sops up liquid, so increasing your fiber intake may deprive your cells of the water they need to perform their daily work. (For more about how your body uses the water you drink, see Chapter 13.) That's why the American Academy of Family Physicians (among others) suggests checking to make sure you get plenty of fluids when you consume more fiber. How much is enough? Back to Chapter 13.

Table 9-2 shows the amounts of all types of dietary fiber — insoluble plus soluble — in a 100-gram (3.5-ounce) serving of specific foods. By the way, nutritionists like to measure things in terms of 100-gram portions because that makes comparing foods at a glance possible.

To find the amount of dietary fiber in your own serving, divide the gram total for the food shown in Table 9-2 (or the appendix) by 3.5 to get the grams per ounce, and then multiply the result by the number of ounces in your portion. For example, if you're having 1 ounce of cereal, the customary serving of ready-to-eat breakfast cereals, divide the gram total of dietary fiber by 3.5; then multiply by one. If your slice of bread weighs ½ ounce, divide the gram total by 3.5; then multiply the result by 0.5 (½).

Or you can just look at the nutrition label on the side of the package because it lists the amounts of the nutrients per serving.

Finally, the amounts on this chart are averages. Different brands of processed products (breads, some cereals, cooked fruits, and vegetables) may have more (or less) fiber per serving.

Table 9-2 Dietary Fiber Content in Common Foods	
Food	Grams of Fiber in a 100-Gram (3.5-Ounce) Serving
Bread	
Bagel	2.1
Bran bread	8.5
Pita bread (white)	1.6
Pita bread (whole wheat)	7.4
White bread	1.9
Cereals	
Bran cereal	35.3
Bran flakes	18.8
Cornflakes	2.0
Oatmeal	10.6
Wheat flakes	9.0
Grains	
Barley, pearled (minus its outer covering), raw	15.6
Cornmeal, whole grain	11.0
De-germed	5.2
Oat bran, raw	6.6
Rice, raw (brown)	3.5
Rice, raw (white)	1.0–2.8
Rice, raw (wild)	5.2
Wheat bran	15.0

Food	Grams of Fiber in a 100-Gram (3.5-Ounce) Serving
Fruits	
Apple, with skin	2.8
Apricots, dried	7.8
Figs, dried	9.3
Kiwi fruit	3.4
Pear, raw	2.6
Prunes, dried	7.2
Prunes, stewed	6.6
Raisins.	5.3
Vegetables	
Baked beans (vegetarian)	7.7
Chickpeas (canned)	5.4
Lima beans, cooked	7.2
Broccoli, raw	2.8
Brussels sprouts, cooked	2.6
Cabbage, white, raw	2.4
Cauliflower, raw	2.4
Corn, sweet, cooked	3.7
Peas with edible pods, raw	2.6
Potatoes, white, baked, w/ skin	5.5
Sweet potato, cooked	3.0
Tomatoes, raw	1.3
Nuts	
Almonds, oil-roasted	11.2
Coconut, raw	9.0
Hazelnuts, oil-roasted	6.4
Peanuts, dry-roasted	8.0
Pistachios	10.8
Other	
Corn chips, toasted	4.4
Tahini (sesame seed paste)	9.3
Tofu	1.2

Provisional Table on the Dietary Fiber Content of Selected Foods (Washington, D.C.: U.S. Department of Agriculture, 1988)

Fiber and your heart:
The continuing saga of oat bran

Oat bran is the second chapter in the fiber fad that started with wheat bran around 1980. Wheat bran, the fiber in wheat, is rich in the insoluble fibers cellulose and lignin. Oat bran's gee-whiz factor is the soluble fiber beta-glucans. For more than 30 years, scientists have known that eating foods high in soluble fiber can lower your cholesterol, although nobody knows exactly why. Fruits and vegetables (especially dried beans) are high in soluble fiber, but ounce for ounce, oats have more. In addition, beta-glucans are a more effective cholesterol-buster than pectin and gum, which are the soluble fibers in most fruits and vegetables.

By 1990, researchers at the University of Kentucky reported that people who add ½ cup dry oat bran (*not* oatmeal) to their regular daily diets can lower their levels of low density lipoproteins (LDLs), the particles that carry cholesterol into your arteries, by as much as 25 percent (see Chapter 8 for more on cholesterol).

Recently, scientists at the Medical School of Northwestern University, funded by Quaker Oats, enlisted 208 healthy volunteers whose normal cholesterol readings averaged about 200 mg/dl for a study involving oat bran. The volunteers' total cholesterol levels decreased an average of 9.3 percent with a lowfat, low-cholesterol diet supplemented by 2 ounces of oats or oat bran every day. About one-third of the cholesterol reduction was credited to the oats.

Oat cereal makers rounded the total loss to 10 percent, and the National Research Council said that a 10 percent drop in cholesterol could produce a 20 percent drop in the risk of a heart attack.

Do I have to tell you what happened next? Books on oat bran hit the bestseller list. Cheerios elbowed Frosted Flakes aside to become the number one cereal in America. And people added oat bran to everything from bagels to orange juice.

Today scientists know that although a little oat bran can't hurt, the link between oats and cholesterol levels is no cure-all.

As a general rule, a cholesterol level higher than 240 mg/dl is considered to be *high*. A cholesterol reading between 200 and 239 mg/dl is considered *borderline high*. A cholesterol level below 200 mg/dl is considered *desirable*.

If your cholesterol level is above 240 mg/dl, lowering it by 10 percent through a diet that contains oat bran may reduce your risk of heart attack without the use of medication. If your cholesterol level is lower than that to begin with, the effects of oat bran are less dramatic. For example:

✔ If your cholesterol level is below 240 mg/dl, a lowfat, low-cholesterol diet alone may push it down 24 points into the moderately risky range, but doesn't take you into "safe" territory, under 200 mg/dl.

✔ If your cholesterol is already low, say 199 mg/dl or less, a lowfat, low-cholesterol diet plus oats may drop it to 180 mg/dl, but the oats account for only a third of your loss.

Recognizing oat bran's benefits, the Food and Drug Administration now permits health claims on oat product labels. For example, the product label may say: "Soluble fiber from foods such as oat bran, as part of a diet low in saturated fat and cholesterol, may reduce the risk of heart disease."

By the way, the soluble pectin in apples and the soluble beta-glucans (gums) in beans and peas also lower cholesterol levels. The insoluble fiber in wheat bran does not.

Chapter 10

Alcohol: Another Form of Grape and Grain

- -

In This Chapter

▶ Discovering how alcohol is made

▶ Exploring different kinds of alcohol beverages

▶ Digesting alcohol

▶ Evaluating alcohol's effect on health

- -

Alcohol beverages are among mankind's oldest home remedies and simple pleasures, so highly regarded that the ancient Greeks and Romans called wine a "gift from the gods," and when the Gaels — early inhabitants of Scotland and Ireland — first produced whiskey, they named it *uisge beatha* (whis-key-ba), a combination of the words for "water" and "life." Today, although you may share their appreciation for the product, you know that alcohol beverages may have risks as well as benefits.

This chapter refers to beverages made from alcohol as "alcohol beverages" rather than "alcoholic beverages," a term that immediately brings to mind the image of tipsy beer bottles rather than simple beer, wine, or spirits.

Revealing the Many Faces of Alcohol

When microorganisms (yeasts) digest (ferment) the sugars in carbohydrate foods, they make two byproducts: a liquid and a gas. The gas is carbon dioxide. The liquid is *ethyl alcohol*, also known as *ethanol*, the intoxicating ingredient in alcohol beverages.

This biochemical process is not an esoteric one. In fact, it happens in your own kitchen every time you make yeast bread. Remember the faint, beer-like odor in the air while the dough is rising? That odor is from the alcohol the yeasts make as they chomp their way through the sugars in the flour. (Don't worry; the alcohol evaporates when you bake the bread.) As the yeasts digest the sugars, they also produce carbon dioxide, which makes the bread rise.

Whenever you see the word *alcohol,* unless otherwise noted, it means ethanol, the only alcohol used in alcohol beverages.

Creating Alcohol Beverages

Alcohol beverages are produced either through fermentation or through a combination of fermentation plus distillation.

Fermented alcohol products

Fermentation is a simple process in which yeasts or bacteria are added to carbohydrate foods such as corn, potatoes, rice, or wheat, which are used as starting material. The yeasts digest the sugars in the food, leaving liquid (alcohol); the liquid is filtered to remove the solids, and water is usually added to dilute the alcohol, producing — voilà — an alcohol beverage.

Beer is made this way. So is wine. *Kumiss,* a fermented milk product, is slightly different because it's made by adding yeasts and friendly bacteria called *lactobacilli* (lacto = milk) to mare's milk. The microorganisms make alcohol, but it isn't separated from the milk, which turns into a fizzy fermented beverage with no water added.

Distilled alcohol products

The second way to make an alcohol beverage is through *distillation.*

As with fermentation, yeasts are added to foods to make alcohol from sugars. But yeasts can't thrive in a place where the concentration of alcohol is higher than 20 percent. To concentrate the alcohol and separate it from the rest of the ingredients in the fermented liquid, distillers pour the fermented liquid into a *still,* a large vat with a wide column-like tube on top. The still is heated so that the alcohol, which boils at a lower temperature than everything else in the vat, turns to vapor, which rises through the column on top of the still, to be collected in containers where it condenses back into a liquid.

This alcohol, called *neutral spirits,* is the base for the alcohol beverages called spirits or distilled spirits: gin, rum, tequila, whiskey, and vodka. Brandy is a special product, a spirit distilled from wine. Fortified wines, such as Port and Sherry, are wines with spirits added.

The foods used to make beverage alcohol

Beverage alcohol can be made from virtually any carbohydrate food. The foods most commonly used are cereal grains, fruit, honey, molasses, or potatoes. Table 10-1 shows you which foods are used to produce the different kinds of alcohol beverages.

On its own, alcohol provides energy (7 calories per gram) but no nutrients, so distilled spirits, such as whiskey or plain, unflavored vodka, serve up nothing but calories. Beer, wine, cider, and other fermented beverages, such as kumiss (fermented milk), contain some of the food from which they were made, so they contain small amounts of proteins and carbohydrates, vitamins, and minerals.

Table 10-1	Foods Used to Make Alcohol Beverages
Original Food	*Alcohol Beverage Produced*
Fruit and fruit juice	
Agave plant	Tequila
Apples	Hard cider
Grapes and other fruits	Wine
Grain	
Barley	Beer, various distilled spirits, kvass
Corn	Bourbon, corn whiskey, beer
Rice	Sake (a distilled product), rice wine
Rye	Whiskey
Wheat	Distilled spirits, beer
Others	
Honey	Mead
Milk	Kumiss (koumiss), kefir
Potatoes	Vodka
Sugar cane	Rum

How Much Alcohol Is in That Bottle?

No alcohol beverage is 100 percent alcohol. It's alcohol plus water, and — if it's a wine or beer — some residue of the foods from which it was made.

The term ABV on the label shows the amount of alcohol as a percentage of all the liquid in the container. For example, if your container holds 10 ounces of liquid and 1 ounce of that is alcohol, the product is 10 percent ABV — the alcohol content divided by the total amount of liquid.

Proof — an older term to describe alcohol content —is two times the ABV. For example, an alcohol beverage that is 10 percent alcohol by volume is 20 proof.

Alcohol beverages may use the term "organic" on the label so long as they comply with the standards set for all foods (see Chapter 17), but right now, alcohol beverages are the only entries in the food and drink market sold without a Nutrition Facts label. Since 2003, The National Consumers League and the Washington-based Center for Science in the Public Interest have petitioned the Food and Drug Administration to create an ingredients label for alcohol beverages to list the ingredients, the number of standard servings in the container, and the alcohol content and calorie count per serving so you can compare products — and control what you drink. To date: No label.

Moving Alcohol through Your Body

Other foods must be digested before being absorbed by your cells, but alcohol flows directly through your body's membranes into your bloodstream, which carries alcohol to nearly every organ in your body. Here's a road map to show you the route traveled by the alcohol in every drink you take:

✔ **Flowing down from mouth to stomach:** Alcohol is an *astringent;* it coagulates proteins on the surface of the lining of your mouth to make it "pucker." Some alcohol is absorbed through the lining of the mouth and throat, but most of the alcohol you drink spills into your stomach, where an enzyme called *gastric alcohol dehydrogenase* (gADH) begins to metabolize (digest) it.

How much alcohol dehydrogenase your body churns out is influenced by your ethnicity and your gender. For example, Asians, Native Americans, and Inuits appear to secrete less gastric alcohol dehydrogenase than do most Caucasians, and the average woman (regardless of her ethnicity) makes less gADH than the average man does. As a result, more unmetabolized alcohol flows from their stomach into their bloodstream, and they're likely to become tipsy on smaller amounts of alcohol than does an average Caucasian male. In any case, a certain amount of unmetabolized alcohol flows through the stomach walls into the blood-stream and on to the small intestine.

✔ **Stopping at the liver:** Most of the alcohol you drink is absorbed through the *duodenum* (the first part of the small intestine), from which it flows through a large blood vessel (the portal vein) into the liver. There, ADH, an enzyme similar to gADH, metabolizes the alcohol, which is then converted to energy by a coenzyme called *nicotinamide adenine dinucleotide* (NAD). NAD is also used to convert the glucose derived from other carbohydrates (check Chapter 9) to energy, so while NAD is being used for alcohol, glucose conversion grinds to a halt.

The normal, healthy liver can process about ½ ounce of pure alcohol (that's 6 to 12 ounces of beer, 5 ounces of wine, or 1 ounce of spirits) in an hour. The rest flows on to your heart.

✔ **Taking time out to breathe:** When it enters the heart, alcohol reduces the force with which the heart muscle contracts. You pump out slightly less blood for a few minutes, blood vessels all over your body relax, and your blood pressure goes down temporarily. The contractions soon return to normal, but the blood vessels may remain relaxed and blood pressure lower for as long as half an hour.

At the same time, alcohol flows in blood from the heart through the pulmonary vein to the lungs. Now you breathe out a tiny bit of alcohol every time you exhale, and your breath smells of liquor. Then the newly oxygenated, still alcohol-laden blood flows back through the pulmonary artery to your heart, and up and out through the *aorta* (the major artery that carries blood out to your body).

✔ **Rising to the surface:** As it circulates in the blood, alcohol raises the level of high-density lipoproteins (HDLs), although not necessarily the specific *good* ones that carry cholesterol out of your body. (For more about lipoproteins, see Chapter 7.) Alcohol also makes blood less likely to clot, temporarily reducing the risk of heart attack and stroke.

Alcohol makes blood vessels expand, so more warm blood flows up from the center of your body to the surface of the skin. You feel warmer for a while and, if your skin is fair, you may flush and turn pink. (Asians, who tend to make less alcohol dehydrogenase than do Caucasians, often experience a characteristic flushing when they drink even small amounts of alcohol.) At the same time, tiny amounts of alcohol ooze out through your pores, and your perspiration smells of alcohol.

✔ **Creating curves in the road:** Alcohol is a sedative. When it reaches your brain, it slows the transmission of impulses between nerve cells that control your ability to think and move.

Do you feel a sudden urge to urinate? Alcohol reduces your brain's production of *antidiuretic hormones,* chemicals that keep you from making too much urine. You may lose lots of liquid, plus vitamins and minerals. You also grow very thirsty, and your urine may smell faintly of alcohol.

✔ **Ending the process:** This cycle continues as long as you have alcohol circulating in your blood, or in other words, until your liver can manage to produce enough ADH to metabolize all the alcohol you've consumed. How long is that? Most people need an hour to metabolize the amount of alcohol (½ ounce) in one drink. But that's an average: Some people have alcohol circulating in their blood for up to three hours after taking a drink.

Alcohol and Health

Beverage alcohol has benefits as well as side effects. The benefits are strongly linked to what is commonly called *moderate drinking* — no more than one drink a day for a woman, two drinks a day for a man. The risks generally arise from excessive drinking and alcohol abuse.

Moderate drinking: Some benefits, some risks

Moderate amounts of alcohol not only reduce stress but also appear to have beneficial effects on various parts of the human body.

For example:

✔ In March 2010, a study of 2,900 Swiss adults, published in the journal *Arthritis and Rheumatism,* suggested that moderate drinking might slow the progression of rheumatoid arthritis (RA); data from earlier studies had noted a lower risk of RA among adults who drink in moderation.

✔ The American Cancer Society's Cancer Prevention Study 1 followed more than one million Americans in 25 states for 12 years to find that moderate alcohol intake had an "apparent protective effect on coronary heart disease." Translation: Men who drink moderately lower their risk of heart attack. The risk is 21 percent lower for men who have one drink a day than for men who never drink.

✔ A similar analysis of data for nearly 600,000 women in the long-running (Harvard) Nurses' Health Study showed that women who drink occasionally or have one drink a day are less likely to die of heart attack than those who don't drink at all.

✔ In 2010, data from a Wageningen University (The Netherlands) study of 35,625 adults age 20 to 70, published in the *American Journal of Clinical Nutrition,* showed that moderate drinkers (one to two drinks a day) have a lower risk than teetotalers of developing Type 2 (non-insulin dependent) diabetes. This confirms many previous reports including one 2003 article in the Archives of Internal Medicine.

✔ A 2003 study at Tulane University School of Public Health and Tropical Medicine shows that men who drink moderately (two drinks a day) also are less likely to die of clot-related stroke. But because alcohol reduces blood clotting, it increases the risk of *hemorrhagic* stroke (stroke caused by bleeding in the brain). Sorry about that.

That's the good news. Here's the bad news: The same studies that applaud the effects of moderate drinking on heart health are less reassuring about the relationship between alcohol and cancer:

✔ The National Cancer Institute labels alcohol, in conjunction with smoking, as a clear risk factor for cancers of the mouth, throat (esophagus, pharynx, larynx), and liver.

✔ Researchers at the University of Oklahoma say that men who drink five or more beers a day double their risk of rectal cancer.

✔ American Cancer Society (ACS) statistics show a higher risk of breast cancer among women who have more than three drinks a week; some studies suggest this effect may apply only to older women using hormone replacement therapy.

A lot and a little versus the middle

When scientists talk about the relationship between alcohol and heart disease, the words *J-curve* often pop up. What's a J-curve? A statistical graph in the shape of the letter J.

In terms of heart disease, the lower peak on the left of the J shows the risk among teetotalers, the high spike on the right shows the risk among those who drink too much, and the curve in the center shows the risk in the moderate middle. In other words, the J-curve says that people who drink moderately have a lower risk of heart disease than people who drink too much or not at all.

According to a recent report from the Alberta (Canada) Alcohol and Drug Abuse Commission, the J-curve may also describe the relationship between alcohol and stroke, alcohol and diabetes, alcohol and bone loss, and alcohol and longevity. The simple fact is that moderate drinkers appear to live longer, healthier lives than either teetotalers or alcohol abusers. Cheers!

Binge drinking: A behavioral no-no

Binge drinkers have been described as "once-in-a-while alcoholics." They don't drink every day, but when they do indulge, they go so far overboard that they sometimes fail to come back up. In simple terms, binge drinking is downing very large amounts of alcohol in a short time, not for a pleasant lift but to get drunk. As a result, binge drinkers may consume so much beer, wine, or spirits that the amount of alcohol in their blood rises to lethal levels that, in the worst case, may lead to death by alcohol poisoning.

Efforts to stamp out binge drinking, which often occurs on college campuses, may rely on guilt or shame to change behavior, but a 2008 study at the Kellogg School of Management at Northwestern University found that binge drinkers are already uncomfortable with their behavior. Attempting to make them more so doesn't work. Instead, the researchers suggested couching anti-binge messages in simple, intelligent language focusing on how to avoid situations that lead to binge drinking rather that the nasty effects of the overindulgence.

The physical effects of excessive drinking

Alcohol abuse is a term generally taken to mean drinking so much that it interferes with your ability to have a normal, productive life. *Excessive drinking,* including binge drinking (see the sidebar "Binge drinking: A behavioral no-no" later in this chapter), can also make you feel terrible the next day. *The morning after* is not fiction. A hangover is a miserable physical fact:

- ✔ You're thirsty because you lost excess water through copious urination.

- ✔ Your stomach hurts and you're queasy because even small amounts of alcohol irritate your stomach lining, causing it to secrete extra acid and lots of *histamine,* the same immune system chemical that makes the skin around a mosquito bite red and itchy.

- ✔ Your muscles ache and your head pounds because processing alcohol through your liver requires an enzyme — nicotinamide adenine dinucleotide (NAD) — normally used to convert *lactic acid,* a byproduct of muscle activity, to other chemicals that can be used for energy. The extra, unprocessed lactic acid piles up painfully in your muscles.

Alcoholism: An addiction disease

No one knows exactly why some people are able to have a drink once a day or once a month or once a year, enjoy it, and move on, while others become addicted to alcohol. In the past, alcoholism has been blamed on "bad genes," lack of willpower, or even a nasty childhood.

As science continues to unravel the mysteries of body chemistry, it's reasonable to expect that researchers will eventually come up with a rational scientific explanation for the differences between social drinkers and people who can't safely use alcohol. It just hasn't happened yet.

What is clear, however, is that *alcoholics* are people who can't control their drinking. Untreated alcoholism is a life-threatening disease that can lead to death either from an accident or suicide (both are more common among heavy drinkers) or from a toxic reaction (acute alcohol poisoning that paralyzes body organs, including the heart and lungs) or from liver damage (cirrhosis) or from malnutrition.

Alcoholics are often emaciated, with such visible symptoms of malnutrition as problem skin, broken nails, and dull hair; less visible symptoms of vitamin and mineral deficiencies may hide underneath the surface. Why? Because alcohol abuse makes it extremely difficult — if not impossible — for the body to extract essential nutrients from food. That's because

- Alcohol depresses appetite.
- An alcoholic may substitute alcohol for food, getting calories but no nutrients.
- Even when the alcoholic eats, the alcohol in his tissues can prevent the proper absorption of vitamins (notably the B vitamins), minerals, and other nutrients. Alcohol may also reduce the alcoholic's ability to synthesize proteins.

This set of problems cannot be resolved simply by downing a multivitamin with the alcohol; it requires medical attention to understand and treat the primary cause, which is — to put it bluntly — drinking too much, much too often.

Who should not drink

No one should drink to excess. But some people shouldn't drink at all, not even in moderation. They include

- **People who plan to drive or do work that requires both attention and skill.** Alcohol slows reaction time and makes your motor skills — turning the wheel of the car, operating a sewing machine — less precise, which make you more likely to end up with a needle through the hand or a head through the windshield.

- **Women who are pregnant or who plan to become pregnant in the near future.** *Fetal alcohol syndrome* (FAS) is a collection of birth defects including low birth weight, heart defects, retardation, and facial deformities documented only in babies born to female alcoholics.

No evidence links FAS to casual drinking — that is, one or two drinks during a pregnancy or even one or two drinks a week. In fact, for years before FAS was identified and diagnosed, pregnant women were routinely advised to drink beer as a source of nutritious calories.

However, the National Institute on Alcohol Abuse and Alcoholism (NIAAA) says that it is not clear yet whether there is any completely safe level of alcohol during pregnancy and notes that in 2005 the U.S. Surgeon General urged women who are pregnant or may become pregnant to abstain from alcohol.

Finally, the sad but scientific fact is that about 7 percent of the babies born in the United States each year are born with birth defects independent of any parental behavior. The parents of these children may feel guilty, even though their behavior had absolutely nothing to do with the birth defect. Your decision about alcohol should take into consideration the psychological possibility of (misplaced) lifelong guilt caused by having had a drink.

✔ **People who take certain prescription drugs or over-the-counter medication.** Alcohol makes some drugs stronger, increases some drugs' side effects, and renders other drugs less effective. At the same time, some drugs make alcohol a more powerful sedative or slow down the elimination of alcohol from your body.

Table 10-2 shows some of the interactions known to occur between alcohol and some common prescription and over-the-counter drugs. This short list gives you an idea of some of the general interactions likely to occur between alcohol and drugs. But the list is far from complete. Today, by law, drugs that interact with alcohol usually carry a warning on the label, but if you're taking any kind of medication — over-the-counter or prescription — and you're not sure of the possibility of interactions, check with your doctor or pharmacist.

Table 10-2	Drug and Alcohol Interactions
Drug	*Possible Interaction with Alcohol*
Analgesics (acetaminophen)	Increased liver toxicity
Analgesics (aspirin and other nonsteroidal inflammatory drugs — NSAIDs)	Increased stomach bleeding; irritation
Anti-arthritis drugs	Increased stomach bleeding; irritation
Antidepressants	Increased drowsiness/intoxication; high blood pressure (depends on the type of drug — check with your doctor)
Antidiabetes drugs	Excessively low blood sugar
Antihypertension drugs	Very low blood pressure

Drug	Possible Interaction with Alcohol
Antituberculosis medication (isoniazid)	Decreased drug effectiveness; higher risk of hepatitis
Diet pills	Excessive nervousness
Diuretics	Low blood pressure
Iron supplements	Excessive absorption of iron
Sleeping pills	Increased sedation
Tranquilizers	Increased sedation

James W. Long and James J. Rybacki, The Essential Guide to Prescription Drugs 1995 (New York: Harper Collins, 1995)

Alcohol and age

As we grow older, our reaction time slows, we see and hear less clearly, and changes in the body's ability to metabolize food may lower our tolerance for alcohol. Each problem increases the risk of injury associated with drinking more than the body can handle.

On the other hand, moderate drinking remains a pleasant experience for people healthy enough to indulge. It also appears to be beneficial to intellectual health. In 2000, data from a 15-year, 1,700-person heart disease study at the Institute of Preventive Medicine, at Kommunehospitalet in Copenhagen, Denmark, showed that older men and women who regularly consumed up to 21 drinks of wine a week were less likely than teetotalers to develop Alzheimer's disease and other forms of dementia. Similarly, a recent 12-year, 1,488-person survey at Johns Hopkins University in Maryland suggests that regular, moderate drinkers score better over time than teetotalers do on the Mini-Mental State Examination (MMSE), a standard test for memory, reasoning, and decision making.

Advice from the Sages: Moderation

Good advice is always current. The folks who wrote Ecclesiastes (a book in the Bible) centuries ago may have been speaking to you when they said, "Wine is as good as life to man if it be drunk moderately." And it's impossible to improve on this slogan from the Romans (actually, one Roman writer named Terence): "Moderation in all things." Hey, you can't get a message more direct — or more sensible — than that.

The power of purple (and peanuts)

Grape skin, pulp, and seeds contain *resveratrol,* a naturally occurring plant chemical that seems to reduce the risk of heart disease and some kinds of cancer. The darker the grapes, the higher the concentration of resveratrol.

Dark purple grape juice, for example, has more resveratrol than red grape juice, which has more resveratrol than white grape juice. Because wine is made from grapes, it, too, contains resveratrol (red wine has more resveratrol than white wine).

But you don't need to drink grape juice or wine or eat grapes to get resveratrol. You can simply snack on peanuts. A 1998 analysis from the USDA Agricultural Research Service in Raleigh, North Carolina, showed that peanuts have 1.7 to 3.7 micrograms of resveratrol per gram of nuts (boiled peanuts are at the upper end). Compare that to the 0.7 micrograms of resveratrol in a glass of red grape juice or 0.6 to 8.0 micrograms of resveratrol per gram of red wine.

In the body, resveratrol appears to reduce inflammation. This fact may explain why a multitude of studies show a lower risk of heart disease among wine drinkers. In 2010, researchers at Johns Hopkins reported that drinking red wine may also reduce the risk of brain damage after a stroke. When they fed one group of lab mice red grape skin and seeds and then induced a stroke, the animals that had been fed the grape appetizers had less brain damage than did a control group of mice which had not. Whether this applies to human beings and how much resveratrol would be needed to produce the same effect remains to be shown.

Finally, a 2010 article in the *American Journal of Pathology* documents the discovery by Washington University researchers that resveratrol appears to inhibit *angiogenesis* (the formation of new blood vessels). Angiogenesis, which is essential to the formation and growth of tumors, also plays a role in the development of extra blood vessels in the eye leading to macular degeneration and diabetes-related blindness. Once again, whether what happened in lab animals will happen in human beings is an open, but intriguing, question.

Chapter 11

Vigorous Vitamins

• •

In This Chapter

▶ Understanding the value of vitamins

▶ Finding vitamins in food

▶ Considering the consequences of vitamin deficiencies or overdoses

▶ Deciding when extra vitamins make sense

• •

*V*itamins are *organic chemicals,* substances that contain carbon, hydrogen, and oxygen that occur naturally in all living things: both plants and animals, such as flowers, trees, fruits, vegetables, chickens, fish, cows, and you. These natural compounds regulate a variety of bodily functions and are essential for building tissues, such as bones, skin, glands, nerves, and blood. They also assist in metabolizing (digesting) proteins, fats, and carbohydrates so that you can extract energy from food. Finally, they prevent nutritional deficiency diseases, promote healing, and encourage good health.

This chapter tells you where the vitamins are, how to add them to your diet, exactly how much of each you should consume each day, and how to tell how much is more than enough.

Listing the Vitamins Your Body Needs

For optimum health, your body requires at least 11 vitamins: vitamin A, vitamin D, vitamin E, vitamin K, vitamin C, and the members of the B vitamin family — thiamin (vitamin B1), riboflavin (B2), niacin, vitamin B6, folate, and vitamin B12. Two more B vitamins (biotin and pantothenic acid) and one unusual compound (choline) are also valuable.

You need only miniscule quantities of each vitamin for good health. In some cases, the recommended dietary allowances (RDAs), determined by the National Research Council, may be as small as several micrograms — $\frac{1}{1,000,000}$, or one one-millionth of a gram.

The father of all vitamins: Casimir Funk

Vitamins are so much a part of modern life you may have a hard time believing they were first discovered less than a century ago. Of course, people have long known that certain foods contain something special. For example, the ancient Greek physician Hippocrates prescribed liver for night-blindness (the inability to see well in dim light). By the end of the 18th century (1795), British Navy ships carried a mandatory supply of limes or lime juice to prevent scurvy among the men, thus earning the Brits once and forever the nickname limeys. Later on, the Japanese Navy gave its sailors whole grain barley to ward off beriberi.

Everyone knew these prescriptions worked, but nobody knew why — until 1912, when Casimir Funk (1884–1967), a Polish biochemist working first in England and then in the United States, identified "somethings" in food that he called *vitamines* (*vita* = life; *amines* = nitrogen compounds).

The following year, Funk and a fellow biochemist, Briton Frederick Hopkins, suggested that some medical conditions, such as scurvy and beriberi, were simply deficiency diseases caused by the absence of a specific nutrient in the body. Adding a food with the missing nutrient to one's diet would prevent or cure the deficiency disease. What else is there to say except, Eureka!

Which, since Funk was Polish but working in England, is probably exactly what he said.

Nutritionists classify vitamins as either *fat soluble* or *water soluble,* meaning that they dissolve either in fat or in water. If you consume larger amounts of fat-soluble vitamins than your body needs, the excess is stored in body fat. Large amounts of fat-soluble vitamins stored in your body may cause problems (see the section "Fat-soluble vitamins" in this chapter). With water-soluble vitamins, your body simply shrugs its shoulders, so to speak, and urinates away most of the excess.

Medical students often use mnemonic (pronounced *neh-mah-nic*) devices — memory joggers — to remember complicated lists of body parts and symptoms of diseases. Here's one to help you remember which vitamins are fat-soluble: "All Dogs Eat Kidneys." In other words, vitamins A, D, E, and K are fat soluble. All the rest dissolve in water.

Fat-soluble vitamins

Vitamin A, vitamin D, vitamin E, and vitamin K have two characteristics in common: All dissolve in fat, and all are stored in your fatty tissues. But like members of any family, they also have distinct personalities. One keeps your skin moist. Another protects your bones. A third keeps reproductive organs purring happily. And the fourth enables you to make special proteins.

Vitamin A

Vitamin A is the moisturizing nutrient that keeps your skin and *mucous membranes* (the slick tissue that lines the eyes, nose, mouth, throat, vagina, and rectum) smooth and supple. Vitamin A is also the vision vitamin, a constituent of *11-cis retinol,* a protein in the *rods* (cells in the back of your eye that enable you to see even when the lights are low) that prevents or slows the development of age-related *macular degeneration,* or progressive damage to the retina of the eye, which can cause the loss of central vision (the ability to see clearly enough to read or do fine work). Finally, vitamin A promotes the growth of healthy bones and teeth, keeps your reproductive system humming, and encourages your immune system to churn out the cells you need to fight off infection.

Your body gets its vitamin A from two classes of chemicals:

✔ *Retinoids* are compounds whose names all start with *ret:* retinol, retinaldehyde, retinoic acid, and so on. These fat-soluble substances are found in several foods of animal origin: liver (again!) and whole milk, eggs, and butter. Retinoids give you *preformed* vitamin A, the kind of nutrient your body can use right away.

✔ *Carotenoids* are *vitamin A precursors,* chemicals such as beta carotene, a deep yellow carotenoid (pigment) found in dark green, bright yellow, and orange fruits and vegetables. Your body transforms a vitamin A precursor into a retinol-like substance. So far, scientists have identified at least 500 different carotenoids. Only 1 in 10 — about 50 altogether — are considered to be sources of vitamin A.

Traditionally, the recommended dietary allowance of vitamin A is measured in International Units (IU). However, because retinol is the most efficient source of vitamin A, the modern way to measure the RDA for vitamin A is as *retinol equivalents,* abbreviated as RE. One microgram (mcg) RE = 3.3 IU. But a simple trip through the vitamin aisle at the drugstore shows that vitamin products still list the RDA for vitamin A in IUs.

Vitamin D

Calcium is essential for hardening teeth and bones, but no matter how much calcium you consume, without vitamin D, your body can't absorb and use the mineral. Researchers at the Bone Metabolism Laboratory at the Jean Mayer USDA Human Nutrition Research Center on Aging at Tufts University in Boston say vitamin D may also reduce the risk of tooth loss by preventing the inflammatory response that leads to periodontal disease, a condition that destroys the thin tissue (ligaments) that connects the teeth to the surrounding jawbone. And a report in the February 2006 issue of *The American Journal of Public Health* was the first to suggest that vitamin D supplements might cut in half a person's risk of developing some forms of cancer, including cancer of the colon, breast, or ovaries.

These last claims remain to be proven, but the very fact that they exist has made vitamin D supplements hot stuff. According to the market research firm Packaged Facts' market study, *Nutritional Supplements in the U.S.,* 4th Edition, sales of vitamin D rose a whopping 8 percent between 2006 and 2010, almost certainly due to a long list of good-news studies linking adequate doses of D to bone health, heart health, and general all around bounciness.

Vitamin D comes in three forms:

- *Calciferol* occurs naturally in fish oils and egg yolk, and, in the United States, it's added to margarines and milk.

- *Cholecalciferol* is created when sunlight hits your skin and ultraviolet rays react with steroid chemicals in body fat just underneath.

- *Ergocalciferol* is synthesized in plants exposed to sunlight. Cholecalciferol and ergocalciferol justify vitamin D's nickname: the Sunshine Vitamin.

The RDA for vitamin D is measured either in International Units (IUs) or micrograms (mcg) of cholecalciferol: 10 mcg cholecalciferol = 400 IU vitamin D.

Vitamin E

Vitamin E maintains your healthy reproductive system, nerves, and muscles. You get vitamin E from *tocopherols* and *tocotrienols,* two families of naturally occurring chemicals in vegetable oils, nuts, whole grains, and green leafy vegetables — your best natural sources of vitamin E.

Tocopherols, the more important source, have two sterling characteristics: They're anticoagulants and antioxidants that reduce blood's ability to clot, thus reducing the risk of clot-related stroke and heart attack. *Antioxidants* prevent free radicals (incomplete pieces of molecules) from hooking up with other molecules or fragments of molecules to form toxic substances that can attack tissues in your body. In fact, nutrition scientists at Purdue University released a study showing that vitamin E promotes bone growth by stopping free radicals from reacting with polyunsaturated fatty acids (see Chapter 8 for information on fats) to create molecules that interfere with the formation of new bone cells.

Some claims about E's heart health benefits are now considered iffy. True, a recent clinical trial at Cambridge University in England showed that taking 800 IU (International Units) vitamin E, two times the RDA, may reduce the risk of nonfatal heart attacks for people who already have heart disease. And, yes, the federal Women's Health Study found that older women taking 600 IU vitamin E per day had a lower risk of heart attack and a lower risk of death from heart disease. But the Heart Outcomes Prevention Evaluation (HOPE) study showed no such benefits. In fact, people taking 400 IU vitamin E per day were more likely to develop heart failure. No one (and no study) has found similar problems among those taking less vitamin E, say 100 IU/day. Whew.

The best sources of vitamin E are vegetables, oils, nuts, and seeds. The RDA is expressed as milligrams *a-tocopherol equivalents* (abbreviated as *a-TE*).

Vitamin K

Vitamin K is a group of chemicals that your body uses to make specialized proteins found in blood *plasma* (the clear fluid in blood). One such protein is prothrombin, the protein chiefly responsible for blood clotting. You also need vitamin K to make bone and kidney tissues. Like vitamin D, vitamin K is essential for healthy bones, activating at least three different proteins that take part in forming new bone cells. In 2003, a report from the long-running Framingham (Massachusetts) Heart Study showed adults consuming the least vitamin K each day are likely to have the highest incidence of broken bones. Finally, in the spring of 2010, a report from the Mayo Clinic suggested to the 101st Annual Meeting of the American Association for Cancer Research that an adequate intake of vitamin K cut the risk of non-Hodgkin's lymphoma, a cancer of the blood, almost in half.

Vitamin K is found in dark green leafy vegetables (broccoli, cabbage, kale, lettuce, spinach, and turnip greens), cheese, liver, cereals, and fruits, but most of what you need comes from resident colonies of friendly bacteria in your intestines, an assembly line of busy bugs churning out the vitamin day and night.

Water-soluble vitamins

The good news about water-soluble vitamins is that it is virtually impossible to overdose on them without taking enormous amounts of supplements. The bad news is that you have to take enough of these vitamins on a more or less regular schedule to protect yourself against deficiencies. (You don't have to take them every day; you could take less one day and more the next, and over time it evens out.)

Vitamin C

Vitamin C, also known by its chemical name ascorbic acid, is essential for the development and maintenance of connective tissue (the fat, muscle, and bone framework of the human body). Vitamin C speeds the production of new cells in wound healing, protects your immune system, helps you fight off infection, reduces the severity of allergic reactions, and plays a role in the syntheses of hormones and other body chemicals.

Lemons, limes, oranges — and bacon?

Check the meat label. Right there it is, plain as day — vitamin C in the form of *sodium ascorbate, isoascorbate,* or *sodium erythorbate.*

Processed meats such as bacon and sausages are preserved with sodium nitrite, which protects the meat from *Clostridium botulinum,* microorganisms that cause the potentially fatal food poisoning known as botulism.

On its own, sodium nitrite reacts at high temperatures with compounds in meat to form carcinogens called nitrosamines. Antioxidant vitamin C prevents the chemical reaction. It also prevents free radicals (incomplete pieces of molecules) from hooking up with each other to form damaging compounds — in this case *carcinogens,* substances that cause cancer.

Which is why Food and Drug Administration (FDA) and Department of Agriculture/Food Safety and Inspection Service (USDA FISIS) rules require vitamin C in your lunchmeat.

Thiamin (vitamin B1)

Call it thiamin. Call it B1. Just don't call it late for lunch (or any other meal). This sulfur *(thia)* and nitrogen *(amin)* compound, the first of the B vitamins to be isolated and identified, helps ensure a healthy appetite. It acts as a *coenzyme* (a substance that works along with other enzymes) essential to at least four different processes by which your body extracts energy from carbohydrates. Thiamin also is a mild diuretic (something makes you urinate more frequently). This vitamin is found in every body tissue, the highest concentrations are in your vital organs — heart, liver, and kidneys.

The richest dietary sources of thiamin are unrefined cereals and grains, lean pork, beans, nuts, and seeds. In the United States, refined flours, stripped of their thiamin, are a nutritional reality, so most Americans get most of their thiamin from breads and cereals enriched with additional B1.

Riboflavin (vitamin B2)

Riboflavin (vitamin B2), the second B vitamin to be identified, was once called vitamin G. Its present name is derivative of its chemical structure, a carbon-hydrogen-oxygen skeleton that includes *ribitol* (a sugar) attached to a *flavonoid* (a substance from plants containing a pigment called flavone).

Like thiamin, riboflavin is a coenzyme. Without it, your body can't digest and use proteins and carbohydrates. Like vitamin A, it protects the health of mucous membranes — the moist tissues that line the eyes, mouth, nose, throat, vagina, and rectum.

You get riboflavin from foods of animal origin (meat, fish, poultry, eggs, and milk), whole or enriched grain products, brewer's yeast, and dark green vegetables (like broccoli and spinach).

Niacin

Niacin is one name for a pair of naturally occurring nutrients, nicotinic acid and nicotinamide. Niacin is essential for proper growth, and like other B vitamins, it's intimately involved in enzyme reactions. In fact, it's an integral part of an enzyme that enables oxygen to flow into body tissues. Like thiamin, it gives you a healthy appetite and participates in the metabolism of sugars and fats.

Niacin is available either as a preformed nutrient or via the conversion of the amino acid tryptophan. Preformed niacin comes from meat; tryptophan comes from milk and dairy foods. Some niacin is present in grains, but your body can't absorb it efficiently unless the grain has been treated with lime — the mineral, not the fruit. This is a common practice in Central American and South American countries, where lime is added to cornmeal in making tortillas. In the United States, breads and cereals are routinely fortified with niacin. Your body easily absorbs the added niacin.

The term used to describe the niacin RDA is NE (niacin equivalent): 60 milligrams tryptophan = 1 milligram niacin = 1 niacin equivalent (NE).

Vitamin B6 (pyridoxine)

Vitamin B6 is another multiple compound, this one comprising three related chemicals: pyridoxine, pyridoxal, and pyridoxamine. Vitamin B6, a component of enzymes that metabolizes proteins and fats, is essential for getting energy and nutrients from food. It also helps lower blood levels of homocysteine (see Chapter 7), an amino acid produced when you digest proteins.

The American Heart Association calls a high level of homocysteine an independent (but not major) risk factor for heart disease, and the American Journal of Clinical Nutrition reported in 2005 that a high homocysteine level may be associated with an age-related decline in memory. Alas, follow-up studies show no reduction in the risk of heart disease or improvement in memory in those who reduce their blood levels of homocysteine.

The best food sources of vitamin B6 are liver, chicken, fish, pork, lamb, milk, eggs, unmilled rice (rice with the bran intact), whole grains, soybeans, potatoes, beans, nuts, seeds, and dark green vegetables, such as turnip greens. In the United States, bread and other products made with refined grains have added vitamin B6.

Folate

Folate, also known as folacin or folic acid, plays a role in the synthesis of DNA, the metabolism of proteins, and the subsequent synthesis of amino acids used to produce new body cells and tissues. It is vital for normal growth and wound healing, and the vitamin is essential to a pregnant woman's ability to create new maternal tissue as well as fetal tissue. The fetus, too, benefits from her mother's folate consumption: An adequate supply of folate during pregnancy dramatically reduces the risk of neural tube (spinal cord) birth defects such as *spina bifida* (the failure of the bones of the spine to close properly around the spinal cord).

Beans, dark green leafy vegetables, liver, yeast, and various fruits are excellent food sources of folate; all multivitamin supplements — and all grain products — in the United States must now include 400 mcg of folate per dose.

Vitamin B12

Vitamin B12 (cyanocobalamin) is a unique nutrient, the only vitamin that contains a mineral — in this case, cobalt. (Cyanocobalamin, a cobalt compound, is commonly used as vitamin B12 in vitamin pills and nutritional supplements.)

Vitamin B12 makes healthy red blood cells. It protects *myelin,* the fatty material that covers your nerves and enables you to transmit electrical impulses (messages) between nerve cells that make it possible for you to see, hear, think, move, and do all the things a healthy body does each day.

This vitamin cannot be produced by higher plants (the ones that yield our fruits and vegetables), but like vitamin K, vitamin B12 is made by beneficial bacteria living in the small intestine. Meat, fish, poultry, milk products, and eggs are good sources of vitamin B12. Grains don't naturally contain vitamin B12, but like other B vitamins, it's added to grain products in the United States.

Biotin

Biotin is a B-vitamin, a component of enzymes that ferry carbon and oxygen atoms between cells. Biotin helps you metabolize fats and carbohydrates and is essential for synthesizing fatty acids and amino acids needed for healthy growth. And it seems to prevent a buildup of fat deposits that may interfere with the proper functioning of liver and kidneys. (No, biotin won't keep fat from settling in more visible places, such as your hips.)

The best food sources of biotin are liver, egg yolk, yeast, nuts, and beans. If your diet doesn't give you all the biotin you need, bacteria in your gut will synthesize enough to make up the difference. No RDA exists for biotin, but the Food and Nutrition Board has established an Adequate Intake (AI), the safe and effective daily dose for nutrients for which no RDA has been set (see Chapter 5).

Pantothenic acid

Pantothenic acid, another B-vitamin, is vital to enzyme reactions that enable you to use carbohydrates and create steroid biochemicals such as hormones. Pantothenic acid also helps stabilize blood sugar levels, defends against infection, and protects *hemoglobin* (the protein in red blood cells that carries oxygen through the body), as well as nerve, brain, and muscle tissue.

You get pantothenic acid from meat, fish, poultry, beans, whole grain cereals, and fortified grain products. As with biotin, the Food and Nutrition Board has established an Adequate Intake (AI) for pantothenic acid.

Choline

In 1998, 138 years after choline was first identified, the Institute of Medicine (IOM) finally declared it essential for human beings. The IOM had good reasons for doing so. Although choline is neither a vitamin, a mineral, a protein, a carbohydrate, nor a fat, it does help keep body cells healthy. It's used to make *acetylcholine,* a chemical that enables brain cells to exchange messages. It protects the heart and lowers the risk of liver cancer. And new research at the University of North Carolina (Chapel Hill) shows that choline plays a role in developing and maintaining the ability to think and remember, at least among rat pups and other beasties born to lab animals that were given choline supplements while pregnant. Follow-up studies showed that prenatal choline supplements helped the animals grow bigger brain cells. True, no one knows whether this would also be true for human babies, but some researchers advise pregnant women to eat a varied diet, because getting choline from basic stuff like eggs, meat, and milk is so easy.

IOM's Food and Nutrition Board, the group that sets the RDAs, has established an AI (Adequate Intake) for choline.

Hand in hand: How vitamins help each other

All vitamins have specific jobs in your body. Some have partners. Here are some examples of nutrient cooperation:

- Vitamin E keeps vitamin A from being destroyed in your intestines.

- Vitamin D enables your body to absorb calcium and phosphorus.

- Vitamin C helps folate build proteins.

- Vitamin B1 works in digestive enzyme systems with niacin, pantothenic acid, and magnesium.

Taking vitamins with other vitamins may also improve body levels of nutrients. For example, in 1993, scientists at the National Cancer Institute and the U. S. Department of Agriculture (USDA) Agricultural Research Service gave one group of volunteers a vitamin E capsule plus a multivitamin pill; a second group, vitamin E alone; and a third group, no vitamins at all. The people getting vitamin E plus the multivitamin had the highest amount of vitamin E in their blood — more than twice as high as those who took plain vitamin E capsules.

Sometimes, one vitamin may even alleviate a deficiency caused by the lack of another vitamin. People who do not get enough folate are at risk of a form of anemia in which their red blood cells fail to mature. As soon as they get folate, either by injection or by mouth, they begin making new healthy cells. That's to be expected. What's surprising is the fact that anemia caused by *pellagra,* the niacin deficiency disease, may also respond to folate treatment.

Get Your Vitamins Here

One reasonable set of guidelines for good nutrition is the list of Recommended Dietary Allowances (RDAs) established by the National Research Council's Food and Nutrition Board. The RDAs present safe and effective doses for healthy people.

You can find the complete chart of RDAs for adults (ages 19 and up) in Chapter 5. Table 11-1 is the easy alternative, presenting the RDAs for adult men and women (ages 19 to 50) plus a quick guide to food portions that give you at least 25 percent of the recommended dietary allowances of vitamins for healthy adult men and women, ages 25 to 50.

Photocopy this chart. Pin it on your fridge. Tape it to your organizer or appointment book. Stick it in your wallet. Think of it as the truly simple way to see how easy it is to eat healthy.

Table 11-1	Servings That Provide at Least 25% of the RDA
Food	*Serving = 25% of the RDA*
VITAMIN A	**RDA: Women 4,000 IU, Men 5,000 IU***
Breads, cereals, grains	
Oatmeal — instant, fortified	2⅓ cup
Cold cereal	1 ounce
Fruits	
Apricots (dried, cooked)	½ cup
Cantaloupe (raw)	½ cup
Mango (raw)	½ medium
Vegetables	
Carrots, kale, peas and carrots, sweet red pepper (all cooked)	½ cup
Meat, poultry, fish	
Liver — chicken, turkey	½ cup (diced)
Dairy products	
Milk — low-fat, skim	2 cups
VITAMIN D	**RDA: Women 5 mcg/200 IU, Men 5 mcg/200 IU**
Meat, poultry, fish	
Salmon (canned)	1½ ounces
Tuna (canned)	2 ounces

Food	Serving = 25% of the RDA
Dairy products	
Eggs	3 medium
Milk — enriched	1 cup
VITAMIN E	**RDA: Women 15 mg a-TE, Men 15 mg a-TE**
Breads, cereals, grains	
Cold cereal	1 ounce
Wheat germ — plain	2 tbsp.
Fruits	
Apricots, peaches (canned)	1 cup
Vegetables	
Greens (cooked) — dandelion, mustard, turnip	1 cup
Meat, poultry, fish	
Shrimp	3 ounces
Other	
Almonds, hazelnuts/filberts	2 tbsp.
Peanut butter	2 tbsp.
Sunflower seeds	2 tbsp.
VITAMIN C	**RDA: Women 75 mg, Men 90 mg****
Breads, cereals, grains	
Cold cereal	1 ounce
Fruits	
Cantaloupe	½ cup, diced
Grapefruit	½
Mango (raw)	½ medium
Orange	1 medium
Strawberries	½ cup
Grape, orange, or tomato juice	¼ cup
Vegetables	
Asparagus, broccoli, Brussels sprouts, kale, kohlrabi, sweet peppers, snow peas (cooked)	½ cup

(continued)

Table 11-1 *(continued)*

Food	Serving = 25% of the RDA
Sweet potato	1 medium
Meat, poultry, fish	
Liver — beef, pork	3 ounces
THIAMIN (VITAMIN B1)	**RDA: Women 1.1 mg, Men 1.2 mg**
Breads, cereals, grains	
Bagel, English muffin, roll	2 whole
Bread	4 slices
Farina, grits	½ cup
Oatmeal — instant, fortified	⅓ cup
Fruits	
Cantaloupe, honeydew	1 cup
Vegetables	
Corn, peas, peas and carrots (cooked)	1 cup
Meat, poultry, fish	
Ham — roast, smoked, cured, lean	3 ounces
Liver — beef, pork	3 ounces
Pork — all varieties except sausage	3 ounces
Other	
Sunflower seeds (hulled, unroasted)	2 tbsp.
RIBOFLAVIN (VITAMIN B2)	**RDA: Women 1.1 mg, Men 1.3 mg**
Breads, cereals, grains	
Bagel, English muffin, pita	2 whole
Cold cereal	1 ounce
Meat, poultry, fish	
Liver — beef, calf, pork	3 ounces
Liver — chicken, turkey	½ cup, diced
Liverwurst	1 ounce

Food	Serving = 25% of the RDA
Dairy products	
Milk — all varieties	2 cups
Yogurt — lowfat, nonfat	1 cup
NIACIN	**RDA: Women 14 mg NE, Men 16 mg NE**
Breads, cereals, grains	
Bagel, bran muffin, English muffin, pita, roll	2 whole
Cold cereal — fortified	1 ounce
Meat, poultry, fish	
Lamb, pork, veal — lean	3 ounces
Liver — beef, calf, pork	3 ounces
Chicken (no skin)	3 ounces (½ breast)
Mackerel, mullet, salmon, swordfish	3 ounces
Other	
Peanuts, peanut butter	4 tbsp.
VITAMIN B6	**RDA: Women 1.3 mg, Men 1.3 mg**
Breads, cereals, grains	
Oatmeal — instant, fortified	⅓ cup
Cold cereal	1 ounce
Fruits	
Banana (raw)	1 medium
Prunes (dried, cooked)	1 cup
Vegetables	
Plantain (boiled)	1 medium
Meat, poultry, fish	
Chicken (roasted, no skin)	½ breast
Lamb — lean only	1 chop
Liver — beef	3 ounces
FOLATE	**RDA: Women 400 mcg, Men 400 mcg**
Breads, cereals, grains	
Whole wheat English muffin, pita	2 whole
Cold cereal	1 ounce

(continued)

Table 11-1 *(continued)*

Food	Serving = 25% of the RDA
Vegetables	
Asparagus, beets, broccoli, Brussels sprouts, cauliflower, Chinese cabbage, creamed corn, spinach (cooked)	1 cup
Beans (dry, cooked) — black-eyed peas, lentils, red kidney	½ cup
Greens (cooked) — mustard, turnip	1 cup
Meat, poultry, fish	
Liver — beef, calf, pork	3 ounces
VITAMIN B12	**RDA: Women 2.4 mcg, Men 2.4 mcg**
Meat, poultry, fish	
Beef, pork, lamb, veal	3 ounces
Liver — beef, calf, pork	3 ounces
Liver — chicken, turkey	½ cup, diced
Catfish, crabmeat, croaker, lobster, mackerel, mussels, oysters, scallops, swordfish, trout, tuna	3 ounces
Dairy products	
Eggs	2 large
Milk — whole, lowfat, skim	2 cups
Yogurt	2 cups
Food	Serving (mg)
CHOLINE	**Adequate Intake: Women 425 mg, Men 550 mg**
Fruits	
Grape juice (canned)	8 ounces (13 mg)
Vegetables	
Cauliflower (cooked)	1 cup (55 mg)
Potato (baked)	1 medium (18 mg)

Food	Serving = 25% of the RDA
Meat, poultry, fish	
Beef (cooked)	3 ounces (59 mg)
Liver (cooked) — beef	3 ounces (453 mg)
Dairy	
Eggs	1 large (200–300 mg)
Milk — whole	8 ounces (10 mg)
Other	
Peanut butter	2 tbsp. (26 mg)

* Although these remain the "official" RDAs, newer recommendations are 900 mcg RE/3,000 IU per day for men and 700 mcg RE/2,300 IU per day for women (the IU amounts are rounded off).
** The Food and Nutrition Board is debating whether to raise the RDA for vitamin C to 200 mg for both men and women.
"Good Sources of Nutrients" (Washington D.C.: U.S. Department of Agriculture/Human Nutrition Service, 1990); "Nutritive Value of Food" (Washington D.C.: U.S. Department of Agriculture, 1991).

Too Much or Too Little: Avoiding Two Ways to Go Wrong with Vitamins

RDAs are broad enough to prevent vitamin deficiencies and avoid the side effects associated with very large doses of some vitamins. If your diet doesn't meet these guidelines, or if you take very large amounts of some vitamins as supplements, you may be in for trouble.

Vitamin deficiencies

The good news is that vitamin deficiencies are rare among people who have access to a wide variety of foods and know how to put together a balanced diet. For example, the only people likely to experience a vitamin E deficiency are premature and/or low-birth-weight infants and people with a metabolic disorder that keeps them from absorbing fat. A healthy adult may go as long as ten years on a vitamin E-deficient diet without developing any signs of a problem.

Aha, you say, but what's this subclinical deficiency I hear so much about?

Nutritionists use the term *subclinical deficiency* to describe a nutritional deficit not yet far enough advanced to produce obvious symptoms. In lay terms, however, the phrase has become a handy explanation for common but hard-to-pin-down symptoms, such as fatigue, irritability, nervousness, emotional depression, allergies, and insomnia. And it's a dandy way to increase the sale of nutritional supplements.

Simply put, the RDAs protect you against deficiency. If your symptoms linger even after you take reasonable amounts of vitamin supplements, something other than a lack of any one vitamin may be to blame. Don't wait until your patience or your bank account has been exhausted to find out. Check with your doctor. While you're waiting for an appointment, Table 11-2 lists the symptoms of various vitamin deficiencies.

Table 11-2	Vitamin Alert: What Happens When You Don't Get the Vitamins You Need
A Diet Low in This Vitamin	*May Produce These Signs of Deficiency*
Vitamin A	Poor night vision; dry, rough, or cracked skin; dry mucous membranes including the inside of the eye; slow wound healing; nerve damage; reduced ability to taste, hear, and smell; inability to perspire; reduced resistance to respiratory infections
Vitamin D	In children: rickets (weak muscles, delayed tooth development, and soft bones, all caused by the inability to absorb minerals without vitamin D) In adults: osteomalacia (soft, porous bones that fracture easily); fatigue
Vitamin E	Inability to absorb fat
Vitamin K	Blood fails to clot
Vitamin C	Scurvy (bleeding gums; tooth loss; nosebleeds; bruising; painful or swollen joints; shortness of breath; increased susceptibility to infection; slow wound healing; muscle pains; skin rashes)
Thiamin (vitamin B1)	Poor appetite; unintended weight loss; upset stomach; gastric upset (nausea, vomiting); mental depression; an inability to concentrate; fatigue
Riboflavin (vitamin B2)	Inflamed mucous membranes, including cracked lips, sore tongue and mouth, burning eyes; skin rashes; anemia; fatigue

A Diet Low in This Vitamin	May Produce These Signs of Deficiency
Niacin	Pellagra (diarrhea; inflamed skin and mucous membranes; mental confusion and/or dementia); fatigue
A Diet Low in This Vitamin	**May Produce These Signs of Deficiency**
Vitamin B6	Anemia; convulsions similar to epileptic seizures; skin rashes; upset stomach; nerve damage (in infants); fatigue
Folate	Anemia (immature red blood cells); fatigue
Vitamin B12	Pernicious anemia (destruction of red blood cells, nerve damage, increased risk of stomach cancer attributed to damaged stomach tissue, neurological/psychiatric symptoms attributed to nerve cell damage); fatigue
Biotin	Loss of appetite; upset stomach; pale, dry, scaly skin; hair loss; emotional depression; skin rashes (in infants younger than 6 months)

Big trouble: Vitamin megadoses

Can you get too much of a good thing? Yes. In fact, some vitamins are toxic when taken in the very large amounts popularly known as *megadoses.* How much is a megadose? Nobody knows for sure. The general consensus is that a megadose is several times the RDA, but the term is so vague that it isn't even in the 28th edition of Stedman's Medical Dictionary (2006), a tome that's pretty much the gold standard in medical word books.

Nonetheless, it is clear that

- ✔ Megadoses of vitamin A (as retinol) may cause symptoms that make you think you have a brain tumor. Taken by a pregnant woman, megadoses of vitamin A may damage the fetus.

- ✔ Megadoses of vitamin D may cause kidney stones and hard lumps of calcium in soft tissue (muscles and organs), as well as nausea and other gastro discomfort.

- ✔ Megadoses of niacin (sometimes used to lower cholesterol levels) can damage liver tissue.

- ✔ Megadoses of vitamin B6 can cause (temporary) damage to nerves in arms and legs, fingers, and toes.

The interesting fact is that with one exception, the likeliest way to get a megadose of vitamins is to take supplements (see Chapter 6 for more on supplements) since it it's pretty much impossible for you to cram down enough food to overdose on vitamins D, E, K, C, and all the Bs.

The exception? Vitamin A. Liver and fish liver oils are concentrated sources of preformed vitamin A (retinol), the potentially toxic form of vitamin A. Liver contains so much retinol that early 20th century explorers to the South Pole made themselves sick on seal and whale liver. (See Table 11-3 for more on vitamin A toxicity, this time from supplements.) On the other hand, even very large doses of vitamin E, vitamin K, thiamin (vitamin B1), riboflavin (vitamin B2), folate, vitamin B12, biotin, and pantothenic acid appear safe for human beings. Table 11-3 lists the effects of vitamin overdoses.

Table 11-3	Amounts and Effects of Vitamin Overdoses for Healthy People
Vitamin	*Overdose and Possible Effect*
Vitamin A	15,000 to 25,000 IU retinol a day for adults (2,000 IU or more for children) may lead to liver damage, headache, vomiting, abnormal vision, constipation, hair loss, loss of appetite, low-grade fever, bone pain, sleep disorders, and dry skin and mucous membranes. A pregnant woman who takes more than 10,000 IU a day doubles her risk of giving birth to a child with birth defects.
Vitamin D	2,000 IU a day can cause irreversible damage to kidneys and heart. Smaller doses may cause muscle weakness, headache, nausea, vomiting, high blood pressure, retarded physical growth, mental retardation in children, and fetal abnormalities.
Vitamin E	Large amounts (more than 400 to 800 IU a day) may cause upset stomach or dizziness. Similarly, in 2005 a meta-analysis (a study comparing the results of several studies) in the *Annals of Internal Medicine* showed that use of "high dose" (400 IU or more) vitamin E supplements might "increase all causes of mortality [death] and should be avoided."
Vitamin C	1,000 mg or higher may cause upset stomach, diarrhea, or constipation.
Niacin	Doses higher than the RDA raise the production of liver enzymes and blood levels of sugar and uric acid, leading to liver damage and an increased risk of diabetes and gout.
Vitamin B6	Continued use of 50 mg or more a day may damage nerves in arms, legs, hands, and feet. Some experts say the damage is likely to be temporary; others say that it may be permanent.
Choline	Very high doses (14 to 37 times the adequate amount) have been linked to vomiting, salivation, sweating, low blood pressure, and — ugh! — fishy body odor.

Acceptable Exceptions: Taking Extra Vitamins as Needed

Who needs extra vitamins? Maybe you. The RDAs are designed to protect healthy people from deficiencies, but sometimes the circumstances of your life (or your lifestyle) mean that you need something extra. Are you taking medication? Do you smoke? Are you on a restricted diet? Are you pregnant? Are you a nursing mother? Are you approaching menopause? Answer yes to any of these questions, and you may be a person who needs larger amounts of vitamins than the RDAs provide.

I'm taking medication

Many valuable medicines interact with vitamins. Some drugs increase or decrease the effectiveness of vitamins; some vitamins increase or decrease the effectiveness of drugs. For example, a woman who's using birth control pills may absorb less than the customary amount of the B vitamins. For more about vitamin and drug interactions, see Chapter 25.

I'm a smoker

It's a fact — you probably have abnormally low blood levels of vitamin C. More trouble: Chemicals from tobacco smoke create more free radicals in your body. Even the National Research Council, which is tough on vitamin overdosing, says that regular smokers need to take about 66 percent more vitamin C — up to 100 mg a day — than nonsmokers.

I never eat animals

On the other hand, if you're nuts for veggies but follow a vegan diet — one that shuns all foods from animals (including milk, cheese, eggs, and fish oils) — you simply cannot get enough vitamin D without taking supplements. Vegans also benefit from extra vitamin C because it increases their ability to absorb iron from plant food. And vitamin B12–enriched grains or supplements are a must to supply the nutrient found only in fish, poultry, milk, cheese, and eggs.

I'm pregnant

Keep in mind that "eating for two" means that you're the sole source of nutrients for the growing fetus, not that you need to double the amount of food you eat. If you don't get the vitamins you need, neither will your baby.

The RDAs for many nutrients are the same as those for women who aren't pregnant. But when you're pregnant, you need extra

- **Vitamin D:** Every smidgen of vitamin D in a newborn's body comes from his or her mom. If the mother doesn't have enough D, neither will the baby. Are vitamin pills the answer? Yes. And no. The qualifier is how many pills, because although too little vitamin D can weaken a developing fetus, too much can cause birth defects. That's why until new recommendations for vitamin D are issued, the second important *d*-word is "doctor." As in, check with yours to see what's right for you.

- **Vitamin E:** To create all that new tissue (the woman's as well as the baby's), a pregnant woman needs an extra 2 a-TE each day, the approximate amount in one egg.

- **Vitamin C:** The level of vitamin C in your blood falls as your vitamin C flows across the placenta to your baby, who may — at some point in the pregnancy — have vitamin C levels as much as 50 percent higher than yours. So you need an extra 10 milligrams vitamin C each day (½ cup cooked zucchini or 2 stalks of asparagus).

- **Riboflavin (vitamin B2):** To protect the baby against structural defects such as cleft palate or a deformed heart, a pregnant woman needs an extra 0.3 milligrams riboflavin each day (slightly less than 1 ounce of ready-to-eat cereal).

- **Folate:** Folate protects the child against cleft palate and neural tube (spinal cord) defects such as *spina bifida*. As many as 2 of every 1,000 babies born each year in the United States have a neural tube defect such as spina bifida because their mothers didn't get enough folate to meet the RDA standard. Taking 400 micrograms folate daily before becoming pregnant and through the first two months of pregnancy significantly lowers the risk of giving birth to a child with cleft palate. Taking 400 micrograms folate each day through an entire pregnancy reduces the risk of neural tube defects.

- **Vitamin B12:** To meet the demands of the growing fetus, a pregnant woman needs an extra 0.2 micrograms vitamin B12 each day (just 3 ounces of roasted chicken).

I'm breast-feeding

You need extra vitamin A, vitamin E, thiamin, riboflavin, and folate to produce sufficient quantities of nutritious breast milk, about 25 ounces/750 ml each day. You need extra vitamin D, vitamin C, and niacin as insurance to replace the vitamins you lose — that is, the ones you transfer to your child in your milk.

I'm approaching menopause

Information about the specific vitamin requirements of older women is as hard to find as, well, information about the specific vitamin requirements about older men. It's enough to make you wonder what's going on with the people who set the RDAs. Don't they know that everyone gets older? Right now, just about all anybody can say for sure about the nutritional needs of older women is that they require extra calcium to stem the natural loss of bone that occurs when women reach menopause and their production of the female hormone estrogen declines. They may also need extra vitamin D to enable their bodies to absorb and use the calcium.

Gender Bias Alert! No similar studies are available for older men. But adding vitamin D supplements to calcium supplements increases bone density in older people.

The current RDA for vitamin D is set at 5 micrograms/200 IU for all adults, but the new AI (Adequate Intake) for vitamin D is 10 micrograms/400 IU for people ages 51 to 70 and 15 micrograms/600 IU or more for people 71 and older. Some researchers suggest that even these amounts may be too low to guarantee maximum calcium absorption. Check with your doctor before adding vitamin D supplements. In very large amounts, this vitamin can be toxic.

I have very light skin or very dark skin

Sunlight — yes, plain old sunlight — transforms fats just under the surface of your skin to vitamin D. So getting what you need should be a cinch, right? Not necessarily. Getting enough vitamin D from sunlight is hard to do when you have very light skin and avoid the sun for fear of skin cancer. Even more difficult is getting enough vitamin D when you have very dark skin, which acts as a kind of natural sun block.

Chapter 12

Mighty Minerals

Minerals are *elements,* substances composed of only one kind of atom. They're inorganic. (Translation: They don't contain the carbon, hydrogen, and oxygen atoms found in all organic compounds, including vitamins.) And they occur naturally in nonliving things, such as rocks and metal ores. Although minerals also are present in plants and animals, they're imported: Plants absorb minerals from the soil; animals obtain minerals by eating plants.

Most minerals have names that describe where they're found or what they look like. For example, the name calcium comes from *calx,* the Greek word for "lime" (chalk), a source of calcium. The name chlorine comes from *chloros,* the Greek word for "greenish-yellow," which just happens to be the color of the mineral. Other minerals, such as americium, curium, berkelium, californium, fermium, and nobelium, are named for where they were first identified or to honor an important scientist.

This chapter tells you which minerals your body requires, which foods provide what minerals, and how much of each mineral a healthy person needs.

The Minerals You Need

Think of your body as a house. Vitamins (see Chapter 11) are like tiny little maids and butlers, scurrying about to turn on the lights and make sure that the windows are closed to keep the heat from escaping. Minerals are more sturdy stuff, the mortar and bricks that strengthen the frame of the house and the current that keeps the lights running.

An elementary guide to minerals

The early Greeks thought that all material on Earth was constructed of a combination of four basic elements: earth, water, air, and fire. Centuries later, alchemists looking for the formula for precious metals, such as gold, decided that the essential elements were sulfur, salt, and mercury. Wrong again.

In 1669, a group of German chemists isolated phosphorus, the first mineral element to be accurately identified. After that, things moved a bit more swiftly. By the end of the 19th century, scientists knew the names and chemical properties of 82 elements. Today, 112 elements have been identified.

The classic guide to chemical elements is the periodic table, a chart devised in 1869 by Russian chemist Dimitri Mendeleev (1834–1907), for whom mendelevium was named. The table was revised by British physicist Henry Moseley (1887–1915), who came up with the concept of *atomic numbers,* numbers based on the number of *protons* (positively charged particles) in an elemental atom.

The periodic table is a clean, crisp way of characterizing the elements, and if you are now or ever were a chemistry, physics, or premed student, you can testify firsthand to the joy (maybe that's not the best word?) of memorizing the information it provides. Personally, I'd rather be forced to watch reruns of *The Dating Game.*

Nutritionists classify the minerals essential for human life as either *major minerals* (including the principal electrolytes — see Chapter 13) or *trace elements.* Nutritionally speaking, the difference between the two is the amount of the mineral you store in your body and how much you need to take in to maintain a steady supply.

Your body stores more than 5 grams (about ⅙ of an ounce) of each of the major minerals and principal electrolytes. To replace what you lose and maintain a healthy level, you need to consume more than 100 milligrams (3.5 ounces) a day of each major mineral. The quantities for trace elements are smaller. You store less than 5 grams of each trace element and need to take in less than 100 milligrams a day to stay even.

The major minerals

The following major minerals are essential for human beings:

- ✔ Calcium
- ✔ Phosphorus
- ✔ Magnesium

  ✔ Sulfur

  ✔ Sodium

  ✔ Potassium

  ✔ Chloride

Note: Sodium, potassium, and chloride, also known as the principal electrolytes, are covered in Chapter 13.

Although sulfur, a major mineral, is an essential nutrient for human beings, it's almost never included in nutritional books and/or charts. Why? Because it's an integral part of all proteins. Any diet that provides adequate protein also provides adequate sulfur. (For more on proteins, check out Chapter 7.)

Calcium

When you step on the scale in the morning, you can assume that about 3 pounds of your body weight is calcium, most of it packed into your bones and teeth.

Calcium is also present in extracellular fluid (the liquid around body cells), where it performs the following duties:

  ✔ Regulating fluid balance by controlling the flow of water in and out of cells

  ✔ Enabling cells to send messages back and forth from one to another

  ✔ Keeping muscles moving smoothly and preventing cramping

An adequate amount of calcium is important for controlling high blood pressure — and not only for the person who takes the calcium directly. At least one study shows that when a pregnant woman gets a sufficient amount of calcium, her baby's blood pressure stays lower than average for at least the first seven years of life, meaning a lower risk of developing high blood pressure later on.

Your best food sources of calcium are milk and dairy products, as well as fish, such as canned sardines and salmon, which come with bones that have been softened and made edible by processing. (*Caution:* Bones in fresh fish are *not* edible and should not be eaten.) Calcium also is found in dark green leafy vegetables, but the calcium in plant foods is bound into compounds that are less easily absorbed by your body.

Calcium: The bone team player

Like all body tissues, bones are constantly being replenished. Old bone cells break down, and new ones are born. Specialized cells called *osteoclasts* start the process by boring tiny holes into solid bone so that other specialized cells, called *osteoblasts,* can refill the open spaces with fresh bone. At that point, crystals of calcium, the best-known dietary bone builder, hook onto the network of new bone cells to harden and strengthen the bone.

Calcium begins its work on your bones while you're still in your mother's womb. But it's not the only mineral at play. Think iron and zinc. Based on a survey of 242 pregnant women in Peru, where zinc deficiency is common, Johns Hopkins researchers found the babies born to women who got prenatal supplements with iron, folic acid, and zinc had longer, stronger leg bones than did babies born to women who got the same supplement minus the zinc.

Once you're born, calcium continues to build your bones, but only with the help of vitamin D, which produces a calcium-binding protein that enables you to absorb the calcium in milk. To make sure you get your D, virtually all milk sold in the United States is fortified with the vitamin. And because you may outgrow your taste for milk but never outgrow your need for calcium, calcium supplements for adults frequently include vitamin D. (Your body also makes vitamin D when you're exposed to sunlight.)

But vitamin D isn't milk's only contribution. Milk also contains *lactoferrin* (*lacto* = milk; *ferri* = iron), an iron-binding compound that stimulates the production of the cells that promote bone growth.

Finally, note that the word *bones* begins with *b* — as in vitamin B12. The female sex hormone estrogen preserves bone; the male sex hormone testosterone builds new bone. As people age and their supply of sex hormones diminishes, they lose bone faster than they can replace it. One complicating factor may be low levels of vitamin B12. A report in the *Journal of Clinical Endocrinology and Metabolism* says that researchers at the University of California, San Francisco, found that women with lower levels of this vitamin also have less dense hip bones.

To summarize: To protect your bones, you need calcium, zinc, iron, and vitamins D and B12, all found most abundantly in milk, cheese, eggs, and red meat. Which sounds like a cardiologist's nutritional high-fat, high-cholesterol nightmare — except that you certainly will edit the menu to read: skim milk, lowfat cheese, egg whites, and lean beef.

Phosphorus

Like calcium, phosphorus is essential for strong bones and teeth. For tiptop performance, you need about half as much phosphorus as calcium. Phosphorus also enables a cell to transmit the *genetic code* (genes and chromosomes that carry information about your special characteristics) to the new cells created when a cell divides and reproduces. In addition, phosphorus

✔ Helps maintain the pH balance of blood (that is, keeps it from being too acidic or too alkaline)

✔ Is vital for metabolizing carbohydrates, synthesizing proteins, and ferrying fats and fatty acids among tissues and organs

✔ Is part of *myelin,* the fatty sheath that surrounds and protects each nerve cell

Phosphorus is in almost everything you eat, but the best sources are high-protein foods, such as meat, fish, poultry, eggs, and milk. These foods provide more than half the phosphorus in a nonvegetarian diet; grains, nuts, seeds, and dry beans also provide respectable amounts.

Magnesium

Your body uses magnesium to make body tissues, especially bone. The adult human body has about an ounce of magnesium, and three-quarters of it is in the bones. Magnesium also is part of more than 300 different enzymes that trigger chemical reactions throughout your body. You use magnesium to

✔ Move nutrients in and out of cells

✔ Send messages between cells

✔ Transmit the genetic code (genes and chromosomes) when cells divide and reproduce

An adequate supply of magnesium also is heart-healthy because it enables you to convert food to energy using less oxygen.

Plant foods such as bananas, dark green fruits and vegetables (magnesium is part of chlorophyll, the green pigment in plants), whole seeds, nuts, beans, and grains are excellent sources of magnesium.

The trace elements

Trace elements also are minerals, but they're present in much, much smaller amounts. That's why they are called *trace* elements. The list includes

✔ Iron

✔ Zinc

✔ Iodine

✔ Selenium

✔ Copper

✔ Manganese

✔ Fluoride

✔ Chromium

✔ Molybdenum

Iron

Iron is an essential constituent of *hemoglobin* and *myoglobin,* two proteins that store and transport oxygen. You find hemoglobin in red blood cells (it's what makes them red). Myoglobin (*myo* = muscle) is in muscle tissue. Iron also is part of various enzymes.

The best food sources of iron are organ meats (liver, heart, kidneys), red meat, egg yolks, wheat germ, and oysters. These foods contain *heme* (heme = blood) iron, a form of iron that your body can easily absorb.

Whole grains, wheat germ, raisins, nuts, seed, prunes and prune juice, and potato skins contain nonheme iron. Because plants contain substances called *phytates,* which bind this iron into compounds, your body has a hard time getting at the iron. Eating plant foods with meat or with foods that are rich in vitamin C (like tomatoes) increases your ability to split away the phytates and get iron out of plant foods.

Zinc

Zinc protects nerve and brain tissue, bolsters the immune system, and is essential for healthy growth. Zinc is part of the enzymes (and hormones such as insulin) that metabolize food, and you can fairly call it the macho male mineral.

The largest quantities of zinc in the male human body are in the testes, where it's used in making a continuous supply of *testosterone,* the hormone a man needs to produce plentiful amounts of healthy, viable sperm. Without enough zinc, male fertility falters. So, yes, the old wives' tale is true: Oysters — a rich source of zinc — are useful for men (yes, women also need zinc).

In addition to oysters, good sources of zinc are meat, liver, and eggs. Zinc is also plentiful in nuts, beans, miso, pumpkin and sunflower seeds, whole-grain products, and wheat germ. But the zinc in plants, like the iron in plants, occurs in compounds that your body absorbs less efficiently than the zinc in foods from animals.

Iodine

Iodine is a component of the thyroid hormones thyroxine and triiodothyronine, which help regulate cell activities. These hormones are also essential for protein synthesis, tissue growth (including the formation of healthy nerves and bones), and reproduction.

The best natural sources of iodine are seafood and plants grown near or in the ocean, but modern Americans are most likely to get the iodine they need from iodized salt (plain table salt with iodine added).

And here's an odd nutritional note: You may get substantial amounts of iodine from milk because the milk is processed and stored in machines and vessels kept clean and sanitary with iodine-based disinfectants that send tiny trace amounts of iodine into the milk. Iodine compounds are also used as dough conditioners (additives that make dough more pliable), so you're also likely to find some iodine in most commercial breads.

Selenium

Selenium was identified as an essential human nutrient in 1979 when Chinese nutrition researchers discovered that people with low body stores of selenium were at increased risk of *Keshan disease,* a disorder of the heart muscle with symptoms that include rapid heartbeat, enlarged heart, and (in severe cases) heart failure, a consequence most common among young children and women of childbearing age.

Although fruits and vegetables grown in selenium-rich soils are themselves rich in this mineral, the best sources of selenium are seafood, meat and organ meats (liver, kidney), eggs, and dairy products.

Copper

Copper is an antioxidant found in enzymes that deactivate free radicals (pieces of molecules that can link up to form compounds that damage body tissues) and make it possible for your body to use iron. Copper also may play a role in slowing the aging process by decreasing the incidence of *protein glycation,* a reaction in which sugar molecules (*gly* = sugar) hook up with protein molecules in your bloodstream, twist the protein molecules out of shape, and make them unusable. Protein glycation may result in bone loss, high cholesterol, cardiac abnormalities, and a slew of other unpleasantries. In people with diabetes, excess protein glycation may also be one factor involved in complications such as loss of vision.

In addition, copper

- Promotes the growth of strong bones
- Protects the health of nerve tissue
- Prevents your hair from turning gray prematurely. But, no, no, a thousand times, no: Large amounts of copper absolutely will not turn gray hair back to its original color. Worse yet, megadoses of copper are potentially toxic.

You can get the copper you need from organ meats (such as liver and heart), seafood, nuts, and dried beans, including cacao beans (the beans used to make chocolate).

Manganese

Most of the manganese in your body is in your glands (pituitary, mammary, pancreas), organs (liver, kidneys, intestines), and bones. Manganese is an essential constituent of the enzymes that metabolize carbohydrates and synthesize fats (including cholesterol). Manganese is important for a healthy reproductive system. During pregnancy, manganese speeds the proper growth of fetal tissue, particularly bones and cartilage.

You get manganese from whole grains, cereal products, fruits, and vegetables. Tea is also a good source of manganese.

Fluoride

Fluoride is the form of fluorine (an element) in drinking water. Your body stores fluoride in bones and teeth. Although researchers still have some questions about whether fluoride is an essential nutrient, it's clear that it hardens dental enamel, reducing your risk of getting cavities. In addition, some nutrition researchers suspect (but cannot prove) that some forms of fluoride strengthen bones.

All soil, ground water, plants and animal tissue contain small amounts of fluoride, but the most steady supply of fluoride comes from fluoridated drinking water (see Chapter 13).

Chromium

Very small amounts of *trivalent chromium,* a digestible form of the very same metallic element that decorates your car and household appliances, are essential for several enzymes that you need to metabolize fat.

Chromium also partners with glucose tolerance factor (GTF), a group of chemicals that enables insulin (an enzyme from the pancreas) to regulate your use of glucose, the end product of metabolism and the basic fuel for every body cell (see Chapter 3). In a recent joint study by USDA and the Beijing Medical University, adults with non-insulin-dependent diabetes who took chromium supplements had lower blood levels of sugar, protein, and cholesterol, which are all good signs for people with diabetes. In a related study, chromium reduced blood pressure in laboratory rats bred to develop hypertension (high blood pressure), a common complication in diabetes.

Right now, little information exists about the precise amounts of chromium in specific foods. Nonetheless, yeast, calves' liver, American cheese, wheat germ, and broccoli are regarded as valuable sources of this trace element.

Molybdenum

Molybdenum (pronounced mo-*lib*-de-num) is part of several enzymes that metabolize proteins. You get molybdenum from beans and grains. Cows eat grains, so milk and cheese have some molybdenum. Molybdenum also leeches into drinking water from surrounding soil. The molybdenum content of plants and drinking water depends entirely on how much molybdenum is in the soil.

Getting the Minerals You Need

Table 12-1 is a handy guide to foods that provide the minerals and trace elements your body needs. This chart is the easy way to figure out which foods (and how much) provide at least 25 percent of the recommended dietary allowance (RDA) for healthy adults ages 25 to 50.

No muss, no fuss, no calculators. Just photocopy these pages and stick them on the fridge. What an easy way to eat right! Wait! One more important note: When you see "men" or "women" in the following chart, it means "men and women ages 25 to 50" — unless otherwise noted.

Table 12-1 Get Your Minerals Here! — Foods and Serving Sizes	
Food	*Serving*
CALCIUM and PHOSPHORUS	**RDA: Calcium — men and women 1,000 mg** **RDA: Phosphorus — men and women 700 mg**
Breads, cereals, grains	
Bran muffin, English muffin	2 whole
Vegetables	
Broccoli, spinach, turnip greens (cooked)	1 cup
Dairy products	
Natural Gruyère, Romano, Swiss, Parmesan cheeses	1 ounce
Processed cheddar or Swiss cheeses	1½ ounces
Natural blue, brick, Camembert, feta, Gouda, Monterey, mozzarella, Muenster, provolone, Roquefort cheeses	2 ounces
Ricotta cheese	½ cup
Ice cream/ice milk	1 cup
Milk — all varieties, including chocolate	1 cup
Yogurt — all varieties	1 cup (8 ounces)

(continued)

Table 12-1 *(continued)*

Food	Serving
Other	
Tofu	½ cup, cubed
MAGNESIUM	**RDA: Men 400–420 mg,* women 310–320 mg***
Breads, cereals, grains	
Bread — whole wheat	4 slices
Bran muffin, English muffin, pita — whole wheat	2 whole
Cold cereal	2 ounces
Vegetables	
Artichoke	2 medium
Black-eyed peas, chickpeas, soybeans, white beans (dry, cooked)	1 cup
Dairy products	
Milk — chocolate, made with skim milk	2 cups
Yogurt — plain nonfat	2 cups
Other	
Nuts and seeds	2 tbsp.
Tofu	½ cup cubed
IRON	**RDA: Men 8 mg, women 18 mg, 8 mg***
Breads, cereals, grains	
Bagel, bran muffin, pita	2 whole
Farina, oatmeal — instant, fortified	⅓ cup
Cold cereal	1 ounce
Fruits	
Apricots (dried, cooked)	1 cup
Vegetables	
Black-eyed peas, chickpeas, lentils, red and white beans (dried, cooked)	1 cup
Soybeans (cooked)	½ cup
Meat, poultry, fish	
Clams (raw) — meat only	3–4 ounces
Oysters (raw) — meat only	1–2 ounces
Other	

Food	Serving
Pine nuts, seeds — pumpkin or squash	4 tbsp.
ZINC	**RDA: Men 11 mg, women 8 mg**
Breads, cereals, grains	
Cold cereals — fortified	2 ounces
Meat, poultry, fish	
Beef — all varieties, lean	3 ounces
Lamb — all varieties, lean	3 ounces
Tongue (braised)	3 ounces
Veal — roast, lean only	3 ounces
Chicken (no skin)	2 legs
Oysters	3 ounces
Dairy products	
Yogurt — all varieties	2 cups
Other	
Seeds — pumpkin or squash	4 tbsp.
COPPER	**AI: Men and women 900 mg**
Breads, cereals, grains	
Barley (cooked)	⅓ cup
Bran muffin, English muffin, pita	2 whole
Fruits	
Prunes (dried, cooked)	1 cup
Vegetables	
Black-eyed peas, lentils, soybeans (cooked)	1 cup
Meat, poultry, fish	
Liver — beef, calf	3 ounces
Liver — chicken, turkey	½ cup, diced
Crabmeat, lobster, oysters, shrimp	3 ounces
Other	
Almonds, Brazil nuts, cashews, hazelnuts/filberts, peanuts, pistachios, walnuts, mixed nuts	4 tbsp.
Seeds — pumpkin, sesame, squash, sunflower	4 tbsp.

*The lower numbers are for people age 19–30; the higher numbers, for people age 31+.
Good Sources of Nutrients (Washington, D.C.: U.S. Department of Agriculture/Human Nutrition Service, 1990); Nutritive Value of Food (Washington, D.C.: USDA, 1991); DRI reports 1998–2004.*

Did you notice something missing from this list? Right: There are no entries for the essential trace elements chromium, fluoride, iodine, molybdenum, and selenium, because a healthful, varied diet provides sufficient quantities of these nutrients. Iodized salt and fluoridated water are extra insurance.

Too Much and Too Little

The Recommended Dietary Allowances (RDAs) and Adequate Intakes (AIs) for minerals and trace elements are generous allowances, large enough to prevent deficiency but not so large that they trigger toxic side effects. (Read more about RDAs and AIs in Chapter 5.)

Avoiding mineral deficiency

What happens if you don't get enough minerals and trace elements? Some minerals, such as phosphorus and magnesium, are so widely available in food that deficiencies are rare to nonexistent. No nutrition scientist has yet been able to identify a naturally occurring deficiency of sulfur, manganese, chromium, or molybdenum in human beings who follow a sensible diet. Most drinking water contains adequate fluoride, and Americans get so much copper (can it be from chocolate bars?) that deficiency is practically unheard of in the United States.

But other minerals are more problematic:

✔ **Calcium:** Without enough calcium, a child's bones and teeth don't grow strong and straight, and an adult's bones lose minerals and weaken. Calcium is a team player. To protect against deficiency, you also need adequate amounts of vitamin D, the nutrient that allows you to absorb the calcium you get from food or supplements. Milk fortified with vitamin D has done much to eliminate rickets (see Chapter 11 on vitamins).

✔ **Iron:** *Iron deficiency anemia* is not just an old advertising slogan. Lacking sufficient iron, your body can't make the hemoglobin it requires to carry energy-sustaining oxygen to every tissue. As a result, you're often tired and feel weak. Mild iron deficiency may also inhibit intellectual performance. In one Johns Hopkins study, high school girls scored higher verbal, memory, and learning test scores when they took supplements providing Recommended Dietary Amounts of iron.

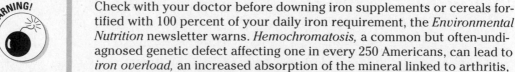

Check with your doctor before downing iron supplements or cereals fortified with 100 percent of your daily iron requirement, the *Environmental Nutrition* newsletter warns. *Hemochromatosis,* a common but often-undiagnosed genetic defect affecting one in every 250 Americans, can lead to *iron overload,* an increased absorption of the mineral linked to arthritis, heart disease, and diabetes, as well as an increased risk of infectious diseases and cancer (viruses and cancer cells thrive in iron-rich blood).

✔ **Zinc:** An adequate supply of zinc is vital for making testosterone and healthy sperm. Men who don't get enough zinc may be temporarily infertile. Zinc deficiency leads to loss of appetite and the ability to taste food. It may also weaken your immune system, increasing your risk of infections. Wounds heal more slowly when you don't get enough zinc. That includes the tissue damage caused by working out. In plain language: If you don't get the zinc you need, your charley horse may linger longer. And, yes, several studies have confirmed that sucking on lozenges containing one form of zinc (zinc gluconate) shortens a cold — by a day or two. Other studies show no effect. Your choice.

✔ **Iodine:** A moderate iodine deficiency leads to *goiter* (a swollen thyroid gland) and reduced production of thyroid hormones. A more severe deficiency early in life may cause a form of mental and physical retardation called *cretinism*.

✔ **Selenium:** Not enough selenium in your diet? Watch out for muscle pain or weakness. To protect against selenium problems, make sure that you get plenty of vitamin E. Some animal studies show that a selenium deficiency responds to vitamin E supplements. And vice versa.

The risks of overdoses

Like any medications, some vitamins and minerals are potentially toxic in large doses. For example:

✔ **Calcium:** Though clearly beneficial in amounts higher than the current RDAs, calcium is not problem-free:

- Constipation, bloating, nausea, and intestinal gas are common side effects among healthy people taking supplements equal to 1,500 to 4,000 milligrams of calcium a day.

- Doses higher than 4,000 milligrams a day may be linked to kidney damage.

- Megadoses of calcium can bind with iron and zinc, making it harder for your body to absorb these two essential trace elements.

✔ **Phosphorus:** Too much phosphorus can lower your body stores of calcium.

✔ **Magnesium:** Megadoses of magnesium appear safe for healthy people, but if you have kidney disease, the magnesium overload can cause weak muscles, breathing difficulty, irregular heartbeat, and/or cardiac arrest (your heart stops beating).

- **Iron:** Overdosing on iron supplements can be deadly, especially for young children. The lethal dose for a young child may be as low as 3 grams (3,000 milligrams) elemental iron at one time. This is the amount in 60 tablets with 50 milligrams elemental iron each. For adults, the lethal dose is estimated to be 200 to 250 milligrams elemental iron per kilogram (2.2 pounds) of body weight. That's about 13,600 milligrams (13.6 g) for a 150-pound person — the amount you'd get in 292 tablets with 50 milligrams elemental iron each. New FDA rules require individual blister packaging for supplements containing more than 30 milligrams iron to foil tiny fingers and prevent accidental overdoses.

- **Zinc:** Moderately high doses of zinc (up to 25 milligrams a day) may slow your body's absorption of copper. Doses 27 to 37 times the RDA (11 mg/males; 8 mg/females) may interfere with your immune function and make you more susceptible to infection, the very thing that normal doses of zinc protect against. Gram doses (2,000 milligrams/2 grams) of zinc cause symptoms of zinc poisoning: vomiting, gastric upset, and irritation of the stomach lining.

- **Iodine:** Overdoses of iodine cause exactly the same problems as iodine deficiency: goiter. How can that be? When you consume very large amounts of iodine, the mineral stimulates your thyroid gland, which swells in a furious attempt to step up its production of thyroid hormones. This reaction may occur among people who eat lots of dried seaweed for long periods of time.

- **Selenium:** Doses as high as 5 milligrams of selenium a day (90 times the RDA) have been linked to thickened but fragile nails, hair loss, and perspiration with a garlicky odor. Extreme megadoses — 27.3 milligrams selenium/436 times the RDA from mislabeled supplements — have been linked to *selenium intoxication* (fatigue, abdominal pain, nausea and diarrhea, and nerve damage). The longer they used the supplements, the worse their symptoms were.

- **Fluoride:** Despite decades of argument, no scientific proof exists that the fluorides in drinking water increase the risk of cancer in human beings. But there's no question that large doses of fluoride — for example from heavily fluoridated well or groundwater in the western United States — leads to *fluorosis* (brown patches on your teeth), brittle bones, fatigue, and muscle weakness. Over long periods of time, high doses of fluoride may also cause *outcroppings* (little bumps) of bone on the spine.

  Fluoride levels higher than 6 milligrams a day are considered hazardous; never take fluoride supplements except as directed by your doctor or dentist.

- **Molybdenum:** Doses of molybdenum two to seven times the Adequate Intake (AI) (45 micrograms) may increase the amount of copper you excrete in urine.

Caution: Interaction ahead

Some minerals interact with other minerals or with medical drugs. For example, calcium binds tetracycline antibiotics into compounds your body can't break apart so that the antibiotic moves out of your digestive tract, unabsorbed and unused. That's why your doctor warns you off milk and dairy products when you're taking this medicine. For more about interactions between minerals and medicines, turn to Chapter 25.

When You May Need More than the RDA

If your diet provides enough minerals to meet the RDAs, you're in pretty good shape most of the time. But a restrictive diet, the circumstances of your reproductive life, and just plain getting older can increase your need for minerals. Here are some scenarios.

You're a strict vegetarian

Vegetarians who pass up fish, meat, and poultry must get their iron either from fortified grain products such as breakfast cereals or commercial breads or naturally from foods such as seeds, nuts, blackstrap molasses, raisins, prune juice, potato skins, green leafy vegetables, tofu, miso, or brewer's yeast. Because iron in plant foods is bound into compounds that are difficult for the human body to absorb, iron supplements are pretty much standard fare.

Vegans — vegetarians who avoid all foods from animals, including dairy products — have a similar problem getting the calcium they need. Calcium is in vegetables, but it, like iron, is bound into hard-to-absorb compounds. So vegans need calcium-rich substitutes. Good food choices are soybean milk fortified with calcium, orange juice with added calcium, and tofu processed with calcium sulfate.

You live inland, away from the ocean

Now here's a story of 20th-century nutritional success. Seafood and plants grown near or in the ocean are exposed to iodine-rich seawater. Freshwater fish, plants grown far from the sea, and the animals that feed on these fish and plants are not exposed to iodine. So people who live inland and get all their food from local gardens and farms cannot get the iodine they need from food.

I'm looking for an iron supplement. What's this "ferrous" stuff?

The iron in iron supplements comes in several different forms, each one composed of elemental iron (the kind of iron your body actually uses) coupled with an organic acid that makes the iron easy to absorb.

The iron compounds commonly found in iron supplements are

- Ferrous citrate (iron plus citric acid)
- Ferrous fumarate (iron plus fumaric acid)
- Ferrous gluconate (iron plus a sugar derivative)
- Ferrous lactate (iron plus lactic acid, an acid formed in the fermentation of milk)
- Ferrous succinate (iron plus succinic acid)
- Ferrous sulfate (iron plus a sulfuric acid derivative)

In your stomach, these compounds dissolve at different rates, yielding different amounts of elemental iron. So supplement labels list the compound and the amount of elemental iron it provides, like this:

Ferrous gluconate 300 milligrams

Elemental iron 34 milligrams

This tells you that the supplement has 300 milligrams of the iron compound ferrous gluconate, which gives you 34 milligrams of usable elemental iron. If the label just says "iron," that's shorthand for elemental iron. The elemental iron number is what you look for in judging the iron content of a vitamin/mineral supplement.

American savvy and technology rode to the rescue in 1924 with the introduction of iodized salt. Then came refrigerated railroad cars and trucks to carry food from both coasts to every inland city and state. Together, modern salt and efficient shipment virtually eliminated goiter, the iodine deficiency disease, in this country. Nonetheless, millions of people worldwide still suffer from chronic iodine deficiency.

You're a man

Just as women lose iron during menstrual bleeding, men lose zinc at ejaculation. Men who are extremely active sexually may need extra zinc. The trouble is, no one has ever written down standards for what constitutes "extremely active." Check this one out with your doctor.

You're a woman

The average woman loses about 2 to 3 teaspoons of blood during each menstrual period, a loss of 1.4 milligrams of iron. Women whose periods are very heavy lose more blood and more iron. Because getting the iron you need from a diet providing fewer than 2,000 calories a day may be virtually impossible, you may develop a mild iron deficiency. To remedy this, some doctors prescribe a daily iron supplement.

Women who use an intrauterine device (IUD) may also be given a prescription for iron supplements because IUDs irritate the lining of the uterus and cause a small but significant loss of blood and iron.

You're pregnant

The news about pregnancy is that women may not need extra calcium. This finding, released late in 1998, is so surprising that it probably pays to stay tuned for more — and definitely check with your own doctor. Meanwhile, pregnant women still need supplements to build not only fetal tissues but also new tissues and blood vessels in their own bodies. Animal studies suggest (but don't prove) that you may also need extra copper to protect nerve cells in the fetal brain. Nutritional supplements for pregnant women are specifically formulated to provide the extra nutrients they need.

You're breast-feeding

Nursing mothers need extra calcium, phosphorus, magnesium, iron, zinc, and selenium to protect their own bodies while producing nutritious breast milk. The same supplements that provide extra nutrients for pregnant women will meet a nursing mother's needs.

Wow — You think that was a hot flash?

Then you need extra calcium. Both men and women produce the sex hormones testosterone and estrogen, although men make proportionately more testosterone, and women, more estrogen. Testosterone builds bone; estrogen preserves it.

At menopause, a woman's production of estrogen drops precipitously, and her bones rapidly become less dense. As men age and their testosterone levels drop, they're also at risk of losing bone tissue, but the loss is less rapid and dramatic than a woman's.

Nutritionists once thought it impossible to reduce the age-related loss of bone density, believing that body ceased to absorb calcium after the mid-20s. Today, that is no longer the case. Regardless of gender, an increased consumption of calcium plus vitamin D appears to help. Not only does vitamin D increase the body's absorption of calcium and protect bones. It may also protect the heart: In 2010, a team of researchers at the University of Auckland (New Zealand) announced that taking calcium supplements alone, without vitamin D, might increase the risk of heart attack.

Chapter 13

Water Works

In This Chapter

▶ Understanding why you need water

▶ Discovering how much water you need

▶ Explaining the nature and functions of electrolytes

▶ Heeding the signs that you need more water

The human body is mostly (50 to 70 percent) water. Exactly how much water your own human body contains depends on how much muscle and fat you have. Muscle tissue has more water than fat tissue, so, because the average male body has proportionately more muscle than the average female body, it also has more water. For the same reason — more muscle — a young body has more water than an older one.

You definitely won't enjoy the experience, but if you have to, you can live without food for weeks at a time, obtaining subsistence levels of nutrients by digesting your own muscle and fat. But water's different. Without it, you'll die in a matter of days — more quickly in a place warm enough to make you perspire and lose water more quickly.

This chapter explains why water is so important and offers some pointers on how to keep your body's water level *level*.

Investigating the Many Ways Your Body Uses Water

Water is a solvent. It dissolves other substances and carries nutrients and other material (such as blood cells) around the body, making it possible for every organ to do its job. You need water to

✔ Digest food, dissolving nutrients so that they can pass through the intestinal cell walls into your bloodstream, and move food along through your intestinal tract

✔ Carry waste products out of your body

✔ Provide a medium in which biochemical reactions, such as metabolism (digesting food, producing energy, and building tissue), occur

✔ Send electrical messages between cells so that your muscles can move, your eyes can see, your brain can think, and so on

✔ Regulate body temperature — cooling your body with moisture (perspiration) that evaporates on your skin

✔ Lubricate your moving parts

Maintaining the Right Amount of Water in Your Body

As much as three-quarters of the water in your body is in *intracellular fluid,* the liquid inside body cells. The rest is in *extracellular fluid,* which is all the other body liquids, such as

✔ Interstitial fluid (the fluid between cells)

✔ Blood plasma (the clear liquid in blood)

✔ Lymph (a clear, slightly yellow fluid collected from body tissues that flows through your lymph nodes and eventually into your blood vessels)

✔ Bodily secretions such as sweat, seminal fluid, and vaginal fluids

✔ Urine

A healthy body must have just the right amount of fluid inside and outside each cell, a situation described as *fluid balance.* Maintaining your fluid balance is essential to life. If there is too little water inside a cell, the cell shrivels and dies. If there's too much water, the cell bursts.

The body maintains its fluid balance through the action of substances called *electrolytes,* mineral compounds that, when dissolved in water, become electrically charged particles called *ions.*

Many minerals, including calcium, phosphorus, and magnesium, form compounds that dissolve into charged particles. But nutritionists generally use the term electrolyte to describe sodium, potassium, and chlorine. The most familiar electrolyte is the one found on every dinner table: sodium chloride — plain old table salt. (In water, its molecules dissolve into two ions: one sodium ion and one chloride ion.)

Fluoridated water: The real Tooth Fairy

Except for the common cold, dental cavities are the most common human medical problem.

You get cavities from *mutans streptococci*, bacteria that live in dental plaque. The bacteria digest and ferment carbohydrate residue on your teeth (plain table sugar is the worst offender) leaving acid that eats away at the mineral surface of the tooth. This eating away is called *decay*. When the decay gets past the enamel to the softer pulp inside of the tooth, your tooth hurts. And you head for the dentist even though you hate it so much you'd almost rather put up with the pain. But almost doesn't count, so off you go.

Brushing and flossing help prevent cavities by cleaning your teeth so that bacteria have less to feast on. Another way to reduce your susceptibility to cavities is to drink *fluoridated water* — water containing the mineral fluorine.

Fluoride — the form of fluorine found in food and water — combines with other minerals in teeth and makes the minerals less soluble (harder to dissolve). You get the most benefit by drinking water containing 1 part fluoride to every 1 million parts water (1 ppm) from the day you're born until the day you get your last permanent tooth, usually around age 11 to 13.

Some drinking water, notably in the American Southwest, is fluoridated naturally when it flows through rocks containing fluorine. Sometimes so much fluoride is in this water that it causes a brownish spotting (or mottling) that occurs while teeth are developing and accumulating minerals. This effect doesn't occur with drinking water artificially supplemented with fluoride at the approved standard of one part fluoride to every million parts of water.

Because fluorides concentrate in bones, some people believe that drinking fluoridated water raises the risk of bone cancers, but no evidence to support this claim has ever been found in human beings. However, in 1990, a U.S. Public Health Service's National Toxicology Program (NTP) study of the long-term effects of high fluoride consumption on laboratory rats and mice added fuel to the fire: Four of the 1,044 laboratory rats and mice fed high doses of fluoride for two years developed *osteosarcoma,* a form of bone cancer.

The study sent an immediate *frisson* (shiver of fear) through the health community, but within a year, federal officials reviewing the study issued an opinion endorsing the safety and effectiveness of fluoridated water.

Here's why: First, the number of cancers among the laboratory animals was low enough to have occurred simply by chance. Second, the cancers occurred only in male rats; no cases were reported in female rats or mice of either sex. Finally, the amount of fluorides the animals ingested was 50 to 100 times higher than what you get in drinking water. To get as much fluoride as those rats did, human beings would have to drink more than 380 8-ounce glasses of fluoridated water a day.

Today, more than half the people living in the United States have access to adequately fluoridated public water supplies. The result is a lifelong 50 percent to 70 percent reduction in cavities among the residents of these communities.

The electrolytes' primary job

Under normal circumstances, the fluid inside your cells has more potassium than sodium and chloride. The fluid outside is just the opposite: more sodium and chloride than potassium. The cell wall is a *semipermeable membrane;*

some things pass through, but others don't. Water molecules and small mineral molecules flow through freely, unlike larger molecules such as proteins.

The process by which sodium flows out and potassium flows in to keep things on an even keel is called the *sodium pump.* If this process were to cease, sodium ions would build up inside your cells. Sodium attracts water; the more sodium there is inside the cell, the more water flows in. Eventually, the cell would burst and die. The sodium pump, regular as a clock, prevents this imbalance from happening so you can move along, blissfully unaware of those efficient, electric ions that tell the water in your body where to go. (See the sidebar "How does water know where to go?")

Other tasks electrolytes perform

In addition to maintaining fluid balance, sodium, potassium, and chloride (the form of chlorine found in food) ions create electrical impulses that enable cells to send messages back and forth between themselves so you can think, see, move, and perform all the bioelectrical functions that you take for granted.

Sodium, potassium, and chloride are also major minerals (see Chapter 12) and essential nutrients. Like other nutrients, they're useful in these bodily processes:

- Sodium helps digest proteins and carbohydrates and keeps your blood from becoming too acidic or too alkaline.

- Potassium is used in digestion to synthesize proteins and starch and is a major constituent of muscle tissue.

- Chloride is a constituent of hydrochloric acid, which breaks down food in your stomach. It's also used by white blood cells to make *hypochlorite,* a natural antiseptic.

Getting the Water You Need

Because the body doesn't store water, you need to take in a new supply every day, enough to replace what you lose when you breathe, perspire, urinate, and defecate. On average, this adds up to 1,500 to 3,000 milliliters (50 to 100 ounces; 6 to 12.5 cups) a day. Here's how:

- 850 to 1,200 milliliters (28 to 40 ounces) is lost in breath and perspiration.

- 600 to 1,600 milliliters (20 to 53 ounces) is lost in urine.

- 50 to 200 milliliters (1.6 to 6.6 ounces) is lost in feces.

How does water know where to go?

Osmosis is the principle that governs how water flows through a semipermeable membrane (one that lets only certain substances pass through) such as the one surrounding a body cell.

Here's the principle: Water flows through a semipermeable membrane from the side where the liquid solution is least dense to the side where it's denser. In other words, the water, acting as if it has a mind of its own, tries to equalize the densities of the liquids on both sides of the membrane.

How does the water know which side is more dense? Now that one's easy: Wherever the sodium content is higher. When more sodium is inside the cell, more water flows in to dilute it. When more sodium is in the fluid outside the cell, water flows out of the cell to dilute the liquid on the outside.

When The Ancient Mariner complained, "Water, water everywhere, and not a drop to drink," he wasn't kidding. He was talking about osmosis. Drink seawater, and liquid flows out of your cells to dilute the salty solution in your intestinal tract. The more seawater you drink, the more water you lose. In other words, when you drink seawater, you're literally drinking yourself into dehydration.

Of course, the same thing happens — though certainly to a lesser degree — when you eat salted pretzels or nuts. The salt in your mouth makes your saliva saltier, drawing liquid out of the cells in your cheeks and tongue, which feel uncomfortably dry. Solution: A glass of water!

Toss in some extra ounces for a safe margin, and you get the current recommendations that women age 19 and up consume about 11 cups of water a day and men age 19 and up, about 15.

Not all that water must come in a cup from the tap. About 15 percent of the water that you need is created when you digest and metabolize food. The end products of digestion and metabolism are carbon dioxide (a waste product that you breathe out of your body) and water composed of hydrogen from food and oxygen from the air that you breathe. The rest of your daily water comes directly from what you eat and drink. You can get water from, well, plain water. Eight 10-ounce glasses give you 2,400 milliliters, approximately enough to replace what your body loses every day, so everyone from athletes to couch potatoes knew that a healthy body needed eight full glasses of water a day.

Or at least they *thought* they knew. But then Dartmouth Medical School kidney specialist Heinz Valtin turned off the tap with one simple question: "Who says that all the water you need has to come from water?"

Valtin's report in the *American Journal of Physiology* (2003) notes that some of the water you require is right there in your food. Fruits and vegetables are full of water. Lettuce, for example, is 90 percent water. Furthermore, you get water from foods that you'd never think of as water sources: hamburger (more than 50 percent), cheese (the softer the cheese, the higher the water content — Swiss cheese is 38 percent water; skim milk ricotta, 74 percent), a plain, hard bagel (29 percent water), milk powder (2 percent), and even butter and margarine (10 percent). Only oils have no water.

In 2008, the National Institutes of Health agreed, issuing new recommendations saying that women appear to get enough water from about 91 ounces (2.7 liters) of water a day from all sources; men, about 125 ounces (3.7 liters) a day. And the usual qualifier holds: Every body is individual, so these are only guidelines.

It is important to recognize that not all liquids are equally liquefying. The caffeine in coffee and tea and the alcohol in beer, wine, and spirits are *diuretics,* chemicals that make you urinate more copiously. Although caffeinated and alcohol beverages provide water, they also increase its elimination from your body — which is why you feel thirsty the morning after you've had a glass or two of wine.

In other words (actually in Valtin's words), a healthy adult in a temperate climate who isn't perspiring heavily can get enough water simply by drinking only when he or she is thirsty.

Bottle battle

Most people in the United States get their drinking water straight from the tap, but a steadily growing number of Americans get theirs in plastic bottles.

Most people who buy the bottles say the liquid inside just tastes better. Others think the bottled stuff is safer, even though municipal water systems are subject to more rigorous regulation than water bottlers, and some plastic water bottles contain BPA (bisphenola), a potential carcinogen that you can avoid by looking for a triangle and the number 7 stamped on the bottom, indicating that the bottle is BPA-free.

Exactly how many people buy exactly how many bottles of water may vary a bit from source to source, but one 2009 report in *Bottled Water Reporter* says that from 2000 to 2008, the total amount of bottled water sold in the United States climbed from 4,725,000,000 gallons to 8,665,600,000. That number translates to nearly 29 gallons of bottled water per year for every man, woman, and child in the country.

Those gallons don't come cheap. The National Resource Defense Council estimates that bottled water costs anywhere from 240 to 10,000 (!) times as much as safe tap water. They're also expensive for the environment. According to the Environmental Protection Agency, Americans tossed away 2,480,000 tons of plastic bottles and jars in 2008 to live forever in landfills or make their way out to sea. Worldwide, the United Nations estimates that every single square mile of ocean on the planet contains 48,000 pieces of floating plastic to drift on the water for years and years and years and years until the plastic finally degrades. Or doesn't.

Container recycling laws, local bans on bottled water, and newly reusable bottles offer hope of some relief from the tons of plastic garbage. So does new technology suggesting that ultraviolet light and heat may render plastic bottles degradable.

Until then, buy a thermos and carry tap water. Your wallet and your planet will thank you.

Taking in Extra Water and Electrolytes As Needed

In the United States, most people regularly consume much more sodium than they need. In fact, some people who are sodium-sensitive may end up with high blood pressure that can be lowered if they reduce their sodium intake. For more about high blood pressure, check out *High Blood Pressure For Dummies* (published by Wiley) by Alan L. Rubin, MD.

Potassium and chloride are found in so many foods that here, too, a dietary deficiency is a rarity. In fact, the only recorded case of chloride deficiency was among infants given a formula liquid from which the chloride was inadvertently omitted.

In 2004, the Adequate Intake (AI) for sodium, potassium, and chloride were set at one-size-fits-all averages for a healthy adult age 19–50 weighing 70 kilograms (154 pounds; see Chapter 5 for more on AI):

✔ **Sodium:** 1,500 milligrams

✔ **Potassium:** 4,700 milligrams

✔ **Chloride:** 2,300 milligrams

Most Americans get much more as a matter of course, and sometimes you actually need extra water and electrolytes. The next sections tell you when.

You're sick to your stomach

Repeated vomiting or diarrhea drains your body of water and electrolytes. Similarly, you also need extra water to replace the liquid lost in perspiration when you have a high fever.

When you lose enough water to be dangerously dehydrated, you also lose the electrolytes you need to maintain fluid balance, regulate body temperature, and trigger dozens of biochemical reactions. Plain water doesn't replace those electrolytes. Check with your doctor for a drink that will hydrate your body without upsetting your tummy.

When plain water is too plain

Serious dehydration calls for serious medicine, such as the World Health Organization's handy-dandy, two-tumbler electrolyte replacement formula.

Caution: If you're reading this while lying in bed exhausted by some variety of *turista,* the traveler's diarrhea acquired from impure drinking water, do not make the formula without absolutely clean glasses, washed in bottled water. Better yet, get paper cups.

Now here's what you need:

Glass No. 1

8 ounces orange juice

A pinch of salt

½ teaspoon sweetener (honey, corn syrup)

Glass No. 2

8 ounces boiled or bottled or distilled water

¼ teaspoon baking soda

Take a sip from one glass, then the other, and continue until finished. If diarrhea continues, contact your doctor.

You're exercising or working hard in a hot environment

When you're warm, your body perspires. The moisture evaporates and cools your skin so that blood circulating up from the center of your body to the surface is cooled. The cooled blood returns to the center of your body, lowering the temperature (your *core temperature*) there, too.

If you don't cool your body down, you continue losing water. If you don't replace the lost water, things can get dicey because not only are you losing water, you're also losing electrolytes. The most common cause of temporary sodium, potassium, and chloride depletion is heavy, uncontrolled perspiration.

Deprived of water and electrolytes, your muscles cramp, you're dizzy and weak, and perspiration, now uncontrolled, no longer cools you. Your core body temperature begins rising, and without relief — air conditioning or a cool shower, plus water, ginger ale, or fruit juice — you may progress from heat cramps to heat exhaustion to heat stroke. The latter is potentially fatal.

But drinking *too much* water while exercising can also be hazardous to your health. Flooding your body with liquid dilutes the sodium in your bloodstream. This may cause body tissues, including your brain, to swell, a condition known as *hyponaturemia,* or "water intoxication." The New Rule from the American College of Sports Medicine is to drink just enough water to maintain your body weight while working out. How much is that? Step on a scale before exercising. Exercise for an hour. Step back on the scale. You need 16 ounces of water to replace every pound lost in your one hour's exercise. Lose one pound, drink 16 ounces. Lose ½ pound, drink 8 ounces.

You're on a high-protein diet

You need extra water to eliminate the nitrogen compounds in protein. This is true of infants on high-protein formulas and adults on high-protein weight-reducing diets. See Chapter 7 to find out why too much protein may be so harmful.

You're taking certain medications

Because some medications interact with water and electrolytes, always ask whether you need extra water and electrolytes whenever your doctor prescribes

- **Diuretics:** These drugs increase the loss of sodium, potassium, and chloride.
- **Neomycin (an antibiotic):** This medicine binds sodium into insoluble compounds, making it less available to your body.
- **Colchicine (an antigout drug):** This medicine lowers your body's absorption of sodium.

Dehydration: When the Body Doesn't Get Enough Water

Every day, each of us loses an amount of water equal to about 4 percent of our total weight. If we don't take in enough water to replace it, warning signals go off loud and clear.

First signs

Early on, when you've lost just a little water, equal to about 1 percent of your body weight, you feel thirsty. If you ignore thirst, it grows more intense.

When water loss rises to about 2 percent of your weight, your appetite fades. Your circulation slows as water seeps out of blood cells and blood plasma.

And you experience a sense of emotional discomfort, a perception that things are, well, not right.

Worsening problems

By the time your water loss equals 4 percent of your body weight (5 pounds for a 130-pound woman; 7 pounds for a 170-pound man), you're slightly nauseated, your skin is flushed, and you're very, very tired. With less water circulating through your tissues, your hands and feet tingle, your head aches, your temperature rises, you breathe more quickly, and your pulse quickens.

Really bad trouble

After this, things go downhill more quickly. When your water loss reaches 10 percent of your body weight, your tongue swells, your kidneys start to fail, and you're so dizzy that you can't stand on one foot with your eyes closed. In fact, you probably can't even try: Your muscles are in spasm.

When you lose enough water to equal 15 percent of your body weight, you're deaf and pretty much unable to see out of eyes that are sunken and covered with stiffened lids. Your skin has shrunk, and your tongue has shriveled.

The crash

When you've lost water equal to 20 percent of your body weight, your body is at the limit of its endurance.

Deprived of life-giving liquid, your skin cracks, and your organs grind to a halt. And so do you.

Ave atque vale, or as the Romans say when in the United States, Canada, Great Britain, Australia, or any place where English is the mother tongue: "Hail and Farewell."

Water words

Chemically speaking, H_2O (one molecule hydrogen, two molecules oxygen) is a queer duck, the only substance on earth that exists as a liquid (water) and a solid (ice) — but never as a bendable plastic material. (No, as chemistry teachers explain each year to first-year chemistry students, snow is not plastic water. It's a collection of solids [ice crystals]).

Semantically speaking, water is also challenging.

For starters, water may be hard or soft, but these terms have nothing to do with how the water feels on your hand. They describe the liquid's mineral content:

✔ *Hard water* has lots of minerals, particularly calcium and magnesium. This water rises to the Earth's surface from underground springs, picking up calcium carbonate as it moves up through the ground.

✔ *Soft water* has fewer minerals. In nature, soft water is surface water, the runoff from rain-swollen streams or rainwater that falls directly into reservoirs. *Water softeners* are products that attract and remove the minerals in water.

What you get at the supermarket is another list of water words:

✔ *Distilled water* is tap water that has been *distilled,* or boiled until it turns to steam, which is then collected and condensed back into a liquid free of impurities, chemicals, and minerals. The term *distilled* is also used

to describe a liquid produced by *ultrafiltration,* a process that removes everything from the water except water molecules. Distilled water makes clean, clear ice cubes and serves as a flavor-free mixer or base for tea and coffee. It won't clog a steam iron, and it's valuable for chemical and pharmaceutical processing.

✔ *Spring water* is water from springs relatively near the Earth's surface. This water has fewer mineral particles and what some people describe as a "cleaner taste" than mineral water.

✔ *Mineral water* is water from deeper down; it picks up minerals on its journey upwards. Mineral spring water is naturally alkaline, which makes it a natural antacid and a mild diuretic.

✔ *Still water* is spring water that flows up to the surface on its own. *Sparkling water* is pushed to the top by naturally occurring gases in the underground spring. So, you ask, what's the big difference? Sparkling water has bubbles; still water doesn't.

✔ *Springlike* or *spring fresh* are terms designed to make the water in the bottle seem more prestigious. Products labeled with these terms aren't spring water; they're most likely to be filtered tap water, the liquid that flows out when you turn on the faucet (see *distilled water,* earlier in this list).

Part III
Healthy Eating

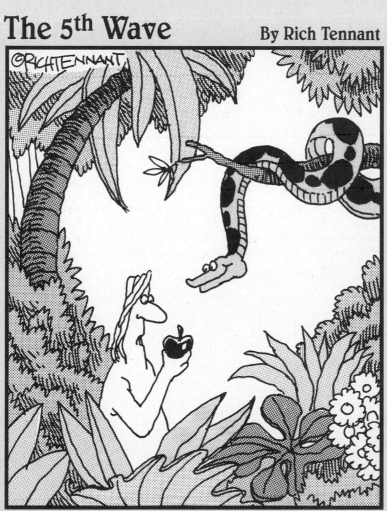

The 5th Wave   By Rich Tennant

"This isn't some sort of fad diet, is it?"

In this part . . .

Want to know how to put foods together to build a healthful diet? Step right up to this part whose chapters are chock-full of guidelines from the *Dietary Guidelines for Americans 2010,* with strategies for making selections that enhance your body while pleasing your palate. Plus, you can read an explanation of why you get hungry and why you find some foods more appetizing than others — an important factor in creating a nutritious diet. (Hey, if it doesn't taste good, why would you want to eat it?)

Chapter 14

Why You Eat When You Eat

Because you need food to live, your body is no slouch at letting you know that it's ready for breakfast, lunch, dinner, and maybe a few snacks in between. This chapter explains the signals your body uses to get you to the table, to the drive-through of your favorite fast-food joint, or to the vending machine down the hall.

Understanding the Difference between Hunger and Appetite

People eat for two basic reasons. The first is hunger; the second is appetite. Hunger and appetite are *not* synonyms. In fact, hunger and appetite are entirely different processes.

Hunger is the need for food. It is

✔ A physical reaction that includes chemical changes in your body related to a naturally low level of glucose in your blood several hours after eating

✔ An instinctive, protective mechanism that makes sure that your body gets the fuel it requires to function reasonably well

---

Pavlov's performing puppies

Ivan Petrovich Pavlov (1849–1936) was a Russian physiologist who won the Nobel Prize in physiology/medicine in 1904 for his research on the digestive glands. Pavlov's Big Bang, though, was his identification of respondent conditioning — a fancy way of saying that you can train people to respond physically (or emotionally) to an object or stimulus that simply reminds them of something that they love or hate.

Pavlov tested respondent conditioning on dogs. He began by ringing a bell each time he offered food to his laboratory dogs so that the dogs learned to associate the sound of the bell with the sight and smell of food.

Then he rang the bell without offering the food, and the dogs responded as though food were on tap — salivating madly, even though the dish was empty.

Respondent conditioning applies to many things other than food. For example, it can make a winning Olympic athlete teary at the sight of the flag that represents his country. Food companies are great at using respondent conditioning to encourage you to buy their products: When you see a picture of a deep, dark, rich chocolate bar, doesn't your mouth start to water, and. . . . Hey, come back! Where are you going?

Appetite is the desire for food. It is

- A sensory or psychological reaction (looks good! smells good!) that stimulates an involuntary physiological response (salivation, stomach contractions)
- A conditioned response to food (see the sidebar on Pavlov's dogs)

The practical difference between hunger and appetite is this: When you're hungry, you eat one hot dog. After that, your appetite may lead you to eat two more hot dogs just because they look appealing or taste good.

In other words, appetite is the basis for the familiar saying: "Your eyes are bigger than your stomach." Not to mention the well-known advertising slogan: "Bet you can't eat just one." Hey, these guys know their customers.

Refueling: The Cycle of Hunger and Satiety

Your body does its best to create cycles of activity that parallel a 24-hour day. Like sleep, hunger occurs at pretty regular intervals, although your lifestyle may make it difficult to follow this natural pattern — even when your stomach loudly announces it's empty!

Recognizing hunger

The clearest signals that your body wants food, right now, are the physical reactions from your stomach that let you know it's definitely time to put more food in your mouth.

An empty belly has no manners. If you do not fill it right away, it will issue an audible, sometimes embarrassing, call for food. This rumbling signal is called a *hunger pang*.

Hunger pangs are muscle contractions. When your stomach's full, these contractions and their continual waves down the entire length of the intestine — known as *peristalsis* — move food through your digestive tract (see Chapter 2 for more about digestion). When your stomach's empty, the contractions just squeeze air, and that makes noise.

This phenomenon was first observed in 1912 by an American physiologist named Walter B. Cannon. (Cannon? Rumble? Could you make this up?) Cannon convinced a fellow researcher to swallow a small balloon attached to a thin tube connected to a pressure-sensitive machine. Then Cannon inflated and deflated the balloon to simulate the sensation of a full or empty stomach. Measuring the pressure and frequency of his volunteer's stomach contractions, Cannon discovered that the contractions were strongest and occurred most frequently when the balloon was deflated and the stomach empty. Cannon drew the obvious conclusion: When your stomach is empty, you feel hungry.

Identifying the hormones that say, "I'm hungry" and "I'm full"

Like so many other body functions, hunger is influenced by hormones — in this case, *ghrelin, insulin, PYY* (peptide tyrosine tyrosine), and *leptin.* These natural chemicals act on the satiety center in your brain to make sure that you get enough to eat — and (perhaps) know when to stop.

✔ **Ghrelin:** Ghrelin (pronounced *grel-in*) is a hormone secreted primarily by cells in the lining of the stomach; smaller amounts are secreted by the hypothalamus (see Figure 14-1). Ghrelin is an appetite stimulant that elicits messages from your brain that say, "I'm hungry." If you're fasting or simply cutting back on food in order to lose weight, your body responds by producing more than normal amounts of ghrelin, triggering a higher than normal desire to eat. This is one way to explain why dieters find it difficult to stick to a reduced-calorie regimen.

✔ **Insulin:** Every time you eat, your pancreas secretes *insulin,* a hormone that enables you to transform the food you eat into *glucose,* the simple sugar on which the body runs, and then to move the glucose into body cells. The higher level of insulin temporarily suppresses appetite, but when the amount of glucose circulating in your blood declines again, you may feel empty, which prompts you to eat. Most people experience the natural rise and fall of glucose — and the consequent secretion of insulin — as a relatively smooth pattern that lasts about four hours. *Note:* People with Type 1 (insulin dependent) diabetes do not produce the insulin needed to process glucose, which continues to circulate around the body and is eventually excreted in sugary urine.

✔ **PYY (peptide tyrosine-tyrosine):** After you've eaten, this hormone, secreted by your small intestine and in lesser amounts by cells in other parts of your digestive tract, acts as an appetite suppressant that cancels out ghrelin's appetite stimulating effects. PYY's message? You're full; stop eating.

✔ **Leptin:** Leptin, identified in 1995 at Rockefeller University in New York, is produced in the body's fat cells, a source of stored energy. Leptin is an appetite suppressant; if your body loses a lot of fat, you also lose leptin. The result? An increase in the desire for food to increase your store of body fat.

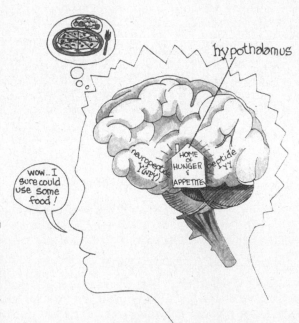

Figure 14-1:
Your hypo-
thalamus is
in charge
of your
appetite!

Beating the four-hour hungries

Throughout the world, the cycle of hunger (glucose and insulin rising and falling as described in the preceding section) prompts a feeding schedule that generally provides four meals during the day: breakfast, lunch, a mid-afternoon snack, and supper.

In the United States, a three-meal-a-day culture forces people to fight this natural eating pattern by going without food from lunch at around noon to supper at 6 p.m. or later. The unpleasant result is that when glucose levels go south around 4 p.m. (and people in other countries are enjoying afternoon tea), many Americans get really testy, growl at their coworkers, make mistakes they'll correct the next day, or try to satisfy their natural hunger by grabbing the nearest food, usually a high-fat, high-calorie snack.

The better way: Five or six small meals

More than 20 years ago, David Jenkins, MD, PhD, and Tom Wolever, MD, PhD, of the University of Toronto, set up a "nibbling study" designed to test the idea that if you even out digestion — by eating several small meals rather than three big ones — you can spread out insulin secretion and keep the amount of glucose in your blood on an even keel all day long.

The theory turned out to be right. People who ate five or six small meals rather than three big ones felt better and experienced an extra bonus: lower cholesterol levels. After two weeks of nibbling, the people in the Jenkins-Wolever study showed a 13.5 percent lower level of low-density lipoproteins (LDL) than people who ate exactly the same amount of food divided into three big meals. As a result, some diets designed to help you lose weight now emphasize a daily regimen of several small meals rather than the basic big three. To be fair about it, though, several studies show no beneficial effect, so this is an if-it-works-for-you-do-it issue.

Maintaining a healthy appetite

The best way to deal with hunger and appetite is to recognize and follow your body's natural cues.

If you're hungry, eat — in reasonable amounts that support a realistic weight. (Read about that topic in Chapter 4.) And remember: Nobody's perfect. Make one day's indulgence guilt-free by reducing your calorie intake proportionately over the next few days.

A little give here, a little take there, and you'll stay on target overall.

What meal is this, anyway?

Breakfast and lunch leave no doubt. The first comes right after you wake up in the morning; the second, in the middle of the day, sometime around noon.

But when do you eat dinner? And what about supper?

According to *Webster's New International Dictionary of the English Language* (2nd Edition, 1941 — 15 pounds, including the new binding I put on when the old one crumbled after I dropped the darned thing on its spine once too often), dinner is the main meal of the day, usually eaten around midday, although (get this) some people, "especially in cities," have their dinner between 6 p.m. and 8 p.m. — which probably makes it their supper, because Webster's calls that a meal you eat at the end of the day.

In other words, dinner is lunch except when it's supper. Help!

Responding to Your Environment on a Gut Level

Your physical and psychological environments definitely affect appetite and hunger, sometimes leading you to eat more than normal, sometimes less.

Baby, it's cold outside

Think of the foods that tempt you in winter — stews, roasts, thick soups — versus those you find pleasing on a simmering summer day — salads, chilled fruit, simple sandwiches.

This difference is no accident. Food gives you calories. Calories keep you warm. Yes, you will need more energy if you're running a marathon in the summer than if you're sitting quietly all day in front of the TV while the snow piles up outside.

But as a general rule, to get the energy it needs to keep you warm, your body will say, "I'm hungry" more frequently when it's cold outside. In addition, you process food faster in a cold environment. Your stomach empties more quickly as food speeds along through the digestive tract, which means those old hunger pangs show up sooner than expected, which, in turn, means that you eat more and stay warmer and . . . well, you get the picture.

Exercising more than your mouth

Everybody knows that working out gives you a big appetite, right? Well, everybody's wrong. People who exercise regularly are definitely likely to have a healthy (read: normal) appetite, but they're rarely hungry immediately after exercising because

> ✔ Exercise pulls stored energy — glucose and fat — out of body tissues, so your glucose levels stay steady and you don't feel hungry.

> ✔ Exercise slows the passage of food through the digestive tract. Your stomach empties more slowly, and you feel fuller longer.

> *Caution:* If you eat a heavy meal right before heading for the gym or the stationary bike in your bedroom, the food sitting in your stomach may make you feel stuffed. Sometimes, you may develop cramps. Or — as Ken DeVault, MD, and I explain in *Heartburn & Reflux For Dummies* (Wiley) — heartburn.

> ✔ Exercise (including mental exertion) reduces anxiety. For some people, that means less desire to reach for a snack.

Taking medicine that changes your appetite

Some drugs affect your appetite, leading you to eat more (or less) than usual. This side effect is rarely mentioned when doctors hand out prescriptions, perhaps because it isn't life-threatening and usually disappears when you stop taking the drug or simply because your doc doesn't know about it. Hey, it happens.

Some examples of appetite uppers are certain antidepressants, antihistamines (allergy pills), diuretics (drugs that make you urinate more frequently), steroids (drugs that fight inflammation), and tranquilizers (calming drugs). Medicines that may reduce your appetite include some antibiotics, anticancer drugs, antiseizure drugs, blood pressure medications, and cholesterol-lowering drugs.

Be warned that not every drug in a particular class of drugs has the same effect on appetite. For example, the antidepressant drug amitriptyline (Elavil) increases your appetite and may cause weight gain, while fluoxetine (Prozac) usually does not.

Unhealthy Relationships with Food

This chapter, as the title says, is about why you eat when you eat. Up until this point, the reasons have been physiological: Your hormones say you're hungry or full, or perhaps the weather says you need more food (or less) for energy. But sometimes, the decision to eat or not eat is triggered by an *eating disorder,* a psychological illness that leads you to eat either too much or too little, or to regard food as your enemy or your savior.

Indulging in a hot fudge sundae or two once in a while is not an eating disorder. Neither is dieting for three weeks so that you can fit into last year's dress this New Year's Eve. Nor is the determination to eat a healthful diet.

The difference between these behaviors and an eating disorder is that the first are medically acceptable while the second are potentially life-threatening illnesses that require immediate medical attention.

For some people, food is not simply a meal. It is the object of love or loathing, a way to relieve anxiety or an anxiety provoker. As a result, human beings may experience various eating disorders: *Obesity, anorexia nervosa, bulimia, binge eating,* and a new candidate for inclusion on this list, *orthorexia.*

Obesity

Although many recent studies document an alarming worldwide increase in obesity (details in Chapter 4), not everyone who is larger or heavier than the current ideal body has an eating disorder. Human bodies come in many different sizes, and some healthy people are just naturally larger or heavier than others. But an eating disorder may be present, though, when

- A person continually confuses the desire for food (appetite) with the need for food (hunger)

- A person who has access to a normal diet experiences psychological distress when denied food

- A person uses food to relieve anxiety provoked by what he or she considers a scary situation — a new job, a party, ordinary criticism, or a deadline

Traditionally, doctors find it difficult to treat obesity, but recent research suggests that some people overeat in response to irregularities in the production of chemicals that regulate satiety (your feeling of fullness). This research may open the path to new kinds of drugs that can control extreme appetite, thus reducing the incidence of obesity-related disorders such as arthritis, diabetes, high blood pressure, and heart disease.

Anorexia nervosa

Anorexia, the eating disorder that sidelined Mary-Kate Olsen in 2004, is voluntary starvation. As you might expect, anorexia is virtually unknown in places where food is hard to come by. Instead, anorexia seems to be an affliction of affluence, most likely to strike the young and well-to-do, more common among young women than among young men.

The signs of anorexia are weighing less than 85 percent of the normal weight, a fear of gaining weight, an obsession with one's appearance, and the belief that one is fat regardless of the true weight. For young women, the absence of three menstrual cycles due to extreme weight loss is another sign.

Up to 40 percent of people with anorexia will develop *bulimia nervosa;* up to 30 percent will develop *binge eating disorder.* (I describe both disorders in the next two sections.) Left untreated, anorexia nervosa may be fatal.

Bulimia nervosa

Unlike people with anorexia, individuals with bulimia don't refuse to eat, but they don't want to hold on to the food they've consumed. They may use laxatives to increase defecation, or they may simply retire to the bathroom after eating to take *emetics* (drugs that induce vomiting) or stick their fingers into their throats to make themselves throw up. Like anorexics, bulimics may develop *binge eating disorder* (see the next section).

Either way, danger looms. Repeated regurgitation can severely irritate or even tear through the lining of the esophagus (throat); the acid stomach contents also damage teeth. (Dentists are often the first medical personnel to identify a bulimic.) In addition, the continued use of emetics may result in a life-threatening loss of potassium that triggers irregular heartbeat or heart failure.

Binge eating disorder

The criterion for a diagnosis of binge eating disorder is consuming enormous amounts of food — a whole chicken, several pints of ice cream, an entire loaf of bread — in one sitting twice a week for up six months. Some binge eaters become overweight; others stay slim by regurgitating. Either way, binge eating, like other eating disorders, is hazardous behavior.

Binge eaters who regurgitate experience adverse effects similar to those associated with bulimia. Binge eaters who do not regurgitate risk not only obesity but, paradoxically, malnutrition. Why? Because the foods they choose may be high in calories but low in vital nutrients. (Think hot fudge sundae again. And again. And again.) More dramatically, the enormous quantities of food they consume may dilate or even rupture the stomach or esophagus, a potentially fatal medical emergency.

Orthorexia nervosa

Orthorexia is a term coined by Steven Bratman, MD, and David Michael Knight in their book *Health Food Junkies* (Broadway Books). This behavior is characterized by an obsession with the need to eat only the *right* foods. The condition isn't a formally recognized eating disorder, but its rigid approach to dining will be familiar to anyone with a friend who spends an inordinate number of hours each day planning perfect meals or who refuses to eat even a smidgen of something that is not organic or has been grown more than a fixed distance from home base. The orthorexic's food choices may actually be healthful; his rigidity and guilt at the possibility of falling off the health food wagon are not.

And the conclusion is . . .

Eating disorders are serious, potentially life-threatening conditions. If you (or someone you know) experience any of the signs and symptoms just described, the safest course is to seek immediate medical advice and treatment.

For more info about eating conditions, contact the National Eating Disorders Association, 603 Stewart St., Suite 803, Seattle, WA 98101; phone 206-382-3587; e-mail info@NationalEatingDisorders.org; Web site www.national eatingdisorders.org.

Chapter 15

Why You Like the Foods You Like

*N*utritionally speaking, *taste* is the ability to perceive flavors in food and beverages. *Preference* is the appreciation of one food and distaste of another. Decisions about taste are physical reactions that are dependent on specialized body organs called taste buds. Although your culture has a decided influence on what you think is good to eat, decisions about food preferences may also depend on your genes, your medical history, and your personal reactions to specific foods.

Tackling Taste: How Your Brain and Tongue Work Together

Your *taste buds* are sensory organs that enable you to perceive different flavors in food — in other words, to taste the food you eat.

Taste buds (also referred to as *taste papillae*) are tiny bumps on the surface of your tongue (see Figure 15-1). Each one contains groups of receptor cells that anchor an antenna-like structure called a *microvillus,* which projects up through a gap (or pore) in the center of the taste bud, sort of like a thread sticking through the hole in Life Savers candy. (For more about the microvilli and how they behave in your digestive tract, see Chapter 2.)

The microvilli in your taste buds transmit messages from flavor chemicals in the food along nerve fibers to your brain, which translates the messages into perceptions: "That's good," or "That's awful."

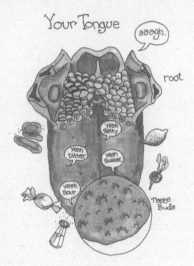

Figure 15-1:
Your tongue
up close.

The five (maybe six) basic flavors

Your taste buds recognize five basic flavors: *sweet, sour, bitter, salty,* and *umami,* a Japanese word describing richness or a savory flavor associated with glutamate (or glutamic acid), the amino acid responsible for the distinctive flavor of soy products (soybeans, tofu, tempeh).

At first, scientists believed that people had specific taste buds for specific flavors: sweet taste buds for sweets, sour taste buds for sour, and so on. The modern theory is that groups of taste buds work together so that flavor chemicals in food link up with chemical bonds in taste buds to create patterns that you recognize as sweet, sour, bitter, and salty. The technical term for this process is *across-fiber pattern theory of gustatory coding.* Receptor patterns for the sweet, sour, bitter, and salty have been tentatively identified, but the pattern for umami remains elusive.

Nutrition researchers now propose that there are also taste bud patterns to recognize the flavor of fatty acids, and some even suggest that there are patterns to recognize the flavor of calcium. Right now, these proposals are nutrition lore rather than nutrition law.

The nose knows — and the eyes have it

Your nose is important to your sense of taste. Just like the taste of food, the aroma of food also stimulates sensory messages. Think about how you sniff your brandy before drinking and how the wonderful aroma of baking bread warms the heart and stirs the soul — not to mention the salivary glands. When you can't smell, you can't really taste. As anyone who's ever had a cold knows, when your nose is stuffed and your sense of smell is deadened, almost everything tastes like plain old cotton. Don't have a cold? You can test this theory by closing your eyes, pinching your nostrils shut, and having someone put a tiny piece of either a raw onion or a fresh apple into your mouth. Bet you can't tell which is which without looking — or sniffing!

Food color is also an important clue to what you'll enjoy eating. Repeated studies show that when testers change the expected color of foods, people find them (the foods, not the testers) less appealing. For example, blue mashed potatoes or green beef lose to plain old white mashed potatoes and red meat every time.

As my technical editor Alfred Bushway notes, one of the most famous food experiments is performed with gelatin whose flavor does not match its color. Without even thinking twice, more than half the volunteers in the test will say the gelatin tastes like the flavor associated with its color — for example, green gelatin tastes like lime and orange like oranges — even when the flavors are actually the opposite.

Your health and your taste buds

Some illnesses and medicines alter your ability to taste foods. The result may be partial or total *ageusia* (the medical term for loss of taste). Or you may experience *flavor confusion* — meaning that you mix up flavors, translating sour as bitter, or sweet as salty, or vice versa.

Table 15-1 lists some medical conditions that affect your sense of taste.

Table 15-1	These Things Make Tasting Food Difficult
This Condition	*May Lead to This Problem*
A bacterial or viral infection of the tongue	Secretions that block your taste buds
Injury to your mouth, nose, or throat	Damage to the nerves that transmit flavor signals
Radiation therapy to mouth and throat	Damage to the nerves that transmit flavor signals

Shaking the salt

Some people are sensitive to sodium; a diet high in salted foods may increase their risk of hypertension (high blood pressure). But salty is not only a flavor on its own; it also intensifies other flavors so people find it difficult to cut back on salt and still enjoy their meals. However, as Jay Schulkin of Georgetown University School of Medicine explains in *Calcium Hunger* (Cambridge University Press), in a series of studies during the 1980s, scientists identified a link between calcium deprivation and salt craving in both laboratory animals and animals living in the wild.

Although no controlled studies have been performed with humans, some researchers suggest a similar phenomenon among women, particularly during pregnancy. Therefore, rather than banishing the salt shaker from every table, the better way to help folks cut back on salt might be to offer a milkshake instead. Lowfat, of course.

Tricking your taste buds

Combining foods can short-circuit your taste buds' ability to identify flavors correctly. For example, when you sip wine (even an apparently smooth and silky one), your taste buds taste something sharp. Take a bite of cheese first, though, and the wine tastes smoother (less acidic) because the cheese's fat and protein molecules coat your receptor cells so that acidic wine molecules cannot connect.

A similar phenomenon occurs during serial wine tastings (sampling many wines, one after another). Try two equally dry, acidic wines, and the second seems mellower because acid molecules from the first one fill up space on the chemical bonds that perceive acidity. Drink a sweet wine after a dry one, and the sweetness often is more pronounced.

Here's another way to fool your taste buds: Eat an artichoke. The meaty part at the base of the artichoke leaves contains *cynarin,* a sweet-tasting chemical that makes any food you taste after the artichoke taste sweeter.

Determining Deliciousness

When it comes to deciding what tastes good, all human beings and most animals have four things in common: They like sweets, crave salt, go for the fat, and avoid the bitter (at least at first).

These choices are rooted deep in biology and evolution. In fact, you can say that whenever you reach for something that you consider good to eat, the entire human race — especially your own individual ancestors — reaches with you.

Listening to your body

Here's something to chew on: The foods that taste good — sweet foods, salty foods, fatty foods — are essential for a healthy body.

✔ Sweet foods are a source of quick energy because their sugars can be converted quickly to glucose, the molecule that your body burns for energy. (Check out Chapter 9 for an explanation of how your body uses sugars.)

Better yet, sweet foods make you feel good. Eating them tells your brain to release natural painkillers called *endorphins.* Sweet foods may also stimulate an increase in blood levels of *adrenaline,* a hormone secreted by the adrenal glands. Adrenaline sometimes is labeled the *fight-or-flight hormone* because it's secreted more heavily when you feel threatened and must decide whether to stand your ground — *fight* — or hurry away — *flight.*

✔ Salt is vital to life. As Chapter 13 explains, salt enables your body to maintain its fluid balance and to regulate chemicals called electrolytes that give your nerve cells the power needed to fire electrical charges that energize your muscles, power up your organs, and transmit messages from your brain.

✔ Fatty foods are even richer in calories (energy) than sugars. So the fact that you want them most when you're very hungry comes as no surprise. (Chapters 3 and 8 explain how you use fats for energy.)

✔ Which fatty food you want may depend on your sex. Several studies suggest that women like their fats with sugar (think chocolate). Men, on the other hand, seem to prefer their fat with salt (think fries).

Former Food and Drug Administration commissioner David A. Kessler believes that one explanation for the increase in obesity among Americans (see Chapter 4) may be the food industry's manipulating our natural desire for rich foods by creating layered products: sugar on top of fat on top of salt. Or vice versa. Need proof? Look no further than the diabolically delicious 2010 newbie, pretzel M&Ms — sugar coating on top of fatty chocolate on top of salty pretzel.

Loving the food you're with: Geography and taste

Marvin Harris was an anthropologist with a special interest in the history of food. In a perfectly delightful book called *Good to Eat: Riddles of Food and Culture* (Simon & Schuster), Harris posed this interesting situation:

Creepy crawly nutrients

Who's to say grilled grasshopper is less appetizing than a lobster? After all, both have long skinny bodies and plenty of legs. But the difference is in the nutrients: The bug beats the lobster hands (legs?) down.

Food 3.5 oz	Protein (g)	Fat (g)	Carbohydrates (g)	Iron (mg)
Water beetle	19.8	8.3	2.1	13.6
Red ant	13.9	3.5	2.9	5.7
Cricket	12.9	5.5	5.1	9.5
Small grass-hopper	14.3	3.3	2.2	3.0
Large grass-hopper	20.6	6.1	3.9	5.0
Lobster	22	<1	<1	0.4
Blue crab	20	<1	0	0.8

USDA and Iowa State University (www.ent.iastate.edu/misc/insectnutrition.html).

Suppose that you live in a forest where someone has pinned $20 and $1 bills to the upper branches of the trees. Which will you reach for? The $20 bills, of course. But wait. Suppose that only a couple of $20 bills are pinned to branches among millions and millions of $1 bills.

Now, substitute chickens for $20 bills and large insects for $1 bills, and you can see why people who live in places where insects far outnumber the chickens spend their time and energy picking off the plentiful high-protein bugs rather than chasing after the occasional chicken — although they wouldn't turn it down if one fell into the pot.

Therefore, the first rule of food choice appears to be that people tend to eat and enjoy what is easily available, which explains the differences in cuisines in different parts of the world.

Here's a second rule: For a food to be appealing (good to eat), it must be both nutritious *and* relatively easy or economical to produce.

A food that meets one test but not the other is likely to be off the list. For example:

✔ The human stomach cannot extract nutrients from grass. So even though grass grows here, there, and everywhere, under ordinary circumstances, it never ends up in your salad.

✔ Cows are harder to raise than plants, especially under the hot South Asian sun; pigs eat what people do, so they compete for your food supply. In other words, although they're highly nutritious, sometimes neither the cow nor the pig is economical to produce, a reasonable — though not the only — explanation for why some cultures have prohibited the use of pigs and cows as food.

Taking offense to tastes

Virtually everyone instinctively dislikes bitter foods, at least at first tasting. This dislike is a protective mechanism. Bitter foods are often poisonous, so disliking stuff that tastes bitter is a primitive but effective way to eliminate potentially toxic food.

According to Linda Bartoshuk, PhD, Professor of Community Dentistry and Behavioral Science, University of Florida, Gainesville, about two-thirds of all human beings carry a gene that makes them especially sensitive to bitter flavors. This gene may have given their ancestors a leg up in surviving their evolutionary food trials.

People with this gene can taste very small concentrations of a chemical called phenylthiocarbamide (PTC). Dr. Bartoshuk tests for the trait by having people taste a piece of paper impregnated with 6-n-propylthiouracil, a thyroid medication whose flavor and chemical structure are similar to PTC. People who say the paper tastes bitter are called *PTC tasters*. People who taste only paper are called *PTC nontasters*. It is interesting to note that more women than men are PTC tasters.

If you're a PTC taster, you're likely to find the taste of saccharin, caffeine, the salt substitute potassium chloride, and the food preservatives sodium benzoate and potassium benzoate really nasty. The same is true for the flavor chemicals common to cruciferous vegetables — members of the mustard family, including broccoli, Brussels sprouts, cabbage, cauliflower, and radishes.

No such ambivalence exists among people who've gotten truly sick — I'm talking nausea and vomiting here — after eating a specific food. When that happens, you'll probably come to like its flavor less. Sometimes, says psychologist Alexandra W. Logue, author of *The Psychology of Eating and Drinking,* your revulsion may be so strong that you'll never try the food again — even when you know that what actually made you sick was something else entirely, like riding a roller coaster just before eating, or having the flu, or taking a drug whose side effects upset your stomach.

If you're allergic to a food or have a metabolic problem that makes digesting it hard for you, you may eat the food less frequently, but you'll enjoy it as much as everyone else does. For example, people who cannot digest *lactose,* the sugar in milk, may end up gassy every time they eat ice cream, but they still like the way the ice cream tastes.

Does digestion depend on whether you like your food? To some extent, it does. The simple act of putting food into your mouth needs to stimulate the flow of saliva and the secretion of enzymes that you need to digest the food. Some studies suggest that if you really like your food, your pancreas may release as much as 30 times its normal amount of digestive enzymes.

However, if you truly loathe what you're eating, your body may refuse to take it in. No saliva flows; your mouth becomes so dry that you may not even be able to swallow the food. If you do manage to choke it down, your stomach muscles and your digestive tract may convulse in an effort to be rid of the awful stuff.

Changing the Menu: Adapting to Exotic Foods

New foods are an adventure. As a rule, people may not like them the first time around, but in time — and with patience — what once seemed strange can become just another dish at dinner.

Learning to like unusual foods

Exposure to different people and cultures often expands your taste horizons. Some taboos — horsemeat, snake, dog — may simply be too emotion-laden to be overcome. Others with no emotional baggage fall to experience. On first taste, most people dislike very salty, very bitter, very acidic, or very slippery foods, such as caviar, coffee, Scotch whisky, and oysters; but many later learn to enjoy them.

Coming to terms with these foods can be both physically and psychologically rewarding:

- Several bitter foods, such as coffee and unsweetened chocolate, are relatively mild stimulants that temporarily improve mood and physical performance.

- Strongly flavored foods, such as salty caviar, offer a challenge to the taste buds.

- Foods such as oysters, which may seem totally disgusting the first time you see or taste them, are symbols of wealth or worldliness. Trying them implies a certain sophistication in the way you face life.

Happily, an educated, adventurous sense of taste can be a pleasure that lasts as long as you live. Professional tea tasters, wine tasters, and others who develop the ability to discern even the smallest differences among flavors continue to enjoy their gift well into old age as long as they continue to provide stimuli in the form of tasty, well-seasoned food.

In other words, as they say about adult life's other major sensory delight, "Use it or lose it."

Stirring the stew: The culinary benefits of immigration

If you're lucky enough to live in a place that attracts many immigrants, your dining experience is flavored by the favorite foods of other people (meaning the foods of other cultures). In the United States, for example, the *melting pot* is not an idle phrase. American cooking literally bubbles with contributions from every group that's ever stepped ashore in what President Lyndon Baines Johnson used to call the "good ole U. S. of A."

Table 15-2 lists some of the foods and food combinations characteristic of specific ethnic/regional cuisines. Imagine how few you might sample living in a place where everybody shares exactly the same ethnic, racial, or religious backgrounds. Just thinking about it is enough to make you stand up and shout, "Hooray for diversity at the dinner table!" (Check out Figure 15-2 for the visuals!)

Table 15-2	Geography and Food Preference
If Your Ancestors Came From	*You're Likely to Be Familiar with This Flavor Combination*
Central and Eastern Europe	Sour cream and dill or paprika
China	Soy sauce plus wine and ginger
Germany	Meat roasted in vinegar and sugar
Greece	Olive oil and lemon
India	Cumin and curry
Italy	Tomatoes, cheese, and olive oil
Japan	Soy sauce plus rice wine and sugar
Korea	Soy sauce plus brown sugar, sesame, and chile
Mexico	Tomatoes and chile peppers
Middle Europe	Milk and vegetables
Puerto Rico	Rice and fish
West Africa	Peanuts and chile peppers

A. W. Logue, The Psychology of Eating and Drinking, 2nd Edition (New York: W. H. Freeman and Company, 1991).

Noshing in the neighborhood

Miami loves Latin; San Francisco, Asian; and Chicago, middle European. But New York is where America comes to eat all around the world.

In a city that speaks more than 170 languages, Zagat's restaurant roster includes 60 different ethnic and regional cuisines ranging from A (Afghan, African, Argentinean, Asian, Australian, Austrian) through P (Persian, Peruvian, Polish, Portuguese, Puerto Rican), and maybe on to Z, if one of the African restaurants on the list serves dishes native to Zambia, Zimbabwe, or Zaire.

Naturally, New York foodies have written the books you need to bring the good stuff home to your own kitchen. A small sampling (in alphabetical order):

The Arthur Avenue Cookbook (Ecco), by Ann Volkwein, celebrates a Bronx neighborhood many call "the real Little Italy" with the recipes for such dishes as baked ziti, osso buco, ricotta cheesecake and cannoli, plus portraits of the restaurateurs, cooks, and marketers who make this area gourmet heaven.

Chinatown, New York (Collins Design), also by Ann Volkwein, does the honors for the largest Chinese community in the Western hemisphere, with special mention to special restaurants and recipes for fresh seafood, a variety of pork dishes, dim sum delicacies, and, of course, the ubiquitous Chinese dumpling. Pictures, too.

The Go Green East Harlem Cookbook/El Librio de Cocina Viva Verde East Harlem (Jones Books), edited by Manhattan Borough President Scott M. Stringer, comes in English if you start reading at one end and Spanish if you turn the book and start from the other cover. Either way, the recipes — contributed by members of the largest Puerto Rican community outside Puerto Rico — are updated to bring traditional dishes into line with modern nutrition guidelines: less fat, more fiber, fresh foods at every turn.

The New Brooklyn Cookbook (William Morrow Cookbooks), by Melissa Vaughn and Brendan Vaughn, with photographs by Michael Turkell, tracks the evolving menu in a part of New York whose best-known culinary triumph was once the Nathan's Hot Dog. The Vaughns' research turns up recipes for such dishes as steak and eggs Korean style, tofu with broad beans and chili bean paste, spaghetti alla vongole, and beef sauerbraten with braised red cabbage and pretzel dumplings, spiced with interviews and profiles of cheesemakers, picklers, chocolatiers, and other local food people.

Sylvia's Family Soul Food Cookbook: From Hemingway, South Carolina, To Harlem (William Morrow Cookbooks), by Sylvia Woods. The mistress of the world famous Sylvia's in Harlem is a treasure trove of American Southern cooking: Oven-fried chicken, chitlins, catfish stew, candied yams soufflé, collard greens, and, of course, hush puppies.

The Veselka Cookbook: Recipes and Stories from the Landmark Restaurant in New York's East Village (Thomas Dunne Books), by Tom Birchard and Natalie Danford, offers up recipes from a Ukrainian restaurant on Manhattan's Lower East Side, once home to a large contingent of Eastern Europeans (vesalka means rainbow in Ukrainian). The collection includes such classics as pierogi, five different kinds of borsht, grilled kielbasa, and poppy seed cake. As a bonus, Veselka owner Birchard tells (pleasant) tales of celebrity customers.

For even more ethnic neighborhood cookbooks, check out Kitchen Arts and Letters, 1436 Lexington Avenue, New York, NY 10128; phone 212-876-5550; e-mail ketters@kitchen artsandletters.com.

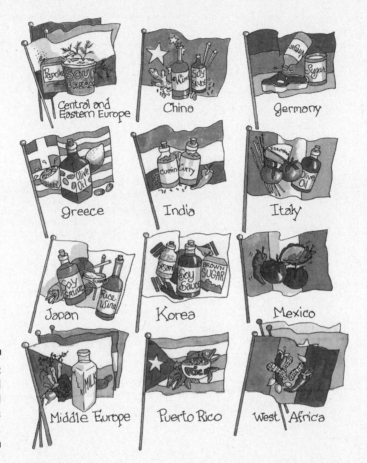

Figure 15-2:
Ethnic and regional cuisines abound.

Of course, enjoying other people's foods doesn't mean Americans don't have their own cuisine. Table 15-3 is a list of made-in-America taste sensations, many created by immigrant chefs whose talents flowered in America's kitchens.

Table 15-3	Foods Born in the United States
This Food Item	*Was Born Here*
Baked beans	Boston (Pilgrim adaptation of Native American dish)
Clam chowder	Boston (the word chowder comes from the French *la chaudière,* the large copper soup pot used by fishermen to make a communal soup)
Hamburger	Everywhere (originally called a Hamburg steak by everyone except the citizens of Hamburg, Germany)

(continued)

Table 15-3 *(continued)*

This Food Item	Was Born Here
Jambalaya	Louisiana (combination of French Canadian [Cajun] with native coastal cookery)
Potato chips	Saratoga Springs, New York (credited to George Crum, a Native American/African American chef at the Moon Lake Lodge resort in Saratoga Springs, New York, in 1853)
Spoon bread	Southern United States (adapted from Native American corn pudding)
Vichyssoise	New York (commonly attributed to Louis Diat, chef at the Ritz Carlton Hotel in New York in 1917, who is said to have named the cold potato-and-cream soup in honor of the city of his birth, Vichy, France)

James Trager, The Foodbook (New York: Grossman Publishers, 1970); About.com, http://cooking fortwo.about.com/od/soupssaladssandwiches/r/Vichyssoise.htm.

Chapter 16

Building a Healthful Diet

The American Heart Association says to edit your consumption of fats and cholesterol. The American Cancer Society says to eat more fruits and veggies. The National Research Council says to watch out for fats, sugar, and salt. The American Diabetes Association says to eat regular meals so your blood sugar stays even. The Food Police say if it tastes good, forget it!

The U.S. Departments of Agriculture and Health and Human Services have incorporated virtually all these rules into the *Dietary Guidelines for Americans 2010* — and added some advisories of their own. But in the end, creating and enjoying the food choices that make a body better is up to you. So this chapter lays out some, yes, *guidelines*.

What Are The Dietary Guidelines for Americans?

The Dietary Guidelines for Americans is a collection of reality-based, sensible nutrition suggestions first published by the U.S. Departments of Agriculture and Health and Human Services (USDA/HHS) as a skinny, 20-page booklet in 1980. Since then, USDA/HHS have published six revised editions (1985, 1990, 1995, 2000, 2005, 2010), with the latest weighing in at a hefty 110 pages, with so many words, sentences, and paragraphs — some repeated several times — that it was not released until January 31, 2011, one month into the timetable for the *Dietary Guidelines 2015*.

The most user-friendly of the seven sets of Guidelines is the 2000 version, which seems to have been written by real people who actually like real food. You could see this philosophy right up front in the first sentence in the first paragraph: "Eating is one of life's greatest pleasures."

Contrast that with the first sentence of the *Dietary Guidelines for Americans 2005*: "The *Dietary Guidelines for Americans*, first published in 1980, provides science-based advice to promote health and reduce risk for chronic disease through diet and physical activity." Alas, what you saw was what you got: A frankly cranky, bare-bones, chilly presentation of the facts.

The 2010 edition is a verbose but directed pull-up-your-bootstraps-and-get-with-the-program document with a single-minded focus on the fact that too many Americans weigh too much (see Chapter 4). The take-away message could not be more clear: *Control what you eat to control your weight to control your health.*

Note: Throughout this chapter, when you read "see Chapter X," it means the chapter in this book, not in the Guidelines.

What's New in 2010

The 2010 Guidelines sets its goal in the first paragraph of the Executive Summary: "Eating and physical activity patterns that are focused on consuming fewer calories, making informed food choices, and being physically active can help people attain and maintain a healthy weight, reduce their risk of chronic disease, and promote overall health."

The fat-fighting recommendations are organized into 6 stand-alone chapters, 16 appendixes, 8 tables, and 11 figures, with a bonus of 2 blank pages for note-taking.

In general, the changes in the Guidelines over the years can be tracked in subtle shifts in emphasis. For example, from 1980 to 1995, the Guidelines offered the simple admonition to "Eat a variety of foods." Then in 2000, that was expanded to suggest using the Food Guide Pyramid (see Chapter 17) to make nutritious choices including a variety of grains, fruits and vegetables.

While the new Guidelines continue this kind of change, some new things are in the mix:

- Cut back dramatically on sodium.
- Lower the percentage of saturated fat in your diet from 10 percent to 7 percent if possible while avoiding *artificial* trans fats entirely.
- Don't eat so many foods with *added* sugars.
- Get enough vitamin D, calcium, potassium, iron, and vitamin B12.
- Eat 8 ounces of seafood a week.
- Investigate a vegetarian diet.

> ✔ Exercise enough to meet the standards set by the 2008 Physical Activity Guidelines for Americans (available online at www.health.gov/paguidelines).
>
> ✔ Keep food safe

More specific data about these new recommendations is (where else?) in the following sections.

Take this with fewer grains of salt

In 1980, the Guidelines advised consumers to "Avoid too much sodium" (1980). By 2000, that had mutated to "Choose and prepare foods with less salt." In 2010, the advice is (some say) draconian.

Most Americans consume about 3,400 mg (1.5 teaspoons) sodium a day. The Guidelines say, "Enough already" and advise everyone to cut that to 2,300 mg/day, about 1 teaspoon of table salt. If you are older than 51 or are African American or have hypertension (high blood pressure), diabetes, or chronic kidney disease, the recommendation is even more stringent. People in this group, which includes about half of all Americans, should take in no more than 1,500 mg sodium per day, about ⅔ teaspoon table salt.

These recommendations have stirred some serious discussion because most people have no problems with sodium. They eat a lot one day, a little less the next, and their bodies adjust. Others, however, don't react so evenly. For them, a high-sodium diet appears to increase the risk of high blood pressure. When you already have high blood pressure, you can tell fairly quickly whether lowering the amount of salt in your diet lowers your blood pressure. But no test is available to predict whether someone who doesn't have high blood pressure will develop it by consuming a diet that's high in sodium. That begs the question: Should medical advice that works for some people be applied to *all* people?

Interestingly enough, moderating your salt intake may have an unadvertised benefit: Lowering your weight a bit. Why? Because sodium is *hydrophilic* (*hydro* = water; *philic* = loving). Sodium attracts and holds water. When you eat less salt, you retain less water, you're less bloated, and you feel thinner.

Don't reduce salt intake drastically without first checking with your doctor. Remember, sodium is an essential nutrient. That's why the Guidelines advocate moderate use, not *no* use at all.

Factoring fats

Nothing is new about nutrition advice advising less fat. Right from the start in 1980, the Guidelines said to "Avoid too much fat, saturated fat, and cholesterol." Keeping daily cholesterol intake under 300 mg has been standard advice almost as long, and the advice to consume a diet "moderate in total fat" showed up in 2000, as did the advice to keep saturated fats to less than 10 percent of total calories.

So what's new here? This:

- Hold your total fat consumption at 20 to 35 percent of daily calories.

- Reduce your intake of sat fats to less than 7 percent of your total daily calories.

- Push your consumption of artificial ("synthetic" or "industrial") trans fats, also called partially hydrogenated fatty acids, as far down as possible. (The naturally occurring trans fats in some foods from animals such as milk and cheese are not included because cutting them from your diet would eliminate lots of important nutrients.)

- Keep cholesterol consumption to less than 300 mg/day; 200 mg/day is even better.

Word to the fat-wise #1: You can reduce your intake of solid fats in food, and thus your intake of sat fats, simply by wielding a sharp knife to cut away as much visible fat as possible from meat and poultry, as well as stripping off the fat-laden poultry skin.

Word to the fat-wise #2: Liquid fats, otherwise known as oils, are mixtures of sat fats and unsaturated fats. Table 8-1, in Chapter 8, shows which oils are high in saturated fatty acids and which are not.

Subtract the added sugar

Yes, this means editing your diet to reduce foods to which sugar is added, such as cakes and cookies, *not* foods such as fruits with naturally occurring sugars. And for the first time, the Guidelines specifically mention sugar-rich soft drinks, suggesting that you substitute water, fat-free milk, 100 percent fruit juice, or unsweetened tea and coffee.

Did you catch what drink is missing from that calorie-free list? Right: No diet sodas. Why? Because some studies suggest that rather than helping you lose weight, these drinks actually lead to weight gain, perhaps by leading you to eat things you wouldn't otherwise have chosen ("I had a diet soda, so I can have a brownie").

In 2005, a team of researchers at the University of Texas Healthy Science Center, San Antonio, released data from an 8-year, 1,550 person study showing that among people drinking sodas sweetened with sugar, the risk of becoming overweight or even obese was

- 26 percent for those drinking up to ½ can daily

- 30.4 percent at ½ to 1 can daily

- 32.8 percent at 1 to 2 cans daily

- 47.2 percent at more than 2 cans daily

No surprise there. But look at the risk for people drinking diet soft drinks:

36.5 percent for those drinking up to ½ can daily

37.5 percent at ½ to 1 can daily

54.5 percent at 1 to 2 cans daily

57.1 percent at more than 2 cans daily

In others words, statistically speaking, the risk for gaining lots of weight rose 41 percent for each can of diet drink a day. Water looks better and better, doesn't it?

Get adequate essential nutrients

For various reasons, even an adequate diet may be deficient in specific nutrients. One example is the fact that as we age, our bodies may be less able to absorb vitamin B12 from food, meaning that supplements are sensible.

This edition of the Guidelines stresses the need to obtain adequate amounts of seven specific nutrients:

- **Potassium:** The potassium in your food can counter the effects of sodium on blood pressure while lowering your risk of kidney stones and loss of bone density.

- **Dietary fiber:** This indigestible food component helps reduce the risk of cardiovascular disease and gastrointestinal problems such as constipation.

- **Calcium:** Bones. Bones. Bones. Get the message?

- **Vitamin D:** More bones, bones, bones (vitamin D enables your body to absorb calcium), plus a host of yet-to-be-proven health benefits such as breast health.

✔ **Iron and folate:** Essential for women who may become pregnant; the first protects the woman's health, and the second protects that of her developing fetus.

✔ **Vitamin B12:** Important for older folk who may be able to absorb less from food.

For the recommended amounts of each nutrient, as well as a more detailed explanation of their benefits, check out Chapter 9 (dietary fiber), Chapter 11 (vitamins), and Chapter 12 (minerals).

Fish for good food

Finding a balance in what fish to eat and how much can be challenging. On the one hand, fish provides undeniably beneficial omega-3 fatty acids (see Chapter 8). On the other hand, some fish is contaminated with methylmercury, a toxic metal that can wreak neurological and cardiovascular havoc particularly in the fetus and in children.

Taking this into account, the Guidelines recommend that

✔ Children and women who are of child-bearing age, pregnant, or nursing avoid *all* King mackerel, shark, swordfish, and tile fish, species widely acknowledged to be highly contaminated.

✔ These individuals eat no more than 12 ounces of fish a week, including no more than 6 ounces of canned albacore tuna.

With these caveats, the Guidelines recommend increasing your intake of fish and seafood from the current per person average of 3.5 ounces/week to at least 8 ounces/week with choices from the list of low-mercury seafood. The Guidelines makes this a cinch with Appendix 11, a chart showing methylmercury content of various types of fish. To access the chart, click `www.cnpp.usda.gov/Publications/DietaryGuidelines/2010/PolicyDoc/Appendices.pdf` and scroll down to Appendix 11, stopping on the way to check out any subject that piques your interest.

Bring on the veggies

In 1980, the first Guidelines directed consumers to "Eat foods with adequate starch and fiber." By 1990, that had become "Choose a diet with plenty of vegetables, fruits, and grain products." Today, the new, direct directive is to make half of your plate vegetables and fruits. Maybe the whole plate: The Guidelines say right out, no mincing words here, those vegetarian-style diets are associated with a variety of health benefits including lower weight, a lower risk of heart disease, and — best of all — a longer life.

Finally, two new charts, Appendix 8 and Appendix 9, detail (respectively) "Lacto-ova Adaptations of USDA Food Patterns" (meal planning for vegetarians who eat dairy products) and "Vegan Adaptations of USDA Food Patterns" (for people who eat only plant foods).

Be active

True, the Guidelines have always suggested moving vigorously every day. What's new this time is the advice to follow the recommendations of the U.S. Health and Human Services' *2008 Physical Activity Guidelines for Americans* (available online at www.health.gov/paguidelines/pdf/paguide.pdf).

Exercise and weight

When you take in more calories from food than you use up running your body systems (heart, lungs, brain, and so on) and doing a day's physical work, you end up storing the extra calories as body fat. In other words, you gain weight. The reverse also is true. When you spend more energy in a day than you take in as food, you pull the extra energy you need out of stored body fat, and you lose weight.

You don't have to be a mathematician to reduce this principle to two simple equations in which E stands for energy (in calories), > stands for greater than, < stands for less than, and W stands for the change in weight:

> If E in > E out: E total = +W
>
> If E in < E out: E total = –W

It's not Einstein's theory of relativity, but you get the picture.

For real-life examples of how the energy-in, energy-out theory works, stick your bookmark in this page and go to Table 3-1 in Chapter 3 to find out how to calculate the number of calories a person can consume each day without pushing up the poundage.

Even being mildly active increases the number of calories you can wolf down without gaining weight. The more strenuous the activity, the more plentiful the calorie allowance. Suppose that you're a 25-year-old man who weighs 140 pounds. The formula in Table 3-1 shows that you require 1,652 calories a day to run your body systems. Clearly, you need more calories for doing your daily physical work, simply moving around, or exercising.

Other reasons to exercise

The Guidelines are correct: Weight control is a good reason to step up your exercise level. But it isn't the only one. Here are four more:

✔ **Exercise increases muscles.** When you exercise regularly, you end up with more muscle tissue than the average bear. Because muscle tissue weighs more than fat tissue, athletes (even weekend-warrior types) may end up weighing more than they did before they started exercising to lose weight. But a higher muscle-to-fat ratio is healthier and more important in the long run than actual weight in pounds. Exercise that changes your body's ratio of muscle to fat gives you a leg up in the longevity race.

✔ **Exercise reduces the amount of fat stored in your body.** People who are fat around the middle as opposed to the hips (in other words an apple shape versus a pear shape) are at higher risk of weight-related illness. Exercise helps reduce abdominal fat and thus lowers your risk of weight-related diseases. Use a tape measure to identify your own body type by comparing your waistline to your hips (around the buttocks). If your waist (abdomen) is bigger, you're an apple. If your hips are bigger, you're a pear.

✔ **Exercise strengthens your bones.** Osteoporosis (thinning of the bones that leads to repeated fractures) doesn't happen only to little old ladies. True, on average, a woman's bones thin faster and more dramatically than a man's, but after the mid-30s, everybody — male and female — begins losing bone density. Exercise can slow, halt, or in some cases even reverse the process. In addition, being physically active develops muscles that help support bones. Stronger bones equal less risk of fracture, which, in turn, equals less risk of potentially fatal complications.

✔ **Exercise increases brainpower.** You know that aerobic exercise increases the flow of oxygen to the heart, but did you also know that it increases the flow of oxygen to the brain? When a rush job (or a rush of anxiety) keeps you up all night, a judicious exercise break can keep you bright until dawn. According to nutrition research scientist Judith J. Wurtman, PhD, when you're awake and working during hours that you'd normally be asleep, your internal body rhythms tell your body to cool down, even though your brain is racing along. Simply standing up and stretching, walking around the room, or doing a couple of sit-ups every hour or so speeds up your metabolism, warms up your muscles, increases your ability to stay awake, and, in Dr. Wurtman's words, "prolongs your ability to work smart into the night." Eureka!

How to exercise

The Guidelines describe three basic types of activity to strengthen heart and lungs, muscles, and bones.

✔ **Aerobic activity** increases heart rate and breathing. Moderate aerobic activity includes walking briskly, bicycling on a level path, and dancing. Intense aerobic activity includes jogging, playing single tennis, or bicycling uphill.

✔ **Muscle-strengthening activity,** such as resistance training, increases the mass and strength of skeletal muscles — that is your arms, legs, back, and so on.

✔ **Bone-building activity** is any exercise, such as running or lifting weights, that makes an impact on your bones.

How much exercise does your body really need?

After you decide to start moving, the Guidelines say, do it every day. How much should you do? Table 16-1 shows the basic recommendations for everyone older than 6; healthy adults may benefit from longer or more intense activity.

Table 16-1   Working Out the Rules for Working Out

Age (Male & Female)	Overall (All Types of Exercise)	Aerobic*	Muscle-Building	Bone-Building
6–17	60 min/day	Every day; intense, at least 3 days/week	At least 3 days/week	At least 3 days/week
18–64	Any activity is beneficial; more is better	2.5 hours/week (moderate); 75 min/week (intense)	2+ days a week	
65+	The adult regimen; any activity within physical limitations is beneficial; older adults should include exercises that improve balance			

Aerobic activity should be done in 10-minute segments.

Keep your food safe

In 2010, the Centers for Disease Control and Prevention (CDC) estimated that spoiled or contaminated food causes between 29 and 71 million illnesses a year in the United States, as many as 215,000 of them serious enough to require hospitalization, with up to 5,000 deaths.

Clearly, keeping food safe to eat is an important goal, important enough to repeat the Guidelines advice here, as well as in Chapters 19, 20, and 21. Having four chapters in one book with info about one subject tells you how important it is, doesn't it?

This equation is one any clean food cook can rely on:

Clean stores + clean hands + clean kitchen + proper storage + proper temperature = safe food

Right now, raw is popular but not — as the Guidelines explain — necessarily healthful. To reduce your risk of picking up an icky bacterial disease along with dinner, the Guidelines advise avoiding "raw" (unpasteurized) milk or any products made from unpasteurized milk (such as cheeses); raw or partially cooked eggs or any dish containing raw eggs; raw or undercooked meat and poultry; unpasteurized juices; and raw sprouts.

Not everybody can — or should — run right out and start chopping down trees or throwing touchdown passes to control his or her weight. In fact, if you have gained a lot of weight recently, have been overweight for a long time, haven't exercised in a while, or have a chronic medical condition, you need to check with your doctor before starting any new regimen. (***Caution:*** Check out of any health club that puts you right on the floor without first checking your vital signs — heartbeat, respiration, and so on.)

Do the Guidelines Work?

Yes. No. Maybe. And who knows?

On the plus side, the Guidelines offer a template for building a healthful diet.

On the down side, not many people take the time to do the building. It is indisputable that the obesity that so worries the authors of the 2010 Guidelines exploded in the years during which the Guidelines were available. Because it is impossible to prove a negative, there is no way to say whether there would be even more overweight Americans without the Guidelines.

As a result, the release of the 2010 Guidelines, like the publication of the six previous editions, has triggered specific criticisms from various corners of the food and nutrition world. In general, the critiques echo four broad complaints:

- ✔ **First:** These are nice rules, but nobody follows them. Proof? The 2005 Guidelines said to eat at least 2.5 cups of fruits and veggies a day, but studies show that only an infinitesimal 4 percent of us — 4 out of every 100 Americans — does that.

- ✔ **Second:** There's still too much emphasis on foods from animals (meat, fish, poultry, dairy products), reflecting a bow to the food industry. Of course, the industry groups see this from the other side, which is why the Salt Institute argues that, "No modern society consumes so little salt, making this proposal [to reduce salt intake even further] as nothing less than a call for an uncontrolled experiment on more than 300 million Americans."

- ✔ **Third:** The authors write off scientific studies with which they do not agree. For example, The Metabolism Society, a group of nutrition researchers and medical professionals, contends USDA/HHS ignore evidence pointing to the benefits of a low-carbohydrate diet for weight loss, insulin regulation, and protection against chronic disease.

✔ **Fourth:** The emphasis on food components such as fats, carbs, vitamins, and minerals contradicts the fact that real people eat food, not nutrients. People who espouse this point of view want the guidelines to recommend specific foods — maybe even specific menus — not theoretical nutrition concepts.

So, with all that, are the Guidelines worth the trouble?

Probably.

Life is not a test. No one loses points for failing to follow the USDA/HHS advice every single day of the year. Nobody's perfect, and these rules can certainly be broken — once in a while.

For example, ideally you should hold your daily intake of cholesterol to less than 300 mg/day. But you can bet that you'll exceed that amount this Saturday when you stroll by the buffet at your best friend's wedding and see Camembert cheese (2 wedges = 54 mg cholesterol), sirloin steak (7 oz = 192 mg cholesterol), salad with Thousand Island dressing (4 tbsp = 45 mg cholesterol), and 3.5 ounces vanilla ice cream (44 mg cholesterol).

Proving the proposition

Unlike previous Guidelines whose claims were simply set out for you to read and adapt or adopt, the 2010 version actually gives you standards by which to evaluate the authors' advice.

✔ **Strong evidence** describes advice based on lots of well-designed studies that include a broad range of consumers. Example: "Research has shown that when larger portion sizes are served, people tend to consume more calories. In addition, *strong evidence* shows that portion size is associated with body weight, such that being served and consuming smaller portions is associated with weight loss."

✔ **Moderate evidence** means that the evidence is pretty good but not up to the standard set by studies showing strong evidence. For example: "*Moderate evidence* shows that adults who eat more whole grains, particularly those higher in dietary fiber, have a lower body weight compared to adults who eat fewer whole grains."

✔ **Limited evidence** means that the evidence comes from smaller or less reliable studies and may not be consistent. For example: ". . . *limited evidence* suggests that increased intake of 100 percent juice has been associated in higher body weight in children and adolescents who are overweight or obese."

Needless to say, many nutritionists and food manufacturers disagree on exactly what studies fit which category. But for now, these standards are a start at something more than simply saying, "Do it because I tell you to." The next Guidelines, scheduled for 2015, will tell whether they were right.

Is this a crisis? Should you stay home? Must you keep your mouth shut tight all night? Are you kidding? Here's the Real Rule: Let the good times roll every once in a while. After the party's over, compensate.

For the rest of the week, go back to your exercise regimen and back to your healthful menu emphasizing lots of the nutritious, delicious, low- or no-fat foods that should make up most of your regular diet.

In the end, you're likely to have averaged out to a desirable amount with no fuss and no muss and be right in line with that headline from the first page of the 2000 Guidelines that I mention at the beginning of this chapter: "Eating is one of life's greatest pleasures."

And the Guidelines, imperfect though they may be, offer some, well, guidelines, on how to make that your nutritionally healthful mantra.

Where to find the Guidelines

To read and/or download the *Dietary Guidelines for Americans 2010* or the Executive Summary, go to www.health.gov/dietary guidelines.

To review earlier editions of the Guidelines, scroll down the page and click the appropriate line. To track the evolution of the Guidelines, scroll to the left and click History.

Prefer print? Hard copies of the *Dietary Guidelines for Americans 2010* are available from the U.S. Government Printing Office either by phone at (866) 512-1800 or from http://bookstore.gpo.gov.

Finally, USDA is launching interactive programs on its Web site to make it easier to plan healthy meals, as well as games and apps to promote healthy eating and exercise. Check out some of them at www.appsforhealthykids.com.

Chapter 17

Making Wise Food Choices

This is a chapter devoted to diagrams, specifically the multiple food Pyramids, sets of nutrition building blocks for grown-ups. Instead of letters in the alphabet, these blocks represent food groups that you can put together in various ways to create the picture of a healthful diet.

Choose one, take notes, follow directions, then choose another, create a different pattern, and so on. Any way you play, your reward is likely to be a better body.

Playing with Blocks: Food Pyramids

The essential message of all good guides to healthful food choices is that no one food is either good or bad — how much and how often you eat a food is what counts. With that in mind, a food pyramid delivers three important messages:

✔ **Variety:** The fact that the pyramid contains several blocks tells you that no single food gives you all the nutrients you need.

✔ **Moderation:** Having blocks smaller than others tells you that although every food is valuable, some — such as fats and sweets — are best consumed in small amounts.

✔ **Balance:** You can't build a pyramid with a set of identical blocks. Blocks of different sizes show that a healthful diet is balanced: the right amount from each food group.

Clearly, food pyramids make it possible for you to eat practically everything you like — as long as you follow the recommendations on how much and how frequently (or infrequently) to eat it.

The original USDA Food Guide Pyramid

The first food pyramid was created by the U.S. Department of Agriculture (USDA) in 1992 in response to criticism that the previous government guide to food choices — the Four Food Group Plan (vegetables and fruits, breads and cereals, milk and milk products, meat and meat alternatives) — was too heavily weighted toward high-fat, high-cholesterol foods from animals.

Figure 17-1 depicts the original USDA Food Guide Pyramid. As you can see, this pyramid is based on daily food choices, showing you which foods are in what groups. Unlike the Four Food Group Plan, the pyramid separates fruits and vegetables into two distinct groups and lists the number of servings from each food group that you should have each day. (The number of servings is provided in ranges. The lower end is for people who consume about 1,600 calories a day, and the upper end is for people whose daily dietary intake nears 3,000 calories.)

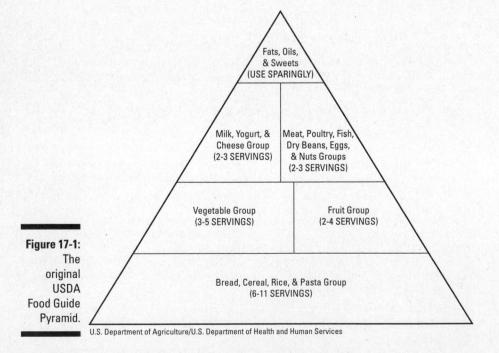

Figure 17-1:
The original USDA Food Guide Pyramid.

Fats, Oils, & Sweets
(USE SPARINGLY)

Milk, Yogurt, & Cheese Group
(2-3 SERVINGS)

Meat, Poultry, Fish, Dry Beans, Eggs, & Nuts Groups
(2-3 SERVINGS)

Vegetable Group
(3-5 SERVINGS)

Fruit Group
(2-4 SERVINGS)

Bread, Cereal, Rice, & Pasta Group
(6-11 SERVINGS)

U.S. Department of Agriculture/U.S. Department of Health and Human Services

Food fight

You might think that once the government came up with this apparently sensible way to decide what's good to eat, everyone in the nutrition establishment would stand up as one to shout, "Huzzah!"

You would be wrong. The complaints began practically the minute the Pyramid hit the street, so to speak.

On the one hand, critics said the Pyramid was indecisive, lumping all fats — good, bad, and in-between — into one category and failing to distinguish between whole grains (good) and refined grains (not great).

On the other hand, critics said the advice was decisive, but in the wrong direction — for example, by allowing more red meat than considered optimal by the real (or at least the emerging) science.

And everybody asked, "How come there's no picture or sentence to tell us to exercise every day to control our weight?"

What to do? Nutritional acrobatics. In 2005, the USDA released a new Food Guide Pyramid which is actually the first Pyramid turned sideways and then stuck into an interactive Web site at www.mypyramid.gov.

This version of the Pyramid has

- Unlabeled sections representing the foods in your daily diet, each identified by color: Orange for grains, green for vegetables, red for fruits, yellow for oils, blue for milk, and purple for meat and beans

- An admonition to eat "lots of different kinds of foods to build a better diet," but no specific servings-per-day recommendations for any food group

- Directions on how to key certain data into a form to find out how many servings of each food group you should eat based on your age, sex, and level of activity, but not — to everyone's surprise — your height and weight

- Steps, actual steps, with a teensy gender-neutral human being climbing up the side of the pyramid to signify (1) physical activity and (2) the fact that you don't have to leap tall buildings in a single bound like Superman (or woman) to improve your nutrition because even small steps can make a big difference

All of which may have been new. But improved? Not so much.

For one thing, all those dietary fats are still stuck together in one category. For another, this Pyramid seemed still to be designed for one perfect person eating one, probably rather boring, "American" diet.

Call me foolish. Call me old-fashioned. Call me a fan of the simplest solution. Which, it seems, is no longer a Pyramid. In May 2011, USDA introduced the new new thing, a plate that shows (sort of) how much of each type of food you should be consuming. More veggies. Fewer meats. So now you can click onto the USDA web site listed above and pull up the latest version of the Totally Official Food Guide Pyramid, sorry, Plate.

Do you disagree? No problem. You can visit www.mypyramid.gov and pull up the latest version of the Totally Official Food Guide Pyramid. Or you can check out one of the following from the Loyal Oppositions.

Pick a perfect Pyramid

Government documents, including Food Guide Pyramids, are often one-size-fits-all — meaning they might not fit you.

Are you a fan of Asian food? Do you like your menu with a Central or South American accent? Does meat turn you off?

Answer yes to any of these questions, and the bad news is that the "official" USDA plate may not be the one for you. The good news is that if you answer yes to any of these questions, there is a special food guide waiting for you.

The Oldways Preservation trust, a Boston-based, internationally known, nonprofit organization devoted to improving our diet with *"positive programs grounded in science, traditions, and delicious foods and drink,"* has created a number of pyramids based on ethnic food plans, perhaps the best known being the Mediterranean Diet Pyramid. The following Oldways pyramids are a guide to good food in various languages (for more about Oldways itself, click www.oldwayspt.org).

The Asian Diet Pyramid

Oldways' partners for this pyramid, introduced at the International Conference on the Diets of Asia in San Francisco in 1995, were the Cornell-China-Oxford Project on Nutrition, Health, and Environment and the Harvard School of Public Health. This pyramid, which you can see at www.oldwayspt.org/asian-diet-pyramid, codifies a primarily vegetarian diet historically linked to the generally low-incidence of cardiovascular disease in Asian countries.

The Vegetarian Diet Pyramid

This pyramid, created by Oldways and the Harvard School of Public Health, was released at the International Conference on Vegetarian Diets in Austin Texas, in 1997. It is a traditional vegetarian plan with fruits, vegetables, grains, and dairy products, but no meat, fish, or poultry, a food plan described as promoting "agricultural sustainability." Translation: Producing these foods takes up less, and thus wastes less, of our natural resources — land, fuel, and water — than modern industrial food production. Good for you; good for the planet.

To see this pyramid, go to www.oldwayspt.org/vegetarian-diet-pyramid.

The Traditional Mediterranean Diet Pyramid

Oldways and the Harvard School of Public Health released the first Mediterranean diet pyramid in 1993; this updated version appeared in 2009. As you can see at www.oldwayspt.org/mediterranean-diet-pyramid, this pyramid has lots of fruits and veggies, poultry and *lean* red meat, olive oil, cheese, and yogurt — all accompanied by moderate amounts of wine. In short, the traditional diet of, yes, the Mediterranean countries circa 1960 when, Oldways explains, "The rates of chronic disease were among the lowest in the world, and adult life expectancy was among the highest, even though medical services were limited." Tastes good, too.

The Latin American Diet Pyramid

Oldways introduced this pyramid, shown at www.oldwayspt.org/latino-diet-pyramid, in 1996 at the Latin American Diet Conference in El Paso, Texas; the updated version appeared in 2009. The food plan in this pyramid is based on the traditional and modern-day diet of Central and South America, which Oldways describes as a melding of three distinct cultures: the indigenous Aztecs, Incas, and Mayans; the 16th-century Spanish explorer; and the Africans brought in first as slaves. The mixture produced a rich blend of local fruit (agave, avocado), vegetables (cassava, chayote), grains (amaranth, maize, quinoa), poultry, and meat (goat), once again accompanied by moderate amounts of alcohol. Plus exercise, of course.

The indulgent vegetarian

The University of Michigan Integrative Medicine, a program that brings together both traditional and complementary medical practices, introduced this pyramid in 2010 (see www.med.umich.edu/umim/food-pyramid). They call it the Healing Foods Pyramid, but you might call it the Semi-Vegetarian Indulgence Pyramid. Yes, it features daily servings of legumes, soy foods, healthy fats (avocados, nuts, seeds, nut butters, and unsaturated oils), an ounce of dark chocolate, and 2 to 4 cups of tea (lower caffeine white or green preferred), plus moderate amounts of alcohol. But it also allows lean meat or poultry in 3-ounce servings, up to three times a week each.

Understanding the Nutrition Facts Labels

Once upon a time, the only reliable consumer information on a food label was the name of the food inside. The 1990 Nutrition Labeling and Education Act changed that forever with a spiffy new set of consumer-friendly food labels that include

- ✔ A mini-nutrition guide that shows the food's nutrient content and evaluates its place in a balanced diet

- ✔ Accurate ingredient listings, with all ingredients listed in order of their weight in the original recipe. For example, the most prominent ingredient in a loaf of bread would be flour

- ✔ Clear identification of ingredients previously listed simply as *colorings* and *sweeteners*

- ✔ Scientifically reliable information about the relationship between specific foods and specific chronic health conditions, such as heart disease and cancer

The Nutrition Facts label is *required by law* for more than 90 percent of all processed, packaged foods, everything from canned soup to fresh pasteurized orange juice. Food sold in really small packages — a pack of gum, for example — can omit the nutrition label but must carry a telephone number or address so that an inquisitive consumer (you) can call or write for the information.

Just about the only processed foods exempt from the nutrition labeling regulations are those with no appreciable amounts of nutrients, those whose content varies from batch to batch, and those from very small food processors:

- ✔ Plain (unflavored) coffee and tea

- ✔ Some spices and flavorings

- ✔ Deli and bakery items prepared fresh in the store where they're sold directly to the consumer, as well as food produced by small companies

- ✔ Food sold in restaurants, unless it makes a nutrition content or health claim (How do you eat well when eating out? Check out Chapter 18.)

Labels are voluntary for fresh raw meat, fish, or poultry and fresh fruits and vegetables, but many markets — perhaps under pressure from customers — have put posters or brochures with generic nutrition information near the meat counter or produce bins.

Just the facts, ma'am

The star of the Nutrition Facts label is the Nutrition Facts panel on the back (or side) of the package. This panel features three important elements: serving sizes, amounts of nutrients per serving, and Percent Daily Value (see Figure 17-2).

Figure 17-2:
A typical
Nutrition
Facts panel.

Nutrition Facts	
Serving Size 1 Cup (240mL)	
Servings Per Container 2	
Amount Per Serving	
Calories 120	Calories from Fat 45
	% Daily Value*
Total Fat 5g	8%
Saturated Fat 3.5g	18%
Trans Fat 0g	
Cholesterol 25mg	8%
Sodium 120mg	5%
Total Carbohydrate 11g	4%
Dietary Fiber 0g	0%
Sugars 11g	
Protein 8g	16%
Vitamin A 10% · Vitamin C 2%	
Calcium 30% · Iron 0% · Vitamin D 25%	
* Percent Daily Values are based on a 2,000 calorie diet. Your daily values may be higher or lower depending on your caloric needs.	

Serving size: This varies from package to package. Serving sizes don't always reflect the typical amount that an adult may eat. In some cases, the serving size may be a very small amount.

Calories: The calories contained in a single serving.

% daily values: The percentage of nutrients that one serving contributes to a 2,000-calorie diet. Parents or children may need more or less than 2,000 calories per day.

Nutrient amounts: The nutritional values of the most important, but not all, vitamins and other nutrients in the product.

Serving size

No need to stretch your brain trying to translate gram-servings or ounce-servings into real servings. This label does it for you, listing the servings in comprehensible kitchen terms such as 1 cup or one waffle or two pieces or 1 teaspoon. It also tells you how many servings are in the package.

The serving size is exactly the same for all products in a category. In other words, the Nutrition Facts chart enables you to compare at a glance the nutrient content for two different brands of yogurt, cheddar cheese, string beans, soft drinks, and so on.

When checking the labels, you may think the suggested serving sizes seem small (especially with so-called low fat items). Think of these serving sizes as useful guides.

Amount per serving

The Nutrition Facts chart tells you the amount (per serving) for several important factors:

✔ Calories

✔ Calories from fat

✔ Total fat (in grams)

✔ Saturated fat (in grams)

✔ Trans fats (in grams)

✔ Cholesterol (in milligrams)

✔ Total carbohydrate (in grams)

✔ Dietary fiber (in grams)

✔ Sugars, those occurring naturally in the food *and* the ones added during preparation (in grams)

✔ Protein (in grams)

Percent Daily Value

The Percent Daily Value enables you to judge whether a specific food is high, medium, or low in fat, cholesterol, sodium, carbohydrates, dietary fiber, sugar, protein, vitamin A, vitamin C, calcium, and iron.

The Percent Daily Value for vitamins and minerals is based on a set of recommendations called the *Reference Daily Intakes (RDI),* which are similar (but not identical) to the Recommended Dietary Allowances (RDAs) for vitamins and minerals discussed in Chapters 11 and 12.

RDIs are based on allowances set in 1973, so some RDIs now may not apply to all groups of people. For example, the Daily Value for calcium is 1,000 milligrams, but many studies — and two National Institutes of Health Conferences — suggest that postmenopausal women who are not using hormone replacement therapy need to consume 1,500 milligrams of calcium a day to reduce their risk of osteoporosis.

The Percent Daily Values for fats, carbohydrates, protein, sodium, and potassium are based on the *Daily Reference Values (DRV).* DRVs are standards for nutrients, such as fat and fiber, known to raise or lower the risk of certain health conditions, such as heart disease and cancer.

Examples of the DRVs are

✔ Saturated fat — less than 10 percent of your calories/9 calories per gram

✔ Carbohydrates — 60 percent of your calories/4 calories per gram

✔ Protein — 10 percent of your calories/4 calories per gram

Sounds authoritative, but the %DV (that's short for Percent Daily Value), as shown on the Nutrition Facts labels, is behind the times. Newer recommendations say

✔ Total fat calories should account for no more than 20 to 35 percent of total daily calories.

✔ No safe level exists for saturated fats or trans fats, thus no %DV is provided for either one. *Note:* The total amount of saturated fat in the portion is the number of grams of sat fat plus the number of grams of trans fat.

✔ Calories from carbs should account for 45 to 65 percent of daily calories.

✔ Women younger than 50 need to consume 25 grams of dietary fiber a day; men younger than 50, 38 grams. After age 51, it's 21 grams for women and 30 grams for men.

✔ Calories from protein should account for about 20 percent of total daily calories.

Will this change the numbers on the Nutrition Facts labels? The sensible answer is, eventually. Are the current Nutrition Facts labels still useful? Absolutely.

Relying on labels: Health claims

Ever since man (and woman) came out of the caves, people have been making health claims for certain foods. These folk remedies may be comforting, but the evidence to support them is mostly anecdotal: "I had a cold. My mom gave me chicken soup, and here I am, all bright-eyed and bushy-tailed. Of course, it did take a week to get rid of the cold completely. . . ."

Is anybody listening?

It may depend on how hungry you are. In 2010, the *Journal of the American Dietetic Association* published a Columbia University report showing that nearly 62 percent of food shoppers read the Nutrition Facts label and that those who read it consume fewer calories, total fat, sat fat, and sugar overall. But in 2011, three years after New York City became the first city in the country to require calorie labeling in fast-food restaurants, a New York University School of Medicine (NYU SOM) study showed that while nearly as many people saw the calorie information as read the Nutrition Facts label, fewer than 10 percent said it influenced their food choices.

Possible conclusion: People who are hungry *right now* pay less attention to nutrition information than people who are buying food to eat when they get hungry later on. Sounds real.

On the other hand, health claims approved by the USDA and the Food and Drug Administration (FDA) for inclusion on the new food labels are another matter entirely. If you see a statement suggesting that a particular food or nutrient plays a role in reducing your risk of a specific medical condition, you can be absolutely 100 percent sure that a real relationship exists between the food and the medical condition. You can also be sure that scientific evidence from well-designed studies supports the claim.

In other words, USDA/FDA-approved health claims are medically sound and scientifically specific. They highlight the known relationships between

- ✔ **Calcium and bone density:** A label describing a food as "high in cal-cium" may truthfully say: "A diet high in calcium helps women maintain healthy bones and may reduce the risk of osteoporosis later in life."

- ✔ **A diet high in fat, saturated fat, and cholesterol and a higher risk of heart disease:** A label describing a food as "low fat, low cholesterol," or "no fat, no cholesterol" may truthfully say: "This food follows the recom-mendations of the American Heart Association's diet to lower the risk of heart disease."

- ✔ **A high-fiber diet and a lower risk of some kinds of cancer:** A label describing a food as "high-fiber" may truthfully say: "Foods high in dietary fiber may reduce the risk of certain types of cancer."

- ✔ **A high-fiber diet and a lower risk of heart attack:** A label describing a food as "high-fiber" may truthfully say: "Foods high in dietary fiber may help reduce the risk of coronary heart disease."

- ✔ **Sodium and hypertension (high blood pressure):** A label describing a food as "low-sodium" may truthfully say: "A diet low in sodium may reduce the risk of high blood pressure."

- ✔ **A fruit-and-vegetable-rich diet and a low risk of some kinds of cancer:** Labels on fruits and vegetables may truthfully say: "A diet high in fruits and vegetables may lower your risk of some kinds of cancer."

- ✔ **Folic acid (folate) and a lower risk of neural tube (spinal cord) birth defects such as spina bifida:** Labels on folate-rich foods may truthfully say: "A diet rich in folates during pregnancy lowers the risk of neural tube defects in the fetus."

Foods with more than 4 grams saturated fat and/or saturated fat plus trans fat per serving cannot have any health claims at all on their labels.

No, you can't say that!

In the summer of 2009, Big Food — a group of brand names familiar to us all — launched a program called Smart Choices. The main objective was to stick a bright green emblem on the front label of certain foods they claimed met Federal nutrition standards, as explained in mind-numbing detail at www.smartchoices program.com/professionals.html.

And that's how a bunch of products including Froot Loops and Cocoa Puffs, formerly regarded as high-sugar *no-no*s, suddenly became health food.

Until the Food and Drug Administration stepped in to say, "No, no," noting that it was planning its very own set of front label info and was definitely not happy to see "misleading" or conflicting nutrition information on the nation's grocery shelves. Or, as Commissioner Margaret Hamburg put it during a phone call with inquiring reporters: "There are products that have gotten the Smart Choices check mark that are almost 50 percent sugar."

In other words, you can stuff yourself with sugared cereals, but you can't pretend they're good to eat.

Ah, well.

How high is high? How low is low?

Today, savvy consumers reach almost automatically for packages labeled "lowfat" or "high fiber." But it's a dollars-to-doughnuts sure bet that hardly one shopper in a thousand knows what "low" and "high" actually mean.

Because these are potent terms that promise real health benefits, the new labeling law has created strict, science-based definitions:

✔ *High* means that one serving provides 20 percent or more of the Daily Value for a particular nutrient. Other ways to say "high" are "rich in" or "excellent source," as in "milk is an excellent source of calcium."

✔ *Good source* means one serving gives you 10 to 19 percent of the Daily Value for a particular nutrient.

✔ *Light* (sometimes written *lite*) is used in connection with calories, fat, or sodium. It means the product has one-third fewer calories or 50 percent less fat or 50 percent less sodium than usually is found in a particular type of product.

- ✔ *Low* means that the food contains an amount of a nutrient that enables you to eat several servings without going over the Daily Value for that nutrient.

    - *Low-calorie* means 40 calories or fewer per serving.

    - *Low fat* means 3 grams of fat or less.

    - *Low saturated fat* means less than 0.5 gram trans fat per serving and 1 gram (or less) saturated fat.

    - *Low-cholesterol* means 20 milligrams or less.

    - Low sodium means 140 mg sodium or less per serving.

- ✔ *Reduced saturated fat* means that the amount of saturated fat plus trans fat has been reduced more than 25 percent from what's normal for the given food product.

- ✔ *Free* means "negligible" — not "none."

    - *Calorie-free* means fewer than 5 calories per serving.

    - *Fat-free* means less than 0.5 gram of fat.

    - *Trans fat-free* means the food has less than 0.5 gram trans fat and 0.5 gram saturated fat per serving.

    - *Cholesterol-free* means less than 2 milligrams of cholesterol or 2 grams or less saturated fat.

    - *Sodium-free* or *salt-free* means less than 5 milligrams of sodium.

    - *Sugar-free* means less than 0.5 gram of sugar.

Notice something missing? Right, there's no definition for "low sodium" per serving. On the other hand, a meal plan with less than 1,000 milligrams sodium per day is considered a low-sodium diet.

Listing what's inside

The extra added attraction on the Nutrition Facts label is the complete ingredient listing, in which every single ingredient is listed in order of its weight in the product, heaviest first, lightest last. In addition, the label must spell out the true identity of some classes of ingredients known to cause allergic reactions:

- ✔ Vegetable proteins (*hydrolyzed corn protein* rather than the old-fashioned *hydrolyzed vegetable protein*)

- ✔ Milk products (*nondairy* products, such as coffee whiteners, may contain the milk protein caseinate, which comes from milk)

- ✔ FD&C yellow No. 5, a full, formal chemical name instead of *coloring*

Organic: The not-quite-finished label term

Organic (as in organic food) is a highly charged food word. But do you know what it means? Don't be embarrassed to say no. Until recently, neither did most health professionals.

To a chemist, *organic* means a substance that contains carbon, hydrogen, and oxygen. By this chemical standard, all foods — and all human beings — are organic.

Yet some people adopted the word *organic* to describe plant foods grown without pesticides or synthetic chemicals, or to describe the poultry, fish, beef, and lamb from animals raised on a diet with no antibiotics or other medicating chemicals to assure healthy and efficiently producing animals.

But these descriptions were not standards regulated by any federal agency. So the USDA set out to create regulations that legally define the term:

✔ In December 1997, the USDA released its first proposal on new standards for organic foods.

✔ In May 1998, after receiving more than 280,000 comments from the public, food growers, and food marketers, the agency announced that although bioengineered and irradiated foods are safe, they're not permitted to carry the organic label.

✔ In October 1998, the USDA issued three more proposals on how animals yielding organic food are to be treated and how the agency will certify producers of organic foods.

✔ In October 2002, the USDA implemented rules saying that foods carrying the organic label must be grown without pesticides or raised without non-organic feed.

✔ In February 2003, Congress passed legislation allowing organic livestock to be given non-organic feed at any time the price of organic feed reaches two times that of the regular stuff, but the organic livestock must be kept in humane conditions.

✔ In 2004, an amendment to an appropriations bill allowed "organic" foods to contain some synthetic ingredients, after which the terms used for organic foods were redefined as follows:

- "100 percent organic" — single ingredient such as a fruit, vegetable, meat, milk, and cheese (excludes water and salt)

- "Organic" — multiple ingredient foods that are 95 to 100 percent organic

- "Made with organic ingredients" — 70 percent of the ingredients are organic (This note can appear on the front of package, naming the specific ingredients.)

- "Contains organic ingredients" — contains less than 70 percent organic ingredients

Will this change again? Probably. For the latest, go to The National Organic Program's "Organic Labeling and Marketing Information" at www.ams.usda.gov/AMSv1.0/getfile?d DocName=STELDEV3004446&acct=no pgeninfo.

Naming the precise source of sweeteners (*corn sugar monohydrate* rather than just *sugar monohydrate*) is still voluntary, but as is true of information about raw meat, fish, and poultry, manufacturers and stores just may respond to consumer pressure.

Choosing Healthful Foods with the Nutrition Facts Label

The Food Guide Pyramid helps balance meals and snacks. In the kitchen, you can increase the nutritional value by thinking of individual dishes as mini food pyramids. At snack time, you can use the Food Guide Pyramid to choose munchies that are a valuable part of your overall daily diet.

For example, although you know that fruits and veggies are good snacks, that doesn't mean that you're stuck with boring carrot sticks or an apple. The food pyramid says "fruits and vegetables," not raw fruits and raw vegetables. Yes, a fresh apple's fine. But so is a baked apple (100 calories), fragrant with cinnamon and decorated with no-fat sour cream (30–45 calories for 2 table-spoons). Carrot strips are okay. So are vegetarian baked beans — yes, baked beans (140 calories plus 26 grams of carbohydrates, 7 grams of protein, 7 grams of dietary fiber, and 2 grams of fat per ½ cup serving), which are con-sidered both veggies *and* a member of the high-protein meat/beans group.

As for the Nutrition Facts label, you can use that as a tool to eat your cake and have it nutritiously by comparing products to choose the best alternatives.

Here's a good example: You find yourself irresistibly drawn to double dark chocolate ice cream (lots of fat, saturated fat, cholesterol, and a whopping 230 calories per ½ cup serving). But then, just as your hand is opening the freezer door, ready to reach for the ice cream, suddenly . . . out of the corner of your eye, you see the Nutrition Facts panel on the label of the no-fat but equally irresistible chocolate sorbet. It says, "No fat, no saturated fat, no cholesterol, and only 90 to 130 calories per serving." When you put the labels side by side, do you need to ask which one comes out the winner?

You — because you get to indulge while protecting your nutrition status. Who could ask for anything more?

Chapter 18

Eating Smart When Eating Out

In This Chapter

▶ Navigating a restaurant menu

▶ Ordering without overdoing

▶ Setting sensible substitutes

▶ Finding nutritious fast-food favorites

*E*ating out is pure pleasure: You don't have to cook, and somebody else washes the dishes. The challenge? To avoid letting luxury lull you into ceding responsibility for your food choices to some chef whose heart belongs to butter.

This chapter lays out strategies for making your adventure nutritionally sound. One trick is to edit a menu in a *white-tablecloth* restaurant (the food professional's description of an upscale eatery) to balance gustatory pleasure with common-sense nutrition. A second is to juggle fast-food choices to fit them into a healthful diet.

No cooking, no dishes, no guilt. Who could ask for anything more?

Interpreting a Restaurant Menu

Restaurants are businesses; they respond to consumer demand. Unfortunately, what consumers have demanded for years are rich foods and big portions. Does that mean you should stop eating out? No. But it does mean you need to use caution when ordering from the menu.

Pinpointing portions

Restaurants don't make friends by serving up teensy little portions. In fact, tiny servings probably sank *nouvelle cuisine,* the 1980s fad that put one string bean, three garden peas, half an artichoke heart, and one sliced cherry tomato on a lettuce leaf and called it the salad course.

Reality dictates that the portions on most restaurant plates rarely come within striking distance of the official serving sizes issued by the U.S. Department of Agriculture. To protect yourself from humongous servings, you need to fix a picture of real-life versions of the recommended portions firmly in your mind.

The task requires an 8-ounce measuring cup, a kitchen scale, and some basic foods.

- ✔ **Meat, fish, and poultry:** Broil a small steak or roast a chicken breast. Use a kitchen scale to weigh a 3-ounce portion. Does the steak look like a deck of cards? How about a small calculator? That's one serving.

- ✔ **Rice and pasta:** Boil some rice or pasta. When it's done, fill the measuring cup to the halfway mark. Take out the rice or pasta and roll it into a tennis ball or a billiard ball. Whatever. That's one serving.

- ✔ **Salads:** Shred some greens. Fill the measuring cup to the 8-ounce mark. Turn the greens out onto a salad plate. That's one serving.

- ✔ **Fruits and veggies:** Dice some fresh apples or carrots or open one can of beets or fruit cocktail. Fill the measuring cup to the halfway mark. Spoon the fruit or vegetables onto a plate. That's one serving.

- ✔ **Beverages:** Open a can of soda or a box of juice. Pour the liquid into the measuring cup, right up to the 8-ounce mark. Pour that into a glass. It's probably more than you get in an upscale restaurant, less than you get at the burger barn. No matter: It's still one serving.

Now that you know what a serving looks like, you can slice away the extra from your restaurant plate — and take it home for lunch or dinner the next day. That's what *doggie bags* are for. (Cat owners will know that doggie bags are called doggie bags because cats are too smart — or, too finicky — to eat someone else's leftovers.)

Asking for proof

When the menu says, "Eat me! I'm healthy," ask for proof. The people who make and market processed foods are required by law to provide detailed ingredient labels on their packages.

In the past few years, legislators have been moving to pass laws that regulate healthful eating in restaurants. For example, chain restaurants must now post the calorie counts and ingredients in their dishes online or at the store. The open listing wave is also lapping at the doors of those chic, white tablecloth establishments.

For the moment, those fancy restaurants still don't have to tell you exactly what's in the beef Stroganoff or vegetable stir-fry. But if any restaurant makes a health claim, writing "low-fat" or "heart-healthy" next to an item on the menu or marking the entry with a little red heart to signify the same thing, the Nutrition Education and Labeling Act says the restaurant has to back up that claim. The law doesn't require an ingredient listing on the menu; the restaurant can comply by making a notebook available that accomplishes at least one of the following tasks:

✔ The notebook can list the nutrient content of each labeled dish or show that the dish was made according to a recipe from an authoritative professional association or dietary group, such as the American Heart Association.

✔ The notebook can show that the nutritional values for the dish are based on a reliable nutrition guide, such as the USDA's voluminous *Agriculture Handbook No. 8,* which is made up of several volumes with perhaps a thousand pages of nutritional analysis for all kinds of food. As with the new, improved labels on food packages, this policy is designed to make sure that any food that claims to be healthy actually is.

For more on the growing move to legislate good nutrition in restaurants as well as grocery stores, see Chapter 18.

Making Smart Menu Choices

From a nutritional point of view, once you get past the serving size, restaurant dining has two other basic pitfalls:

✔ Garnishes and side dishes are too rich.

✔ Meals have too many courses.

Not to worry. The following stratagems solve these two problems.

Starting simple

Set the nutritional tone of dinner right off the bat with your choice of appetizer. You have two possible alternatives. The first alternative is to opt for a really rich, high-density food, such as a cream soup, and then coast downward, calorie-fat-and-cholesterol-wise, for the rest of the meal.

A second alternative is to go the other way, choosing a tasty but low-calorie, lowfat appetizer, such as clear soup, a salad with lemon juice dressing, or shellfish — shrimp cocktail comes in a cost of just 10 to 30 calories per shrimp — with no-fat (catsup/horseradish) sauce, thus allowing yourself richer choices later in the meal.

Elevating appetizers to entrees

For smaller portion sizes or to skip the calorie-laden sides that come with most entrees, order an appetizer as your main course. For example, many restaurants serve an appetizer consisting of a really big bowl of maybe 30 steamed mussels in their shells in a low-oil, fresh tomato sauce with perhaps one crusty piece of French bread underneath to sop it up. When you add a glass of cold, dry white wine and one more piece of bread, this appetizer becomes a meal in itself with fewer calories and less fat than most any entree on the menu.

Less expensive, too.

Skipping the fat on the bread

Don't butter your bread. Don't oil it, either. Many restaurants serve up a dish of flavored olive oil in place of butter. True, the olive oil has less saturated fat than butter, and it has no cholesterol, but the calorie count is exactly the same. All fats and oils (butter, margarine, vegetable oils) give you about 100 calories a tablespoon. And you may get even more calories from the oil if you do a lot of dipping.

Consumer alert: Don't assume that your bread is lowfat just because you didn't butter it. Many different types of breads come already buttered (or oiled). One example is focaccia, the thick, savory Italian bread. Others are popovers and muffins.

To test the fat content of your bread, pick up a piece or put it on your napkin. If your hand feels greasy or the bread leaves an oily spot on your napkin, you have your answer.

Going naked: Undressed veggies

Victorians boiled vegetables practically into oblivion — no color, no texture, no taste. Then came 20th-century butter, cheese, and cream sauces, often burnished under the broiler to a browned crust.

Then *natural* became the watchword, and steaming took over. But in fact, you don't have to settle for boring steamed stuff or for veggies like cauliflower that taste like cardboard when raw. (The difference between raw cauliflower and cauliflower that's been steamed for 15 or 20 minutes and dusted with dill is so vast that people who insist on passing out the stuff cold should be charged with vegetable abuse.)

Today, smart restaurant cooks rely on herbs and spices, *reduced* (boiled down and thickened) fat-free bouillons, unusual salad combinations, and imaginative treatments, such as purees and kabobs, to make their vegetables tasty but trim. The result? Food heaven and nutrition joy as the vegetable flavors come through, and the calories stay very, very, very low.

To reap the low-calorie rewards, simply avoid veggie dishes labeled

- ✔ Au beurre (with butter)
- ✔ Au gratin (with cheese sauce)
- ✔ Batter-dipped (eggs, oil, fried)
- ✔ Breaded (breadcrumbs, oil, fried)
- ✔ Fritters (fried)
- ✔ Fritto (fried)
- ✔ Tempura (battered and fried)

Minimizing the main dish

From a nutritionist's point of view, the most sensible dinner choice may be something broiled, baked, or roasted — without added fat, and with the drippings siphoned off. But you can also lower the fat content of any main dish simply by wielding a mean knife and fork to cut away the vestiges of visible fat on your chops or steak or the skin-on poultry.

Another approach is to order a main course meat dish without the "main" part. That is, order your meat, fish, or poultry as a small-serving appetizer and then ask your waiter for a veggie entree. Or opt for an assortment of the side dishes that usually accompany the meat course instead of a veggie entree.

Demand tiny boiled onions. Baby peas with mint. Pickled beets and red cabbage. Sugared carrots. Sautéed spinach. Darling little boiled or baked potatoes with a crust of paprika or cumin. The more, the merrier. The result may not be entirely fat-free, but it almost certainly has fewer calories, less fat, more dietary fiber, and a wider variety of nutrients than plain meat or poultry.

Sidelining sauces

Dining out is a treat, so treat yourself — within reason. Have your *béarnaise* (egg yolks, butter), *béchamel* (butter, flour, heavy cream), brown sauce (beef drippings, flour), and hollandaise (butter, egg yolks), as long as you have them in reasonable amounts.

Ask the waiter to bring the sauce on the side, take a tablespoonful (about a soup spoonful), and hand back the rest.

When ordering from an Italian menu, the general rule is to avoid the olive-oil-based sauces and choose the tomato-based red sauce because many restaurants now make their red sauces skinny — all tomato, with little or no oil.

Satisfying your sweet tooth

After a heavy meal, your body often craves something sweet. Lower your calories and fat totals by splitting a dessert with your dinner partner. Or pick a rich but fat-free sweetened coffee such as espresso or a Greek or Turkish brew. Or tea. Or a diet cola.

Or, on special occasions, a small after-dinner wine or liqueur, about 100 to 200 calories per ounce, but no fat, thank you.

Discovering the Healthful Side of Fast Food

Fast food can be good food. By choosing carefully, you can enjoy burgers while still meeting recommended daily dietary allowances for all important nutrients plus vitamins and minerals. A fast-food burger on a bun, plus a salad and either a small, lowfat milk shake, an 8-ounce cup of milk, a small cola, or plain old water may not sound like great nutrition, but the version served up in some fast-food restaurants is actually relatively low in fat and relatively high in valuable nutrients.

Choosing wisely at the drive-through

The greatest problem with fast food, as with all restaurant food, is *very* big servings with *very* high calorie counts and *very* scary fat content. Case in point: McDonald's Angus bacon and cheeseburger which clocks in at 790 calories, 39 grams of fat (17 of them artery-clogging sat fat), plus 145 mg cholesterol.

On the other hand, who says you have to choose that burger? Table 18-1 compares the nutrient values of three basic McDonald's meals that qualify as sensible in anyone's diet book.

For the record:

✔ The burger in these three meals is the basic, small, no-frills hamburger just as it comes from the grill.

✔ The salad is a small side salad with one packet of Newman's Own lowfat balsamic vinaigrette dressing.

✔ The parfait is the Fruit 'N Yogurt without granola.

✔ The milk is an 8-ounce container of lowfat (1 percent) milk.

✔ The soda is a small (16-ounce) diet Coke.

All three meals derive less than 30 percent of their calories from fat, are relatively low in cholesterol, and provide respectable amounts of dietary fiber and bone-building calcium.

But nothing's perfect: Each of these combos delivers more than half the day's sodium allowance in one moderately small meal. And substitutes are potential saboteurs. Adding just one small serving of McDonalds fries piles on another 230 calories plus an extra 8 percent DV total fat.

Finally, two notes about Table 18-1:

✔ *Note #1:* The Daily Value, often abbreviated as DV, is a nutritional guideline suggesting how much of each nutrient you need each day on a 2,000-calorie diet. For a detailed explanation of the DV and how it's used on food labels, check out Chapter 17.

✔ *Note #2:* The numbers in this table are accurate as of this writing. But menus and ingredients are subject to change, so check the nutrition brochure at your local burger heaven or online from time to time. You never know when something new — good or not so good — may pop up on your plate.

Table 18-1	Nutritious Fast-Food Meals? Yes!		
Nutrient (% Daily Value/ DV)*	Burger, Salad, Milk (462 Calories)	Burger, Salad, Parfait, Water (440 Calories)	Burger, Salad, Small Diet Cola (270 Calories)
Calories from fat	21%	20%	17%
Saturated fat	24%	21%	16%
Cholesterol	13%	11%	9%
Dietary fiber	12%	12%	12%
Vitamin C	35%	42%	31%
Calcium	42%	32%	12%
Sodium	57%	54%	53%

Source: McDonald's Corporation, as of January 2007, at http://nutrition.mcdonalds.com/nutritionex-change/nutritionfacts.pdf.

Finding fast-food ingredient guides

All fast-food restaurants now make nutrition information widely available — in some cities by law, in others by choice. McDonald's even puts its numbers on the food wrapper.

If your local eatery doesn't have brochures on hand or post them on the wall, don't be shy: Write, call, or click for a copy.

Note: Companies that don't give you a mailing address usually have a "write us" e-mail form on their Web sites.

Arby's
Consumer Affairs Department
1155 Perimeter Center West
Atlanta, GA 30338
Phone 800-487-2729
Web site www.arbys.com (click Nutrition)

Burger King Corporation
5505 Blue Lagoon Dr.
Miami, FL 33126
Phone 305-378-3535
Web site www.bk.com (click Nutrition)

Dunkin' Donuts
Consumer Care
130 Royall St.
Canton, MA 02021
Phone 800-859-5339
Web site www.dunkindonuts.com (select Nutrition under About Us)

KFC (Kentucky Fried Chicken)
P.O. Box 725489
Atlanta, GA 31139
Phone 800-225-5532
Web site www.kfc.com (click Nutrition)

McDonald's
2111 McDonald's Dr.
Oak Brook, IL 60523
Phone 800-244-6227
Web site www.mcdonalds.com (click Food and then click Nutrition)

Pizza Hut
14841 Dallas Pkwy.
Dallas, TX 75254
Phone 800-948-8488
Web site www.pizzahut.com (click Contact Us and then click Nutritional
Information)

Quiznos
1001 17th Street, Suite 200
Denver, CO 80202
Phone: 866-4-TOASTED
Web site www.quiznos.com (click the red box labeled Menu when it appears)

Subway
325 Bic Dr.
Milford, CT 06460
Phone 800-888-4848 or 203-877-4281
Web site www.subway.com (click Menu/Nutrition)

Wendy's
Customer Service Department
4288 W. Dublin-Granville Rd.
Dublin, OH 43017
Phone: 614-764-3100
Web site www.wendys.com (click Food)

Fast facts for fatigued fingers

Too tired to troll through the separate sites for individual fast-food restaurants? Head for www.nutritiondata.com.

On the home page, slide your mouse to the right where you find Nutrition Topics. Run down this list to *Fast-food nutrition facts* for restaurants like *Arby's, Burger King, McDonald's, Starbucks, and more*. Click the Fast-food nutrition facts entry to pull up a long list of dishes, brand-name and generic, each with a complete analysis of nutrients. The data includes a familiar Nutrition Facts Label chart plus charts showing the calorie count per portion, plus fats and fatty acids, protein and amino acids, vitamins, minerals, sterols (the fatty compounds cholesterol, in animal foods, and phytosterols, in plants), and "other" (water and stimulants).

Part IV
Food Processing

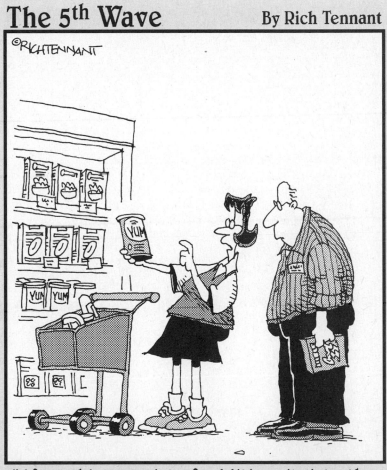

"After this long list of additives, it lists the expiration date. Does that pertain to the product or the person who eats it?"

In this part . . .

Have you ever wondered why canned green beans aren't as green as fresh ones? Or why an originally translucent egg white turns white when you cook it? Or why frozen carrots are mushy when you defrost them? Or — modern technology at its most mysterious — why exposing food to radiation keeps it fresh longer? Wonder no more. Just shift your eyes to the right to find out what happens when you cook, freeze, dry, or zap food.

Chapter 19

What Is Food Processing?

In This Chapter
▶ Preserving foods through processing
▶ Improving flavor, aroma — and nutrition
▶ Introducing substitutes for fat and sugar
▶ Following one bird through the processing process

Say "processed food," and most people think "cheese spread." They're right, of course. Cheese spread is, in fact, a processed food. But so are baked potatoes, canned tuna, frozen peas, skim milk, pasteurized orange juice, and scrambled eggs. In broad terms, food processing is any technique that alters the natural state of food — cooking, freezing, pickling, drying, and so on.

This chapter describes how each form of processing changes food from a living thing (animal or vegetable) into a component of a healthful diet — and at the same time

✔ Lengthens shelf life

✔ Reduces the risk of foodborne illnesses

✔ Maintains or improves a food's texture and flavor

✔ Upgrades the nutritional value of foods

Preserving Food: Five Methods of Processing

When you are talking about food, the term *natural* doesn't necessarily translate as "safe" or "good to eat." Food spoils (naturally) when microbes living (naturally) on the surface of meat, a carrot, a peach, or whatever reproduce (naturally) to a population level that overwhelms the food (naturally).

Sometimes you can see, feel, or smell this happening. You can *see* mold growing on cheese, *feel* how meat or chicken turns slippery, and *smell* when the milk turns sour. The mold on cheese, the slippery slickness on the surface of the meat or chicken, and the odor of the milk are caused by exploding populations of microorganisms. Don't even argue with them; just throw out the food.

Food processing reduces or limits the growth of food's natural microbe population thus lengthening the shelf life of food and lowering the risk of food-borne illnesses.

For simplicity's sake, here's a list of the methods used to extend the shelf life of food:

- Temperature methods
  - Cooking
  - Canning
  - Refrigeration
  - Freezing
- Air control
  - Canning
  - Vacuum-packaging
- Moisture control
  - Dehydration
  - Freeze-drying (a method that combines methods of controlling the temperature, air, and moisture)
- Chemical methods
  - Acidification
  - Mold/bacteria inhibition
  - Salting (dry salt or brine)
- Irradiation
- High-pressure processing

Temperature control

Exposing food to high heat for a sufficiently long period of time reduces the natural population of bacterial spoilers and kills microbes that otherwise may make you sick. For example, *pasteurization* (heating milk or other liquids such as fruit juice to 145 to 154.4 degrees Fahrenheit for 30 minutes) kills nearly all pathogens (disease-causing microorganisms) and most other bacteria, as does high-temperature, short-time pasteurization (161 degrees Fahrenheit for 15 seconds).

Chilling also protects food by slowing the rate of microbial reproduction. For example, milk refrigerated at 50 degrees Fahrenheit or lower may stay fresh for almost a week because the cold prevents organisms that survived pasteurization from reproducing.

Removing the water

Like all living things, the microbes on food need water to survive. Dehydrate the food, and the bugs won't reproduce, which means the food stays edible longer. That's the rationale behind raisins, prunes, and *pemmican,* a dried mix of meat, fat, and berries adapted from East Coast Native Americans and served to 18th- and 19th-century sailors of every national stripe. Dehydration (loss of water) occurs when food is

- ✔ Exposed to air and sunlight
- ✔ Heated for several hours in a very low (250 degrees Fahrenheit) oven or smoked (the smokehouse acts as a very low oven)

Controlling the air flow

Just as microbes need water, most also need air. Reducing the air supply almost always reduces the bacterial population.

Foods are protected from air by vacuum-packaging. A *vacuum* — from *vacuus,* the Latin word for "empty" — is a space with virtually no air. Vacuum-packaging employs a container (generally a plastic bag or a glass jar) from which the air is removed before it's sealed. When you open a vacuum-packed container, the sudden little pop you hear is the vacuum being broken.

Tantalizing tidbit of food nomenclature

Central American Indians dried meat to produce *chaqui,* a name carried north by Spanish explorers who used it to describe the dried meats of the Southwestern Indians, which eventually became — you saw this coming, right? — jerky.

If there's no popping sound, the seal has already been broken, allowing air inside, and that means the food inside may be spoiled or may have been tampered with. Do not taste-test: Throw out the entire package, food and all.

Chemical warfare

About two dozen chemicals are used as *food additives* or *food preservatives* to prevent spoilage. The most common are:

- **Acidifiers:** Most microbes don't thrive in highly acidic settings, so a chemical that makes a food more acidic prevents spoilage. Wine and vinegar are acidifying chemicals, and so are *citric acid,* the natural preservative in citrus fruits, and *lactic acid,* the natural acid in yogurt.

- **Mold inhibitors:** Sodium benzoate, sodium propionate, and calcium propionate slow (but do not entirely stop) the growth of mold on bread. Sodium benzoate also is used to prevent the growth of molds in cheese, margarine, and syrups.

- **Bacteria-busters:** Salt is *hydrophilic* (hydro = water; phil = loving). So is sugar. When you cover fresh meat with salt (or sugar), the salt (or sugar) draws water up and out of the meat — and up and out of the cells of bacteria living on the meat. The bacteria die; the meat dries. And you get to enjoy sugar-cured ham or corned beef (which gets its name from the fact that large grains of salt were once called "corns").

Irradiation

Irradiation is a technique that exposes food to electron beams or to *gamma radiation,* a high-energy light stronger than the X-rays your doctor uses to make a picture of your insides. *Gamma rays* are ionizing radiation, the kind that kills living cells. As a result, irradiation prolongs the shelf life of food by destroying microbes and insects on plants (which also make food safer longer) and slowing the rate at which some plants ripen. For a detailed discussion of the history and effects of irradiation, check out Chapter 21.

Improving Food's Appeal and Nutritional Value

Some food processing really does make your food taste better: A well-broiled steak is generally conceded to taste better than a raw one. Processing also allows you to sample a wide variety of seasonal foods (mostly fruits and vegetables) all year long. And it enables food producers to improve the nutritional status of many basic foods, such as grains and milk, by enriching or altering them to meet the needs of modern consumers.

Intensifying flavor and aroma

One advantage of food processing is that it enables you to enjoy things never seen in nature, such as the ever-popular — and ever-criticized — cheese spread. A more mundane benefit of food processing is that it intensifies aroma and flavor, almost always for the better. Here's how:

- **Drying concentrates flavor.** A prune has a different, darker, more intensely sweet flavor than a fresh plum.

- **Heating heightens aroma by quickening the movement of aroma molecules.** In fact, your first tantalizing hint of dinner usually is the scent of cooking food. Chilling has the opposite effect: It slows the movement of the molecules. To sense the difference, sniff a plate of cold roast beef versus hot roast beef straight from the oven. Or sniff two glasses of vodka, one warm, one icy from the freezer. One comes up scent-free; the other has the olfactory allure of pure gasoline. Guess which is which.

- **Warming foods intensifies flavors.** This development is sometimes beneficial (warm roast beef is somehow more savory than cold roast beef), sometimes not (warm milk is definitely not as popular as the icy-cold version).

- **Changing the temperature changes texture.** Heating softens some foods (butternut squash is a good example) and solidifies others (think eggs). Chilling keeps the fats in pâté firm so the stuff doesn't melt down into a puddle on the plate. Ditto for the gelatin that keeps dessert molds and dinner aspics standing upright.

Adding nutrients

The addition of vitamins and minerals to basic foods has helped eliminate many once-common nutritional deficiency diseases. The practice is so common that you take the following for granted:

- Breads, cereals, and grains are given extra B vitamins to replace the vitamins lost when whole grains are stripped of their nutrient-rich covering to produce white flour or white rice or degermed cornmeal. The vitamin enrichment reduces the risk of the B vitamin–deficiency diseases beriberi and pellagra.

- Breads, cereals, and grains are also fortified with iron to replace what's lost in milling.

✔ All milk sold in the United States contains added vitamin D to reduce the risk of the bone-deforming vitamin D–deficiency diseases rickets (among children) and osteomalacia (among adults).

✔ Added fat-free milk proteins turn *skim milk* — milk from which the fat has been removed — into a creamier liquid with more calcium but less fat and cholesterol than whole milk.

Combining benefits

Adding genes from one food (such as corn) to another food (such as tomatoes) may make the second food taste better and stay fresh longer. You can bet that this is one hot topic; for more about genetic engineering at the dinner table, check out Chapter 22.

Faking It: Food Substitutes

In addition to its many other benefits, food processing offers up some totally fake but widely appreciated substitute fats and sweeteners. Actually, these may be just the tip of the iceberg, so to speak. In 1985, the Brits introduced Quorn, a brand-name meat substitute made from fungi that had become the No. 1 meat substitute worldwide when it was first brought to the United States in 2002. Quorn seems to have slipped back into the nutritional netherworld in the United States, but as processing becomes more adventurous, who knows what strange and wonderful dishes lie just beyond the entrance to the Nutritional Twilight Zone?

Alternative foods No 1: Fat replacers

Dietary fat (the fat found naturally in food) carries flavors and makes food taste and feel "rich." But it's also high in calories, and some fats (the saturated and trans fats described in Chapter 8) can clog your arteries. One way to deal with this problem is to eliminate the fat from food, as in skim milk. Another way is to head for the food lab and create a no- or low-calorie substitute that will not clog your arteries.

Classifying fat replacers

Over the years, food technologists have created three types of fat replacers:

✔ *Carbohydrate-based fat replacers* are complex carbohydrates that thicken food but are not absorbed by the body. (For more on the different types of carbohydrates in plant foods, see Chapter 9.) Examples of natural carb-based fat replacers are carrageenan (a seaweed extract), guar gum (from guar beans), cellulose (insoluble dietary fiber), inulin (from the chicory root), and modified food starches (complex carbohydrates from grains chemically treated to change its texture or make it easier to dissolve and digest). *Oatrim* is a manufactured carb-based fat substitute made from modified oat flour, which is rich in gums called beta-glucans. *Stellar* is a fat substitute made from corn starch. *Z trim* is made from bran (soy, oats, grains, and so on) fiber.

✔ ***Protein-based fat replacers*** are commonly made by heating and blending proteins from egg whites and milk into tiny balls (technical term: *microparticulated protein*) that form a substance that feels and tastes like fat. Simplesse is a protein-based fat substitute. ***Note:*** These products do not provide significant amounts of dietary protein.

✔ ***Fat-based fat replacers*** are made from naturally occurring fats that have been modified so that they are indigestible; they block the body's absorption of other fats. *Olestra* is a fat- (and sugar-) based fat substitute. *Salatrim,* whose name comprises the first letter of the words *short-and long-chain acyl triglyceride molecules* is another fat-based fat substitute. (For more on triglycerides, see Chapter 8.)

Table 19-1 lists several examples of fat replacers currently found in foods.

Table 19-1		Finding the Fake Fats
Fat Replacer	*Calories/ Gram* ₁	*Used in*
Carbohydrate-based		
Natural		
Cellulose	0	Dairy products (such as imitation sour cream)
Gums	0	Baked goods, sauces, and salad dressings
Inulin	1–1.2	Baked goods (including fillings, icing), dairy products (including cheese, whipped cream), meat products
Modified food starch	1–4	Baked goods, salad dressings, various dessert products
Manufactured		
Oatrim	<1	Baked goods, nonfat milks (such as nonfat whipped "cream")
Stellar	1	Baked goods, margarines, salad dressing, commercial soups, processed cheese products

(continued)

Table 19-1 (continued)

Fat Replacer	Calories/ Gram [1]	Used in
Z trim	0	Baked goods, salad dressings, sauces, soups, meat products
Protein-based		
Simplesse [2]	1.3	Cold milk products (ice cream, yogurt), salad dressings (including mayonnaise)
Fat-based		
Olestra (Olean [tm])	0	Snack foods, baked goods
Salatrim (Benefat [tm])	5	Baked goods, "filled" milk products [3]

[1] The carbohydrates and protein in food provide 4 calories per gram; dietary fat has 9 calories per gram.
[2] Simplesse degrades when heated.
[3] Milk whose natural fat is removed and replaced with another.

Evaluating fat replacers

Regardless of their source, the three important nutrition questions about fat replacers are

✔ Do these additives contribute to weigh loss?

✔ Do these additives enhance the nutrient value of food?

✔ Are these additives safe?

Do fat replacers help people lose weight?

Maybe.

One reason food manufacturers use fat replacers is to reduce the amount of fat and therefore the number of calories in ordinarily high-calorie foods such as cakes, cookies, and potato chips. But lowering the fat content may mean increasing calories from other ingredients such as sugar. In the end, the calorie count of the lowfat food may not be much lower than that of the regular product.

On the other hand, even if the calorie count stays the same, simply adding the fat replacer may alter, in a good way, how the food affects your body. In 2008, a team of nutrition researchers from the University of Copenhagen published a report in the *American Journal of Clinical Nutrition* showing that when volunteers were given one of two meals — the first with foods with their normal fats in place, the second with foods whose fats had been replaced with Salatrim — those who got the second meal were less hungry for a longer period of time after eating. Why? The authors explain that Salatrim is not absorbed by the body, and it inhibits the body's absorption of other fats in food. As a result, more food fat stays in the intestines longer, creating the feeling of fullness that decreases appetite.

That being said, calorie control, a balanced diet, and a reasonable amount of exercise remain the most healthful tools for weight loss.

Are fat replacers nutritious?

Carbohydrate-based fat replacers do add carbs to food in the form of soluble or insoluble dietary fiber (Chapter 9, again). But neither protein-based fat replacers nor fat-based fat replacers contribute anything but infinitesimal amounts of nutrients. In addition, because natural food fats help your body dissolve and absorb fat soluble nutrients (see Chapter 11), foods made with these substitute fats commonly contain added vitamin A, vitamin D, vitamin E, and vitamin K.

Are fat replacers safe?

The adverse effects of carb-based fat replacers such as Z Trim are very small and usually limited to minor gastro discomfort such as flatulence (intestinal gas) due to an increase in dietary fiber.

Fat-based replacers are more problematic.

Eating lots of food made with Olestra/Olean may cause diarrhea. When FDA approved Olestra in 1996, the FDA-required label stated that Olestra might cause abdominal cramping and loose stools. In 1998, an 18-member FDA food advisory committee reaffirmed the agency's original decision that Olestra/Olean is safe for use in snack foods and concluded that the fat alternative's gastrointestinal effects did not significantly affect public health. Five years later, following a review of several studies conducted after foods with Olestra/Olean went on sale, the FDA concluded that the statement was no longer required. But the fact is that eating excess amounts of Olestra/Olean-altered food may still lead to uncomfortable results. Be smart: Read labels and limit the chips.

A second fat-based fat replacer, *Simplesse,* is made of milk and egg proteins, which means it may be problematic for people who are

✔ Sensitive to milk (the label on a food with Simplesse must carry the word "milk")

✔ Sensitive to eggs

✔ On low-protein diets (for example, kidney disease patients)

In the end, the American Heart Association has written that while "fat replacers on the market are considered safe by the U.S. Food and Drug Administration (FDA), their long-term benefits and safety are not known. The cumulative impact of using multiple fat replacers as they increase in the marketplace is unknown. Still, within the context of a healthy diet that meets dietary recommendations, fat replacers used appropriately can provide flexibility with diet planning."

Alternative foods No. 2: Substitute sweeteners

Most substitute sweeteners were discovered by accident in laboratories where researchers touched a paper or a pencil and then stuck their fingers in their mouths to discover, "Eureka! It's sweet." As Harold McGee wrote in the first edition of his wonderful *On Food and Cooking* (Collier Books, 1988), "These stories make one wonder about the standards of laboratory hygiene." (Alas, when Mr. McGee updated and expanded his book for the second edition, he took out most of the trenchant observations such as this one. Get the second edition for the details; keep the first for the fun.)

Because substitute sweeteners are not absorbed by your body and don't provide any nutrients, scientists call them by their proper name: *non-nutritive sweeteners.* The best-known (listed in order of their discovery and/or FDA approval) are:

- ✔ **Saccharin (Sweet 'N Low):** This synthetic sweetener was discovered by accident (the fingers-in-the-mouth syndrome) at Johns Hopkins in 1879. A ban on saccharin was proposed in 1977, after it was linked to bladder cancer in rats; however, it's still on the market, and diabetics who have used saccharin for years show no excess levels of bladder cancer. In 1998, the executive committee of the National Toxicology Program (NTP) recommended that saccharin be taken off the list of suspected human carcinogens, but this step has not yet been taken. **Note:** Most people think saccharin is very sweet, but if you hate broccoli, you're likely to think saccharin's bitter. Check out Chapter 15 to see why.

- ✔ **Cyclamates:** These sweeteners, created in 1937 at the University of Illinois, were subsequently linked to cancer in laboratory animals and banned (1969) in the United States. Since then, the FDA has stated that follow-up studies show no such link, but cyclamates — which are legal in Canada and many other countries — remain banned in the United States.

- ✔ **Aspartame (Equal, NutraSweet):** Another accidental discovery (1965), *aspartame* is a combination of two amino acids, aspartic acid and phenylalanine. Aspartame is safe for most healthy people; the exception is those born with *phenylketonuria (PKU),* a metabolic defect characterized by a lack of the enzyme needed to digest phenylalanine. In the body (or when it is exposed to heat), aspartame breaks down into its constituent ingredients, and the excess phenylalanine can pile up in brain and nerve tissue, leading to mental retardation in young children.

- ✔ **Sucralose (Splenda):** *Sucralose,* discovered in 1976, is a no-calorie sweetener made from sugar. But the body doesn't recognize sucralose as a carbohydrate or a sugar, so it zips through the intestinal tract unchanged. More than 100 scientific studies conducted during a 20-year period attest to its safety, and the FDA has approved its use in a variety of foods, including baked goods, candies, substitute dairy products, and frozen desserts.

✔ **Acesulfame-K (Sunett):** The *K* is the chemical symbol for potassium, and this artificial sweetener, with a chemical structure similar to saccharin, is found in baked goods, chewing gum, and other food products. In 1998, the FDA approved its use to prolong the shelf life of soft drinks.

✔ **Neotame:** Neotame is a modified version of aspartame. In 2002, the FDA approved Neotame for use as a tabletop sweetener, as well as for use in jams and jellies, syrups, puddings and gels, fruits, fruit juices, and non-alcohol beverages.

✔ **Stevia (Truvia):** In 2008, the FDA ruled that Truvia, a sweetener made from stevia (a South American plant member of the sunflower family) can be designated GRAS ("generally regarded as safe"). Stevia (Truvia), used to sweeten some carb-free soft drinks, is estimated to be 200 to 300 times sweeter than sugar.

✔ **Tagatose (Naturlose, Shugr):** In 2003, the FDA approved the use of tagatose, a white powder made from lactose (the sugar in milk), in cereal, soft drinks, frozen desserts, candy, chewing gum, and cake frosting. Tagatose may cause gastric upset (gas and diarrhea); paradoxically, it may also act as an aid to digestion.

Table 19-2 compares the calorie content and sweetening power of sugar versus the substitute sweeteners. For comparison, sugar has 4 calories per gram.

Table 19-2   Comparing Substitute Sweeteners to Sugar

Sweetener	*Calories Per Gram*	*Sweetness Relative to Sugar**
Sugar (sucrose)	4	
Tagatose	1.5**	Similar
Cyclamates	0	30–60 times sweeter than sugar
Acesulfame-K	0	150–200 times sweeter than sugar
Aspartame	4**	160–200 times sweeter than sugar
Stevia (Truvia)	0	200–300 times sweeter than sugar
Saccharin	0	200–700 times sweeter than sugar
Sucralose	0	600 times sweeter than sugar
Neotame	0	7,000–13,000 times sweeter than sugar

* The range of sweetness reflects estimates from several sources.
** Aspartame has 4 calories per gram and tagatose 1.5, but you need so little to get a sweet flavor that you can count the calorie content as 0.

A Last Word: Follow That Bird

You can sum up the essence of food processing by following the trail of one chicken from the farm to your table. (Vegetarians are excused from this section.)

A chicken's first brush with processing is, ugh, slaughtering, after which it's plucked and shipped off to the food processor or the supermarket, packed in ice to slow the natural bacterial decomposition. In the food factory, your chicken may be boiled and canned whole, or boiled and cut up and canned in small portions like tuna fish, or boiled into chicken soup to be canned or dehydrated into bouillon cubes, or cooked with veggies and canned as chicken à la king, or fried and frozen in whole pieces, or roasted, sliced, and frozen into a chicken dinner, or . . . you get the picture.

When you buy a fresh (raw) chicken instead of a cooked one, you perform similar rituals in your own kitchen. First, the chicken goes to the refrigerator (or freezer), then to the stove for thorough cooking to make sure that no stray bacteria contaminate your dinner table (or you), and then back to the fridge for the leftovers. In the end, the chicken's been processed. And you have eaten. That's the point of this story.

Sweet alcohols

Polyols—sometimes known as sugar alcohols—are naturally occurring, sweet, sugar-free carbohydrate/alcohol compounds with fewer calories per gram than sucrose (sugar).

Eight polyols — erythritol, hydrogenated starch hydrolysates (including maltitol syrups), isomalt, lactitol, maltitol, mannitol, sorbitol, and xylitol — are currently used in foods such as baked goods, sugar-free candy, and chewing gum, as well as drugs such as toothpaste (polyols do not contribute to tooth decay), mouthwash, and cough syrup.

The polyols are absorbed and converted to energy with little or no insulin, so these sweeteners are most useful for people with diabetes or those on a low carbohydrate, sugar-free diet. However, because they're not completely absorbed in the intestines, if consumed in large amounts, polyols may have laxative effects.

Chapter 20

Cooking and Nutrition

Y ou can bet that the first cooked dinner was an accident involving some poor wandering animal and a bolt of lightning that charred the beast into medium rare sirloin. Then a caveman attracted by the aroma tore off a sizzled hunk and forthwith offered up the first restaurant rating: "Yum."

After that, it was but a hop, a skip, and a jump, anthropologically speaking, to gas ranges, electric broilers, and microwave ovens. This chapter explains how these handy technologies affect the safety, nutritional value, appearance, flavor, and aroma of the foods that you heat.

For more detail on what and how to cook, check out *Cooking Basics For Dummies,* 4th Edition, by Brian Miller, Marie Rama, and Eve Adamson, and then fire up the stove.

What's Cooking?

The dictionary defines cooking as preparing food by heating it. In your kitchen, that means exposing food to the energy created either by fire or electromagnetic waves.

Cooking with fire

Ever since man discovered fire and how to control cooking — rather than having to wait for a passing thunderbolt — the human race has generally relied on three simple ways of heating food:

✔ **An open flame:** You hold the food directly over — or under — the flame or put the food on a griddle on top of the flame. (The electric heating coil is a 20th-century variation on the open flame.)

✔ **Hot air:** You put the food in a closed box (an oven) and heat the air in the oven to create high-temperature dry heat.

✔ **Hot liquid:** You submerge the food in hot liquid or suspend the food over the liquid so that it cooks in the steam escaping from the surface.

Sophisticated cooks may combine two or more of these methods. For example, cooking food in a wrapper, such as aluminum foil or a papaya leaf (see Chapter 29), combines two methods: open fire (the grill) or hot air (the oven) plus the steam from the food's own juices (hot liquid).

The basic methods for cooking with heat generated by fire or an electric coil are

Open Flame	*Hot Air*	*Hot Liquid*
Broiling	Baking	Boiling
Grilling	Roasting	Deep-frying
Toasting		Poaching
		Simmering
		Steaming
		Stewing

Cooking with electromagnetic waves

A gas or electric stove generates thermal energy (heat) that warms and cooks food. A microwave oven generates electromagnetic energy (microwaves) produced by a device called a magnetron.

The energy transmitted from the magnetron excites water molecules in food. The water molecules leap about like hyperactive 3-year-olds, producing friction which produces the heat that cooks the food.

Because the dish on which food sits in a microwave oven has very few water molecules, it generally stays cool. But some dishes or containers do heat up. To be safe, use a potholder when taking a dish out of the microwave

How Cooking Alters Food

Cooking foods changes the way food looks, smells, feels, and tastes. In fact, the appetizing texture of cooked food, its rich color, intense flavor, and fragrant aroma all are products of its having been exposed to heat.

Changing food's texture

Exposure to heat alters the structures of proteins, fats, and carbohydrates, changing their *texture* (the way food particles are linked to make the food feel hard or soft). In other words, cooking can turn crisp carrots soft and tough meat tender.

Protein

Proteins are made of very long molecules that sometimes fold over into accordion-like structures (see Chapter 7 for details about proteins). Although heating food doesn't lower its protein value, it does

- Break protein molecules into smaller fragments
- Cause protein molecules to unfold and form new bonds to other protein molecules
- Make proteins clump together

Need an example? Consider the egg. When you cook one, the long protein molecules in the white unfold, form new connections to other protein molecules, and link up in a network that tightens to squeeze out moisture so that the egg white hardens and turns opaque. The same unfold-link-squeeze reaction turns translucent poultry firm and white and makes gelatin set. The longer you heat proteins, the stronger the network becomes, and the tougher, or more solid, the food will be.

To see this work, scramble two eggs — one beaten and cooked plain and one beaten with milk and then cooked. Adding liquid (milk) makes it more difficult for the protein network to squeeze out all the moisture, so the egg with the added milk cooks up softer than the plain egg.

Grains: Split personality performers

In cooking, grains, such as corn, exhibit split personalities — part protein, part complex carbohydrates. When you boil an ear of corn, the protein molecules inside the kernels do the break-unfold-network dance (the molecules break their links, the protein unfolds, and the molecules form new links). At the same time, carbohydrate starch granules begin absorbing moisture and then soften.

The trick to boiling perfect corn is to control this process, removing the corn from the water when starch granules have absorbed enough moisture to soften the kernels but before the protein network has tightened.

That's why cookbooks advise that corn have only a short stay in the pot. But if you're a person who likes corn chewy, just let it boil away, 15 minutes, 30 minutes — you be the judge.

Fat

Heat melts fat, which may then run off food, lowering the calorie count. In addition, moist cooking methods break down connective tissue — the supporting framework of the body, which includes some adipose (fatty) tissue — thus, making the food softer and more pliable. You can see this most clearly when cooking fish. The fish flakes when it's done because its connective tissue has been destroyed.

When meat and poultry are stored after cooking, their fats continue to change, this time by picking up oxygen from the air. Oxidized fats have a slightly rancid taste, more politely known as *warmed-over flavor.* You can slow — but not entirely prevent — this reaction by cooking and storing meat, fish, and poultry under a blanket of food rich in *antioxidants,* chemicals that prevent other chemicals from reacting with oxygen. Vitamin C is a natural antioxidant, so gravies and marinades made with tomatoes, citrus fruits, or tart cherries slow the natural oxidation of fats in cooked or stored foods.

Carbohydrates

Cooking has different effects on simple carbohydrates and complex ones (more about them in Chapter 9). When heated

- ✔ Simple sugars — such as sucrose or the sugars on the surface of meat and poultry — caramelize, or melt and turn brown. (Think of crème caramel.)

- ✔ Starch, a complex carbohydrate, becomes more absorbent, which is why pasta expands and softens in boiling water.

- ✔ Some dietary fibers (gums, pectins, hemicellulose) dissolve, so vegetables and fruits soften when cooked.

The last two reactions may make the nutrients inside previously fiber-stiffened cells more available to your body.

A less beneficial effect of heat on carbs surfaced early in 2002 when Swedish researchers set off a nutritional hoo-ha with the announcement that exposing starchy carbohydrate foods — such as potatoes and bread — to the high heat of baking or frying produces *acrylamides,* a family of chemicals known to cause cancer in rats. Then things got worse when scientists at the City of Hope Cancer Research Center (Los Angeles) said that acrylamides could trigger cell changes leading to cancer in human beings. But a 2003 analysis of data from a study of 987 cancer patients and 538 healthy "controls" conducted by researchers at Harvard School of Public Health and the Departments of Oncology–Pathology and Medical Epidemiology at Karolinska Institutet in Stockholm showed no evidence of an increased risk of bowel, bladder, or kidney cancer among fans of fries and toast. By 2010, the official FDA position on acrylamides was, essentially, No Big Deal: "FDA's best advice for acrylamide and eating," the agency said, "is that consumers adopt a healthy eating plan, consistent with the Dietary Guidelines for Americans, that emphasizes fruits, vegetables, whole grains, and fat-free or lowfat milk and milk products; includes lean meats, poultry, fish, beans, eggs, and nuts; and is low in saturated fats, *trans* fats, cholesterol, salt (sodium), and added sugars."

Enhancing flavor and aroma

Heat degrades (breaks apart) flavor and aroma chemicals. As a result, most cooked food has a more intense flavor and aroma than raw food.

A good example is what happens when you cook cruciferous vegetables, such as cabbage and cauliflower. These vegetables get their distinctive flavor and aroma from mustard oils, which intensify the longer the vegetables are cooked. But every rule has an exception: Heat destroys *diallyl disulfide,* the chemical that gives raw garlic its bite and bark. So cooked garlic tastes and smells milder than the raw version.

Shading the color palette

Carotenoids — the natural red and yellow pigments that make carrots and sweet potatoes orange and tomatoes red — are practically impervious to heat and the acidity or alkalinity of cooking liquids. No matter how you cook them or how long, these particular pigments stay bright and sunny.

You can't say the same for the other pigments in food, the ones that make other foods naturally red, green, or white. These pigments react — usually for the worse — to heat, acids (such as wine, vinegar, or tomato juice), and basic (alkaline) chemicals (such as mineral water or baking soda and water). Here's a brief rundown on the color changes that you can expect when you cook food:

- Red beets and red cabbage get their colors from pigments called *anthocyanins.* Acids make these pigments redder. Alkaline solutions fade anthocyanins from red to bluish purple.

- Potatoes, cauliflower, rice, and white onions are whitened by pigments called *anthoxanthins.* When anthoxanthins are exposed to alkaline chemicals (mineralized water or baking soda), they turn yellow or brownish. Acids prevent this reaction. Boil cauliflower florets in water, and they darken slightly. Boil them in tomato juice, rinse off the juice, and you'll see — white cauliflower.

- Green veggies are colored by *chlorophyll,* a pigment that reacts with acids in cooking water (or in the vegetable itself) to form *pheophytin,* a brown pigment. The only way to short-circuit this reaction is to protect the vegetables from acids. Old-time cooks added alkaline baking soda, but that increases the loss of certain vitamins (see "Protecting the Nutrients in Cooked Foods" later in this chapter) and softens the vegetables. Fast cooking at high heat or cooking in lots of water (which dilutes acids) lessens these color changes.

✔ The natural red color of fresh meat comes from *myoglobin* in the muscle tissue and *hemoglobin* in blood. When meat is heated, the pigment molecules are *denatured,* or broken into fragments. They lose oxygen and turn brown or — after long cooking — turn the really unappetizing gray characteristic of steam-table meats. This inevitable change is more noticeable in beef than in pork or veal because beef, which contains more myoglobin, starts out naturally redder.

How Pots and Pans Affect Food

A pot is a pot is a pot, right? Wrong. In fact, your choice of pots can affect the nutrient value of food by

✔ Adding nutrients to the food

✔ Slowing the natural loss of nutrients during cooking

✔ Actively increasing the loss of nutrients during cooking

In addition, some pots make the food's natural flavors and aromas more intense, which, in turn, can make the food more — or less — appetizing. Read on to find out how your pot can change your food. And vice versa.

Aluminum

Aluminum is lightweight and conducts heat well. That's good. But the metal

✔ Makes some aroma chemicals smellier (particularly those in the cruciferous vegetables — cabbage, broccoli, Brussels sprouts, and so on)

✔ Flakes off, turning white foods (such as cauliflower or potatoes) yellow or brownish

Early speculation aside, aluminum flaking is not hazardous to your health: Cooking with aluminum pots does not increase your risk for developing Alzheimer's disease. True, cooking salty or acidic foods (wine, tomatoes) in aluminum pots increases the flaking, but even then, the amount of aluminum you get from the pot is less than you get naturally every day from food and water.

Red to blue and back again

The following experiment lets you see colors change right before your very eyes. You will need

☞ 1 small can sliced beets

☞ 1 saucepan

☞ 3 small glass bowls

☞ 1 cup water

☞ 1 teaspoon baking soda

☞ 3 tablespoons white vinegar

Line up the glass bowls on your kitchen counter. Open the can of beets. Remove six slices of beets. Put two slices in the first glass bowl and four slices in the saucepan. Put the rest in a small container and refrigerate for dinner. No sense wasting good beets!

Mix the baking soda into the water and add this alkaline solution to the saucepan. Heat for 4 minutes; don't heat too high — the solution foams. Turn off the heat. Remove the beets from the pan. Put two slices each in the second and third glass bowls.

Ignore the second bowl. Add the vinegar (an acid) to the third bowl. Wait two minutes. Now look: The beets in the first bowl (straight from the can) should still be bright red. Alkaline compounds darken colors, so the beets in the second bowl, straight from the baking soda bath, should be almost navy blue. Acids reverse the reaction, so beets in the third bowl, with added vinegar, should be heading back to bright red. Not yet? Add another tablespoon of vinegar and watch chemistry do its magic....

Copper

Copper pots heat steadily and evenly. To take advantage of this property, many aluminum or stainless steel pots are made with a layer of copper sandwiched into the bottom. But naked copper is a potentially poisonous metal. That's why copper pots are lined with tin or stainless steel. Whenever you cook with copper, periodically check the lining of the pot. If it's damaged — meaning that you can see the orange copper peeking through the silvery lining — have the pot relined or throw it out.

Ceramics

The chief virtue of plain terra cotta (the orange clay that looks like red bricks) is its *porosity,* the fact that it contains millions of tiny pores that allow excess steam to escape while holding in just enough moisture to make food tender.

Copper and egg whites: A chemical team

When you whip an egg white, its proteins unfold, form new bonds, and create a network that holds air in. That's why the runny white turns into stable foam.

You can certainly whip egg whites successfully in a glass or ceramic bowl — chilled, and absolutely free of any fat, including egg yolk, which would prevent the proteins from linking tightly. But the best choice is copper: the ions (particles) flaking off the surface bind with and stabilize the foam. (Aluminum ions stabilize but darken the whites.)

But wait. Isn't copper toxic? (See Chapter 12.) Yes, but the amount you get in an occasional batch of whites is so small it's insignificant, safetywise.

Decorated ceramic vessels are another matter. For one thing, the glaze makes the pot much less porous so that meat or poultry cooked in a covered painted ceramic pan steams instead of roasts, producing a soggy surface rather than a crisp one.

More importantly, some pigments used to paint or glaze the pots contain lead. To seal the decoration and prevent lead from leaching into food, the painted pots are *fired* (baked in an oven). If the pots are fired in an oven that isn't hot enough or if they aren't fired for a long enough period of time, lead will leach from ceramics when in contact with acidic foods, such as fruit juices or foods marinated in wine or vinegar.

Ceramics made in the United States, Japan, and Great Britain generally are considered safe, but for maximum protection, hedge your bets. Unless the pot comes with a tag or brochure that specifically says it's acid-safe, don't use it for cooking or storing foods. And always wash decorated ceramics by hand; repeated passes through the dishwasher can wear down the surface.

Enamelware

Enameled pots are made of metal covered with *porcelain,* a fine translucent china. Enamelware heats more slowly and less evenly than plain metal. A good-quality enameled surface resists discoloration and does not react with food. But it can chip, and it's easily marked or scratched by cooking utensils other than wood or hard plastic. If the surface chips and you can see the metal underneath, discard the pot lest metals flake into your food.

Glass

Glass is a neutral material that does not react with food. However, two cautions apply:

✔ Do not use a glass-and-metal pot in the microwave oven. The metal blocks microwaves. More importantly, it can cause *arcing* — a sudden electrical flare that may damage the oven and scare you out of your wits.

✔ Remember that glass breaks — sometimes all over the floor. Are you a person who often drops things? Pass on the glass.

Iron

Iron conducts heat well and stays hot significantly longer than other pots. It's easy to clean. It lasts forever, and it releases iron ions into food, which may improve the nutritional value of dinner.

In 1985, nutrition researchers at Texas Tech University in Lubbock set out to measure the iron content of foods cooked in iron pots. Among their discoveries: Beef stew (0.7 milligrams of iron per 100 grams/3.5 ounces, raw) can end up with as much as 3.4 milligrams of iron per 100 grams after cooking slightly longer than an hour in an iron pot.

The downside? "Pumping iron" is not a bad way to describe the experience of cooking with iron pots. They're really, really heavy.

Nonstick

Nonstick surfaces are made of plastic (polytetrafluoroethylene; PTFE for short) plus *hardeners* — chemicals that harden and seal the surface. As long as the surface is unscratched and intact, it will not react with food.

To avoid surface scratches, stick to wooden or plastic spoons when using these pots. Otherwise, your pot may end up looking like chickens have been stomping on the surface. Scratched nonstick pots and pans are not a health hazard. If you swallow tiny pieces of the nonstick coating, they pass through your body undigested.

However, when nonstick surfaces get very hot, they may

✔ Separate from the metal to which they're bound (the sides and bottom of the pot)

✔ Emit odorless fumes

If the cooking area is not properly ventilated, you may experience *polymer fume fever* — flu-like symptoms with no known long-term effect. To prevent this, keep the stove flame moderate and the windows open.

Stainless steel

Stainless steel is an *alloy,* a substance composed of two or more metals. Its virtues are hardness and durability; its drawback is poor heat conduction. In addition, stainless steel isn't *really* stainless. When exposed to high heat, stainless steel develops a characteristic multi-hued "rainbow" discoloration. Starchy foods, such as pasta and potatoes, may darken the pot, and undissolved salt can pit the surface. If your stainless steel pot is scratched deeply enough to expose the inner layer under the shiny surface, the metals in the alloy may flake into your food. Toss the pot.

Plastic and paper

Plastic melts and paper burns, so you obviously can't use plastic or paper containers in a stove with an open flame (gas) or heat source (electric). But you can use them in the microwave so long as you pick a proper plastic.

When plastic dishes or plastic wrap are heated in a microwave oven, they may emit potentially carcinogenic compounds that can migrate into your food. To reduce your exposure to these compounds, the U.S. Department of Agriculture's Food Safety and Inspection Service (FSIS) says you need to choose plastic containers labeled "for microwave oven use." Thin plastic storage bags, margarine tubs, and whipped topping bowls are convenient but way, way off-limits. The American Plastic Council also offers three common-sense tips for using the right kind of plastics in the microwave:

- ✔ Follow the directions on the plastic container or package. If it doesn't say "microwaveable," it isn't. For example, Styrofoam and other take-out food carriers rarely are microwaveable, so put the food you've ordered into a different container before reheating it.

- ✔ Trays for microwave meals are meant to be used only once; after you heat the food, toss the tray.

- ✔ When covering food to prevent splatters, use microwave-safe plastic wraps only.

Because the Food and Drug Administration requires microwave-safe plastics to meet strict safety standards, repeated studies show no ill effects from their minimal leakage.

For more about plastics in the microwave, visit the USDA's Food Safety and Inspection Service (FSIS) Web site at www.fsis.usda.gov.

Protecting the Nutrients in Cooked Foods

Myth: All raw foods are more nutritious than cooked ones.

Fact: Some foods (such as meat, poultry, and eggs) are positively dangerous when consumed raw (or undercooked). Other foods are less nutritious raw because they contain substances that destroy or disarm other nutrients. For example, raw dried beans contain enzyme inhibitors that interfere with your body's ability to digest protein. Heating disarms the enzyme inhibitor.

But there's no denying that some nutrients are lost when foods are cooked. Simple strategies such as steaming food fast rather than boiling, or broiling rather than frying, can significantly reduce the loss of nutrients.

Maintaining minerals

Virtually all minerals are unaffected by heat. Cooked or raw, food has the same amount of calcium, phosphorus, magnesium, iron, zinc, iodine, selenium, copper, manganese, chromium, and sodium. The single exception to this rule is potassium, which — although not affected by heat or air — escapes from foods into the cooking liquid.

Those volatile vitamins

Many vitamins are sensitive to and easily destroyed by heat, air, water, or fats (cooking oils). Table 20-1 shows which nutrients are sensitive to these influences.

Table 20-1	What Takes Nutrients Out of Food?			
Nutrient	**Heat**	**Air**	**Water**	**Fat**
Vitamin A	X			X
Vitamin D				X
Vitamin E	X	X		X
Vitamin C	X	X	X	
Thiamin	X		X	
Riboflavin			X	
Vitamin B6	X	X	X	
Folate	X	X		

(continued)

Table 20-1 (continued)

Nutrient	Heat	Air	Water	Fat
Vitamin B12	X		X	
Biotin			X	
Pantothenic acid	X			
Potassium			X	

To avoid specific types of vitamin loss, keep in mind the following tips:

✔ **Vitamins A, E, and D:** To reduce the loss of fat-soluble vitamins A and E, cook with very little oil. For example, bake or broil liver, which is rich in vitamin A, with very little oil. Ditto for fatty fish, one of the few natural food sources of vitamin D.

✔ **B vitamins:** Strategies that conserve protein in meat and poultry during cooking also work to conserve the B vitamins that leak out into cooking liquid or drippings: Use the cooking liquid in soup or sauce. *Caution:* Do not shorten cooking times or use lower temperatures to lessen the loss of heat-sensitive vitamin B12 from meat, fish, or poultry. These foods and their drippings must be thoroughly cooked to ensure that they're safe to eat.

To preserve the Bs in grains, do not rinse the grains before cooking unless the package advises you to do so (some rice does need to be rinsed). Simply rinsing some rices once may take away as much as 25 percent of its thiamin (vitamin B1). Toast or bake cakes and breads only until the crust is light brown to preserve heat-sensitive Bs.

✔ **Vitamin C:** To reduce the loss of water-soluble, oxygen-sensitive vitamin C, cook fruits and vegetables in the least possible amount of water. For example, a series of experiments at Cornell University demonstrated that when you cook 1 cup of cabbage in 4 cups of water, the leaves lose as much as 90 percent of their vitamin C. Reverse the ratio — 1 cup water to 4 cups cabbage — and you hold on to more than 50 percent of the vitamin C.

Another C-saver is to bake or boil root vegetables (carrots, potatoes, sweet potatoes) whole, in their skins. This trick retains about 65 percent of the vitamin C.

Serve cooked vegetables quickly: After 24 hours in the fridge, vegetables lose one-fourth of their vitamin C; after two days, nearly half.

How Cooking Keeps Food Safe

The Centers for Disease Control and Prevention estimates that each year 76,000,000 million Americans sicken, 325,000 are hospitalized, and 5,000 die from foodborne illness caused primarily by pathogens (disease-causing organisms).

Readers who are really good mathematicians will see right away that the National Institute of Diabetes and Digestive and Kidney Disease (NIDDK) is correct in noting that these numbers equal

- 6,333,333 cases of foodborne illness each and every month
- 1,461,538 cases every week
- 208,219 cases every day
- 8,675 cases every hour
- 144 cases every minute
- 2 cases every second

Should these numbers worry you?

Yes.

Although pathogens in food are most dangerous for the very young, the very old, and those whose immune systems have been weakened by illness or medication, the truth is that these microorganisms are equal-opportunity troublemakers — anyone who eats food carrying them may get sick.

Naming the bad guys

Many microorganisms that live naturally in food are harmless or even beneficial.

For example:

- *Lactobacilli* (lacto = milk; bacilli = rod-shaped bacteria) digest sugars in milk and convert the milk to yogurt, acidophilus buttermilk, kefir, koumiss, and Swiss or Ementhal cheese.
- Nontoxic molds convert milk to cheeses such as Brie, Camembert, Gorgonzola, or blue cheese whose blue streaks are safe, edible mold, but molds not part of the cheese-making process can be hazardous. For the USDA's advice on which mold is which and which cheese to use and which to discard once mold appears, go to www.fsis.usda.gov/factsheets/molds_on_food.

Some organisms, however, are decidedly unfriendly.

For example:

- ✔ *Clostridium botulinum (C. botulinum)* thrives in the absence of air (as in low-acid, canned food such as corn or string beans) to churn out a potentially fatal neurotoxin. (***Note:*** In medicine, low doses of purified botulinum toxin are used to weaken or paralyze muscles so as to reduce facial wrinkles or alleviate muscle spasms.)

- ✔ *Campylobacter jejuni (C. jejuni),* which flourishes in raw meat and poultry and unpasteurized milk, has been linked to Guillain-Barré syndrome, a paralytic illness that sometimes follows flu infection.

Table 20-2 lists the common food pathogens and the foods in which they are most likely to be found.

Table 20-2	Disease-Causing Organisms in Food
The Bug	*Where You Find It*
Campylobacter jejuni	Raw meat and poultry, unpasteurized milk
Clostridium botulinum	Underprocessed low-acid canned foods or vacuum-packed smoked fish
Clostridium perfringens	Foods made from poultry or meat
E. coli	Raw beef, precut bagged salads
Listeria monocytogenes	Raw meat and seafood, raw milk, some raw cheeses
Salmonella bacteria	Poultry, meat, eggs, dried foods, dairy products
Staphylococcus aureus	Custards, salads (that is, egg, chicken, and tuna salads)

USDA Meat and Poultry Hotline

How cooking helps make food safe

While cleanliness along the line from field to dinner table is important to controlling food-borne illness, proper cooking is even more so.

Simply heating food to the temperatures shown in Table 20-3 is not a guaranteed protection against food-borne illness, but cooking food thoroughly and keeping it hot (or chilling it quickly) after it has been cooked does incapacitate many dangerous bugs or slows the rate at which they reproduce, thus reducing the risk.

Do not rely on instinct to tell you whether a food has reached safe temperature during cooking. Use a food thermometer. And because some things are more complicated than they seem, read the directions that come with the thermometer to be sure you're doing it right.

Table 20-3	How Hot Is Safe?
This Food . . .	*Is Done (Generally Safe to Eat) When Cooked to This Internal Temperature*
Eggs and Egg Dishes	
Eggs	Cook until yolk and white are firm
Egg dishes	160°F
Ground Meat and Meat Mixtures*	
Turkey, chicken	165°F
Veal, beef, lamb, pork	165°F
Fresh Beef*	
Medium rare	145°F
Medium	160°F
Well-done	170°F
Fresh Pork	
Medium	160°F
Well-done	170°F
Poultry	
Chicken, whole	180°F
Turkey, whole	180°F
Poultry breasts, roasts	170°F
Poultry thighs, wings	Cook until juices run clear
Duck and goose	180°F
Ham	
Fresh (raw)	160°F
Precooked (to reheat)	140°F

* Undercooked hamburger is a major source of the potentially lethal organism E. coli 0157:H7. To be safe, the internal temperature of the meat must read 165°F.
** After the bird is cooked, the stuffing should be removed immediately and stored separately in the refrigerator.
USDA Food Safety and Inspection Service, "A Quick Consumer Guide to Safe Food Handling," Home and Garden Bulletin, No. 248 (August 1995).

Two hours — and you're out!

Microorganisms thrive on food at temperatures between 40 and 140 degrees Fahrenheit, the cooking temperature that inactivates many — though not all — hazardous organisms.

To protect food after cooking, keep it hot or chill it right away.

More questions about food safety? Call or click:

✔ USDA Meat and Poultry Hotline Phone: 1-888-MPHotline (1-888-564-6854) E-mail: mphotline.fsis@usda.gov

✔ FDA Seafood Hotline Phone: 800-332-4010 202-205-4314 in Washington DC

✔ Food Safety and Information Service Phone: 1-888-MPHotline (1-888-674-6854) Web site: www.fsis.usda.gov

✔ Food Safety Network at the University of Guelph (Canada) Phone 866-503-7638 (toll-free in Canada)E-mail: fsnrsn@uoguelph.ca Web site (English): www.foodsafetynetwork.ca/en/

Chapter 21

What Happens When Food Is Frozen, Canned, Dried, or Zapped

Cold air, hot air, no air, and radioactive rays — all can be used to make food safer for longer periods of time by reducing or eliminating damage from exposure to air or organisms (microbes) that live on food.

The methods described in this chapter all have one important thing in common: Used correctly, each process can dramatically lengthen food's shelf life. The downside? Nothing's perfect, so you still have to monitor your food to make sure that the preservation treatment has, well, preserved it. The following pages tell you how.

Cold Comfort: Chilling and Freezing

Keeping food cold, sometimes very cold, slows or suspends the activity of microorganisms bent on digesting your food before you do.

Unlike heat, which kills many of the microbes (see Chapter 20), chilling or freezing food may just reduce the microbial population, sidelining them for a while. For example, *mold spores* (hibernating mold organisms) may sleep inside frozen food like so many hibernating bears inside a wintry cave. When spring comes, the bears bounce back to life; thaw the food, and the mold spores do the same.

How long things stay safe in the refrigerator or freezer varies from food to food and to some extent on the packaging (better packaging, longer freezing time). Table 21-1 provides a handy guide to the limits of safe cool storage for fresh food in a refrigerator/freezer maintaining a constant temperature. If these conditions aren't met, food may spoil more quickly.

Use your common sense: If food seems in any way questionable, *throw it out without tasting.* Or as the catchy saying goes: When in doubt, throw it out. And for more information on the effects of freezing, check out the Food Safety and Inspection Service fact sheet at `www.fsis.usda.gov/factsheets/focus_on_freezing/index.asp#12`.

Table 21-1 How Long Foods Generally Stay Safe in Cold Storage

Food	*Refrigerator (40°F)*	*Freezer (0°F)*
Eggs		
Fresh, in shell	3 weeks	Don't freeze
Raw yolks, whites	2–4 days	1 year
Hard cooked	1 week	Doesn't freeze well
Liquid pasteurized eggs or egg substitutes, opened	3 days	Doesn't freeze well
Liquid pasteurized eggs or egg substitutes, unopened	10 days	1 year
Mayonnaise, Commercial		
Open jar	2 months	Don't freeze
TV Dinners, Frozen Casseroles		
As originally packed, until ready to serve	Don't refrigerate: Keep frozen	3–4 months
Deli and Vacuum-Packed Products		
Prestuffed pork and lamb chops, chicken breasts stuffed with dressing	1 day	Doesn't freeze well
Store-cooked convenience meals	1–2 days	Doesn't freeze well
Commercial brand vacuum-packed dinners with USDA seal, unopened	2 weeks	Doesn't freeze well
Soups and Stews		
Vegetable or meat-added	3–4 days	2–3 months
Ground Meats and Stew Meats		
Hamburger and stew meats	1–2 days	3–4 months

Food	Refrigerator (40°F)	Freezer (0°F)
Ground turkey, veal, pork, lamb, and mixtures of them	1–2 days	3–4 months
Hot Dogs and Lunch Meats***		
Hot dogs, opened	1 week	In freezer wrap, 1–2 months
Hot dogs, unopened	2 weeks	In freezer wrap, 1–2 months
Lunch meats, opened	3–5 days	In freezer wrap, 1–2 months
Lunch meats, unopened	2 weeks	In freezer wrap, 1–2 months
Bacon and Sausage		
Bacon*	7 days	1 month
Sausage, raw — pork, beef, turkey	1–2 days	1–2 months
Smoked breakfast links, patties	7 days	1–2 months
Hard sausage — pepperoni, jerky sticks	2–3 weeks	1–2 months
Ham, Corned Beef		
Corned beef in pouch with pickling juices*	5–7 days	Drained and wrapped, 1 month
Ham, canned, label says to keep refrigerated	6–9 months	Don't freeze
Ham, fully cooked — whole	7 days	1–2 months
Ham, fully cooked — half	3–5 days	1–2 months
Ham, fully cooked — slices	3–4 days	1–2 months
Fresh Meat		
Steaks — beef	3–5 days	6–12 months
Chops — pork	3–5 days	4–6 months
Chops — lamb	3–5 days	6–9 months
Roast — beef	3–5 days	6–12 months
Roast — lamb	3–5 days	6–9 months
Roasts — pork, veal	3–5 days	4–6 months
Variety meats — tongue, brain, kidneys, liver, heart, chitterlings	1–2 days	3–4 months

(continued)

Table 21-1 *(continued)*

Food	Refrigerator (40°F)	Freezer (0°F)
Meat Leftovers		
Cooked meat and meat dishes	3–4 days	2–3 months
Gravy and broth	1–2 days	2–3 months
Fresh Poultry		
Chicken or turkey, whole	1–2 days	1 year
Poultry pieces	1–2 days	2–3 months
Giblets	1–2 days	3–4 months
Cooked Poultry, Leftover		
Fried chicken	3–4 days	4 months
Cooked poultry dishes	3–4 days	4–6 months
Poultry pieces, plain	3–4 days	4 months
Poultry pieces covered with broth or gravy	1–2 days	6 months
Chicken nuggets, patties	1–2 days	1–3 months

* Follow date on package.
*** **Caution:** Even when food is in date and has been properly refrigerated, always boil or broil hot dogs to an internal temperature of 165°F.*
Food Safety and Inspection Service, "A Quick Consumer's Guide to Safe Food Handling," Home and Garden Bulletin, No. 248 (U.S. Department of Agriculture, August 1995).

How freezing affects the texture of food

When food freezes, the water inside each cell forms tiny crystals that can tear cell walls. As the food is thawed, the liquid inside the cell leaks out, leaving thawed food dryer than fresh food.

What's that brown spot on my burger?

Freezer burn is a dry brownish spot left when moisture evaporates from the surface of frozen food. Because freezer burn changes the composition of fats on the surface of foods such as meat and poultry, it will cause some change in flavor, as well.

To prevent freezer burn, wrap food securely in freezer paper or aluminum foil and put the item in a plastic bag. The more air you keep out, the fewer brown spots will develop.

Beef that has been frozen, for example, is noticeably dryer than fresh beef. Dry cheeses, such as cheddar, turn crumbly. Bread dries, too. You can reduce the loss of moisture by thawing the food in its freezer wrap so that it has a chance to reabsorb the moisture that's still in the package.

You can't restore the crispness of vegetables that get their crunch from stiff, high-fiber cell walls. After ice crystals puncture the walls, the vegetable (carrots are a good example) turns mushy. The solution? Remove carrots and other crisp vegetables such as cabbage, before freezing the stew.

Refreezing frozen food

The official word from the U.S. Department of Agriculture is that you can refreeze frozen food — as long as the food still has ice crystals or feels refrigerator-cold to the touch.

The exception may be sauced frozen food, such as frozen macaroni and cheese, because there may be hidden pockets of thawed food where the bacteria are whooping it up as we speak. In other words, partial thaw? Out the door.

Canned Food: Keeping Out Contaminants

Food is canned by heating what goes into the container and then sealing the container to keep out air and microbes. It is then reheated after the can/jar is sealed.

Like cooked food, canned food is subject to changes in appearance and nutritional content. Heating food often changes its color and texture (see Chapter 20). It also destroys some vitamin C. But canning effectively destroys a variety of pathogens, and it deactivates enzymes that might otherwise cause continued deterioration of the food.

A modern variation on canning is the sealed plastic or aluminum bag known as the *retort pouch.* Food sealed in the pouch is heated but for a shorter period than that required for canning. As a result, the pouch method does a better job of preserving flavor, appearance, and heat-sensitive vitamin C.

The sealed can or pouch also protects food from deterioration caused by light or air, so the seal must remain intact. If the seal is broken, air seeps into the can or pouch, carrying microbes that can begin to spoil the food.

A more serious hazard associated with canned food is *botulism,* a potentially fatal form of food poisoning that may result if the food is not heated for a sufficient period of time to a temperature high enough to kill all *Clostridium botulinum* (or *C. botulinum*) spores. *C. botulinum* is an *anaerobic* (an = without; aerobic = air) organism that thrives in the absence of oxygen, a condition nicely fulfilled by a sealed can. If a low-acid food is incorrectly canned, *botulinum* spores not destroyed by high heat during the canning process may produce a toxin that can kill by paralyzing muscles, including the heart muscle and the muscles that enable you to breathe.

To avoid potentially hazardous canned food, do not buy, store, or use any can that is

- ✔ **Swollen.** The swelling suggests that bacteria are growing inside and producing gas.

- ✔ **Damaged, rusted, or deeply dented along the seam.** A break in the can permits air to enter and may promote the growth of organisms other than *C. botulinum*.

Consumer alert: Never, never, *never* taste any food from a swollen or damaged can "just to see if it's all right." ***Remember:*** When in doubt, throw it out.

Dried Food: No Life without Water

Drying protects food by removing the moisture that bacteria, yeasts, and molds need to live.

Drying food the low-tech way means putting it out in the sun and waiting for it to dry on its own, the technique used to produce the famous dates of the Arabian desert and the dried meat of the American plains. Drying food the high-tech, modern commercial way means putting food out on racks and employing fans to quick-dry the food at a low temperature under vacuum pressure. At home, a food dehydrator works similar magic.

Spray drying is a method used to dry liquids, such as milk, by blowing the liquids (in very small droplets) into a heated chamber where the droplets dry into a powder that can be reconstituted (made back into a liquid) by adding water. Instant coffee is a spray-dried product. So are instant teas, powdered milk, and all the various instant fruit beverages.

How drying affects food's nutritional value

As always, exposure to heat and/or air (oxygen) reduces a food's vitamin C content, so dried foods have less vitamin C than fresh foods.

One good example is the plum versus the prune (a dried plum):

- ✔ One fresh, medium-size plum, weighing 66 grams (a bit more than 2 ounces) without the pit, has 6 milligrams vitamin C, 7 to 8 percent of the Recommended Dietary Allowance for a healthy adult.

- ✔ An equivalent amount of uncooked dried (low-moisture) prunes (66 grams) has only 1.3 milligrams vitamin C.

But wait! Before you leap to the conclusion that fresh Is always more nutritious than dried, consider this: Dried fruit has less water than fresh fruit. That means its weight reflects more solid fruit. Although drying destroys some vitamin C, removing water concentrates what's left, along with other nutrients, jamming more calories, dietary fiber, and/or air-resistant vitamins and minerals into a smaller space.

As a result, dried food often has surprisingly more nutritional bounce to the ounce than fresh food. Once again, consider the plum and the prune:

- ✔ A medium-size, pit-free plum weighing slightly more than 2 ounces provides 35 calories, 0.1 milligram iron, and 670 IU (67 RE) vitamin A. (What's IU? What's RE? Check out Chapter 5.)

- ✔ Two ounces of uncooked, low-moisture prunes have about 193 calories, 2 milligrams iron, and 952 IU (72 RE) vitamin A. In other words, if you're trying to lose weight, you need to be aware that although dried fruit is low in fat and rich in nutrients, it's also high in calories.

When dried fruit may be hazardous to your health

Many fruits contain an enzyme (polyphenoloxidase) that darkens the fruit flesh when the fruit is exposed to air. To prevent the fruits from darkening when dried, the fruits are treated with sulfur compounds known as *sulfites*. The sulfites — sulfur dioxide, sodium bisulfite, sodium metabisulfite — can cause potentially serious allergic reactions in sensitive individuals. For more about sulfites, see Chapters 22 and 23.

Irradiation: A Hot Topic

Irradiation is a technique that exposes food to electron beams or *gamma radiation,* a high-energy light stronger than the X-rays your doctor uses to make a picture of your insides. Gamma rays are *ionizing radiation,* the kind of radiation that kills living cells. Ionizing radiation can sterilize food or at least prolong its shelf life by

- ✔ Killing microbes and insects on plants (wheat, wheat powder, spices, dry vegetable seasonings)

- ✔ Killing disease-causing organisms on pork *(Trichinella),* poultry *(Salmonella),* and ground beef (pathogenic *E. coli*)

> ✔ Preventing potatoes from sprouting during storage
>
> ✔ Slowing the rate at which some fruits ripen

Irradiation does not change the way food looks or tastes. It does not change food texture. It does not make food radioactive. It does, however, alter the structure of some chemicals in foods, breaking molecules apart to form new substances called *radiolytic products* (radio = radiation; lytic = break).

About 90 percent of all compounds identified as radiolytic products (RP) are also found in raw, heated, and/or stored foods that have not been exposed to ionizing radiation. A few compounds, called *unique radiolytic products* (URPs), are found only in irradiated foods.

You can get answers to the most commonly asked questions about food irradiation at the Web site maintained by the Centers for Disease Control (CDC):

www.cdc.gov/nczved/divisions/dfbmd/diseases/irradiation_food

Are irradiated foods harmful?

Food irradiation has been declared safe and effective in controlling microbial food poisoning and preserving food quality by the United States Department of Health and Human Services, the United States Public Health Service, the American Medical Association, the National Association of State Departments of Agriculture, the American Dietetic Association, and the World Health Organization.

Some consumers, however, remain leery of the process, fearful that it may expose them to radiation or that compounds produced only when foods are irradiated may eventually turn out to be harmful.

In fact, irradiated foods do not emit radiation. But the story of irradiating foods is still unfolding, a situation that makes many people uneasy. For example, the FDA's 2003 decision to allow irradiated ground beef into the National School Lunch Program has triggered debates in many school districts; several — including Los Angeles and the District of Columbia — have simply banned irradiated foods from their menus.

Around the world, all irradiated food is identified with this international symbol.

Just in case that isn't enough to get the message across, the package must also carry the words "treated by irradiation" or "treated with irradiation." The only exceptions are spices and commercially produced food that contains some irradiated ingredients, such as spices. The symbol and/or wording isn't required, for example, on the packaging for a frozen pizza that's seasoned with irradiated oregano.

Table 21-2 lists the foods approved for irradiation in the United States.

Table 21-2   Foods Approved for Irradiation in the U.S.

Food	Approval Date
Wheat, wheat flour	1964
White potatoes	1964
Garlic powder, onion powder, dried spices	1983, 1985
Dried enzyme preparations (such as milk protein clotting enzymes used in making cheese)	1985
Pork	1985
Fruit and vegetables (fresh)	1986
Herbs, herbal teas, spices, vegetable seasonings	1986
Poultry (fresh, frozen)	1990 (FDA), 1992 (USDA)*
Beef, lamb, pork, horsemeat, & byproducts	1997 (FDA), 2000 (USDA)*
Ready-to-eat, unrefrigerated meat/poultry products	1999
Fresh eggs (in shell)	2000
Seeds for sprouting	2000
Fruit & vegetable juices	2000
Imported fruits and vegetables	2002
Meat for the National School Lunch program	2002
Fresh spinach and iceberg lettuce	2008
Fresh or frozen mollusks (oysters, clams, mussels, scallops)	2009
Ready-to-eat foods (cold cuts [sliced or packaged], frozen foods, packaged salads)	Pending
Fresh or frozen crustacean (shrimp, crabs, lobster)	Pending
Unrefrigerated beef, lamb, pork, horse meat, & byproducts	Pending

* Both the FDA and the USDA must approve treatment of meat and poultry.
Sources: Federal Centers for Disease Control; Food and Drug Administration; Food Safety and Inspection Services, U.S. Department of Agriculture.

Is that food still good to eat?

Understanding the dating terms on food package labels can help you figure out whether the food inside is still safe and tasty — or ready to be discarded. Here's what the words mean:

✔ **Sell by:** The last date on which the food can be offered for sale. Stored properly, most perishable foods like milk and packaged meats are safe for a few days past the sell-by date.

✔ **Best if used by or Use by:** Refers to the food's flavor and quality, not its safety; the manufacturer's recommendation of the last date on which the food is likely to taste best.

✔ **Expires or Do not use after:** The last date on which a product either provides the highest nutritional value or works best (for example, the last date yeast is likely to make bread rise).

✔ **Packing date:** Used on eggs from USDA; written as a number from 1 (January 1) to 365 (December 31 — except in a leap year, naturally). Eggs from USDA-inspected plants may also carry an expiration date.

Chapter 22

Better Eating through Chemistry

*I*f the title of this chapter turns you off, you're not alone. Many people think that when you're talking about food, natural's good, and chemical's bad. Period. But in fact, every single thing in the world is made of chemicals: your body, the air you breathe, the paper on which this book is printed, and the glasses through which you read it, not to mention every single bite of food you eat and every ounce of beverage you drink.

This chapter is about the naturally occurring *and* the added natural or synthetic chemicals in your food and the technological processes that help make food more nutritious; enhance its appearance, flavor, and texture; and keep it fresh on the shelf longer. More to the point, this chapter explains that without these products and processes, human beings would still have to gather (or kill) dinner fresh each day to serve it up fast before it spoils.

Finally, this chapter talks about new and unusual processes, such as genetic engineering (which is discussed in the section "Looking Beyond Additives: Foods Nature Never Made").

Nature's Beneficial Chemistry

The same plant foods that yield carbohydrates (see Chapter 9) are also the source of *phytochemicals,* natural compounds other than vitamins manufactured only in plants (*phyto-* is the Greek word for plant).

Phytochemicals, such as coloring agents and antioxidants, are the substances that produce many of the beneficial effects associated with a diet rich in fruits, vegetables, beans, and grains. The best source of phytochemicals are highly colored vegetables and fruits. Best example: Deep green leafy veggies. *Note:* Plants don't manufacture minerals; they absorb them from the soil. Therefore, minerals aren't phytochemicals.

In fact, the undeniable value of phytochemicals is one reason the *Dietary Guidelines for Americans* urges you to have as many as nine servings of fruits and vegetables and several servings of grains every day.

The most interesting phytochemicals in plant foods appear to be antioxidants, hormonelike compounds, and enzyme-activating sulfur compounds. Each group plays a specific role in maintaining health and reducing your risk of certain illnesses.

Antioxidants

Antioxidants are named for their ability to prevent a chemical reaction called *oxidation,* which enables molecular fragments called *free radicals* to join together, forming potentially carcinogenic (cancer-causing) compounds in your body.

Antioxidants also slow the normal wear-and-tear on body cells, so some researchers noted that a diet rich in plant foods (fruits, vegetables, grains, and beans) seems likely to reduce the risk of chronic conditions, such as heart disease, and maybe reduce the risk of some kinds of cancer.

However, recent studies show that although a diet rich in fruits and veggies is healthful as all get-out, stuffing yourself with the antioxidant vitamins A and C has no effect on the risk of heart disease.

Hormonelike compounds

Many plants contain compounds that behave like *estrogens,* the female sex hormones. Because only animal bodies can produce true hormones, these plant chemicals are called *hormonelike compounds* or *phytoestrogens* (plant estrogen). Seems fair.

The three kinds of phytoestrogens are

- ✔ Isoflavones, in fruits, vegetables, and beans
- ✔ Lignans, in grains
- ✔ Coumestans, in sprouts and alfalfa

The most studied phytoestrogens are the isoflavones known as *daidzein* and *genistein* (found in soy), two compounds with a chemical structure similar to *estradiol,* which is the estrogen produced by mammalian ovaries. Like natural or synthetic estrogens, phytoestrogens hook onto sensitive spots in reproductive tissue (breast, ovary, prostate, and so on), but the plant estrogen-like compounds are weaker so researchers once suggested that they might provide postmenopausal women with the benefits of estrogen (stronger bones and relief from hot flashes) without the higher risk of reproductive cancers associated with hormone replacement therapy (HRT). But recent animal and human studies suggested that, like natural and synthetic hormones, the plant compounds may stimulate tumor growth while having little effect on menopausal symptoms such as hot flashes. Bottom line? According to the International Food Information Council, "Further clinical studies will continue to increase understanding of the role of soy in maintaining and improving health." Couldn't have said it better myself.

Sulfur compounds

Slide an apple pie in the oven, and soon the kitchen fills with an aroma that makes your mouth water and your digestive juices flow. But boil some cabbage and — what is that awful smell? It's sulfur, the same chemical that identifies rotten eggs.

Cruciferous vegetables (named for the Latin word for "cross," in reference to their *x*-shaped blossoms), such as broccoli, Brussels sprouts, cauliflower, kale, kohlrabi, mustard seed, radishes, rutabaga, turnips, and watercress, all contain stinky sulfur compounds. The group includes sulforaphane glucosinolate (SGSD), glucobrassicin, gluconapin, gluconasturtin, neoglucobrassicin, and sinigrin.

These natural chemicals seem to tell your body to rev up its production of enzymes that inactivate and help eliminate carcinogens. For example, in animal studies at Johns Hopkins University School of Medicine, rats given chemicals known to cause breast tumors were less likely to develop tumors when they were given broccoli sprouts, a food that's unusually high in sulforaphane. In 2005, a human trial conducted in China by researchers from Johns Hopkins, Qidong Liver Cancer Institute, Jiao Tong University (Shanghai), and the University of Minnesota Cancer Center showed that the sulforaphane-rich sprouts appear to help the body defang *aflatoxins,* toxic compounds produced by molds that grow on grains such as rice. Aflatoxins, which damage cells and raise the risk of cancer, may be linked to the high incidence of stomach and liver cancers in China where fermented foods are common. Further studies are in the planning phases.

While you're waiting for final analyses, the best nutrition advice is to enjoy your phytochemicals. Dig into those veggies, fruits, and grains — and turn to Chapter 13 to find out why you need to wash them down with plenty of cold, clear water.

Exploring the Nature (And Science) of Food Additives

Food additives may be natural or synthetic. For example, vitamin C is a natural preservative. Butylated hydroxyanisole (BHA) and butylated hydroxytoluene (BHT) are synthetic preservatives. To ensure your safety, both the natural *and* synthetic food additives used in the United States come only from the group of substances known as the *Generally Recognized as Safe (GRAS)* list.

All additives on the GRAS list

- ✔ Are approved by the Food and Drug Administration (FDA), meaning that agency is satisfied that the additive is safe and effective

- ✔ Must be used only in specifically limited amounts

- ✔ Must be used to satisfy a specific need in food products, such as protection against molds

- ✔ Must be effective, meaning that they must actually maintain freshness and safety

- ✔ Must be listed accurately on the label

Adding nutrients

Vitamin D, which is added to virtually all milk sold in the United States, is one example of a clearly beneficial food additive. Most U.S. bread and grain products are fortified with added B vitamins, plus iron and other essential minerals to replace what's lost when whole grains are milled into white flour for white bread. Some people say that we'd be better off simply sticking to whole grains. But adding vitamins and minerals to white flours enhances a product that many people prefer.

Some nutrients also are useful preservatives. For example, vitamin C is an antioxidant that slows food spoilage and prevents destructive chemical reactions. In the United States, manufacturers must add a form of vitamin C *(isoascorbic acid* or *sodium ascorbate)* to bacon and other luncheon meats to prevent the formation of potentially cancer-causing compounds.

Adding colors and flavors

Colors, flavoring agents, and flavor enhancers make food look and taste better. Like other food additives, these three may be either natural or synthetic.

Colors

Coloring agents, which may be natural or synthetic, make food look better. An example of a natural coloring agent is *beta carotene,* the natural yellow pigment in many fruits and vegetables. Beta carotene is used to make margarine (which is naturally white) look like creamy yellow butter. Other natural coloring agents are *annatto,* a yellow-to-pink pigment from a tropical tree; *chlorophyll,* the green pigment in green plants; *carmine,* a reddish extract of *cochineal* (a pigment from crushed beetles); *saffron,* a yellow herb; and *turmeric,* a yellow spice.

An example of a synthetic coloring agent is FD&C Blue No. 1, a bright blue pigment made from coal tar and used in soft drinks, gelatin, hair dyes, and face powders, among other things. And, yes, as scientists have discovered more about the effects of coal-tar dyes, including the fact that some are carcinogenic, many of these coloring agents have been banned from use in food in one country or another but are still allowed in cosmetics.

Flavors and flavor enhancers

Every cook worth his or her spice cabinet knows about natural flavor ingredients, especially the most basic natural ones: salt, sugar, vinegar, wine, and fruit juices.

Artificial flavoring agents reproduce natural flavors. For example, a teaspoon of fresh lemon juice in the batter lends cheesecake a certain *je ne sais quoi* (French for "I don't know what" — a little something special), but artificial lemon flavoring works just as well. You can sweeten your morning coffee with natural sugar or with the artificial sweetener saccharin. (For more about substitute sweeteners, see Chapter 19.)

Alphabet soup: Understanding artificial colors

When you read the label on a food, drug, or cosmetic product containing artificial colors, you may see the letters *F, D,* and *C* — as in FD&C Yellow No. 5. The *F* stands for food. The *D* stands for drugs. The *C* stands for cosmetics. An additive whose name includes all three letters can be used in food, drugs, and cosmetics. An additive

without the *F* is restricted to use in drugs and cosmetics or is for external use only (translation: You don't take them by mouth). For example, D&C Green No. 6 is a blue-green coloring agent used in hair oils and pomades. FD&C Blue No. 2 is a bright blue coloring agent used in hair rinses, as well as mint jellies, candies, and cereals.

What color is your cauliflower?

This is not a frivolous question. In addition to basic white, cauliflower now comes in lime green, purple, and a smashing new orange variety bred at the New York State Agricultural Experiment Station in Geneva (NY).

Whether orange cauliflower is prettier than white, green, or purple is a personal decision, but there's no question that it's more nutritious. The orange color comes from beta-carotene, the yellow carotenoid, the body converts to vitamin A. As Michael Dickson, Professor Emeritus at Cornell University and former head of the Geneva facility, explains, orange cauliflower has the most vitamin A, about 25 times more than white.

Carotenoids are vital to phytosynthesis, the process by which plants convert light to energy, because they are antioxidants, compounds that protect the chlorophyll from being attacked and destroyed by oxygen in the air. They may also be vital to human beings because when we eat foods with carotenoids or other antioxidant plant pigments, such as the red and blue anthocyanins in blueberries, beets, and strawberries, the yellow zeaxanthins in corn, spinach, and persimmons, and the white anthoxanthins in white potatoes, cauliflower, rice, and white onions, the pigments become *chemopreventers*, substances that stop trouble before it starts. Carotenoids may keep molecular fragments called free radicals from hooking up to form compounds that can damage cells, causing changes that may lead to heart disease, cancer, and other age-related degenerative diseases.

This is such a valuable effect that from time to time people have tried to take the carotenoid out of the plant and put it and its benefits into a pill. It rarely works: In one famous incident in the late 1980s, people who took beta carotene supplements to lower their risk of various kinds of cancer turned out to raise their risk instead.

To get the goods, you have to eat the food. Which illustrates another benefit of natural plant pigments: They make food look inviting. Orange may not be natural to cauliflower, but it is a natural plant food color, and as Dr. Dickson notes, some cooks will like the orange cauliflower because it contrasts nicely with white foods such as rice, fish, and potatoes.

On the other hand, colors that aren't natural to food can be definite turn-offs. In psychological studies, the classic "yuck" food has always been mashed potatoes tinted blue with food coloring. But when JetBlue dishes out bags of blue (get it?) potato chips made from a naturally blue variety of potatoes. They go like hot cakes. Go figure.

Flavor enhancers are a slightly different kettle of fish. They intensify a food's natural flavor instead of adding a new one. The best-known flavor enhancer is *monosodium glutamate (MSG)*, which is widely used in Asian foods. MSG may trigger headaches and other symptoms in people sensitive to the seasoning.

Adding preservatives

Food spoilage is a totally natural phenomenon. Milk sours. Bread sprouts mold. Meat and poultry rot. Vegetables lose moisture and wilt. Fats turn rancid. The first three kinds of spoilage are caused by *microbes* (bacteria, mold, and yeasts). The last two happen when food is exposed to *oxygen* (air).

All preservative techniques — cooking, chilling, canning, freezing, drying — prevent spoilage either by slowing the growth of the organisms that live on food or by protecting the food from the effects of oxygen. Chemical preservatives do essentially the same thing:

- *Antimicrobials* are natural or synthetic preservatives that protect food by slowing the growth of bacteria, molds, and yeasts.

- *Antioxidants* are natural or synthetic preservatives that protect food by preventing food molecules from combining with oxygen (air).

Table 22-1 is a representative list of some common preservative chemicals and the foods in which they're found.

Table 22-1	Preservatives in Food
Preservative	*Found in . . .*
Ascorbic acid*	Sausages, luncheon meats
Benzoic acid	Beverages (soft drinks), ice cream, baked goods
BHA (butylated hydroxyanisole)	Potato chips and other foods
BHT (butylated hydroxytoluene)	Potato chips and other foods
Calcium propionate	Breads, processed cheese
Isoascorbate*	Luncheon meats and other foods
Sodium ascorbate*	Luncheon meats and other foods
Sodium benzoate	Margarine, soft drinks

* A form of vitamin C
Ruth Winter, A Consumer's Dictionary of Cosmetic Ingredients (New York: Crown, 1996)

Naming some other additives in food

Food chemists use a variety of the following types of natural and chemical additives to improve the texture of food, to keep it smooth, or to prevent mixtures from separating:

✔ *Emulsifiers,* such as lecithin and polysorbate, keep liquid-plus-solids, such as chocolate pudding, from separating into, well, liquid and solids. They can also keep two unfriendly liquids, such as oil and water, from divorcing so that salad dressing stays smooth.

✔ *Stabilizers,* such as the alginates (alginic acid) derived from seaweed, make food such as ice cream feel smoother, richer, or creamier in your mouth.

✔ *Thickeners* are natural gums and starches, such as apple pectin or corn-starch, that add body to foods.

✔ *Texturizers,* such as calcium chloride, keep foods such as canned apples, tomatoes, or potatoes from turning mushy.

Although many of these additives are derived from foods, their real benefit is aesthetic (the food looks and tastes better), not nutritional.

Determining the Safety of Food Additives

The safety of any chemical approved for use as a food additive is based on whether it is

✔ Toxic

✔ Carcinogenic

✔ Allergenic

Defining toxins

A *toxin* is a poison. Some chemicals, such as cyanide, are toxic (poisonous) in very, very small doses. Others, such as sodium ascorbate (a form of vitamin C), are nontoxic even in very large doses. All chemicals on the GRAS list are considered nontoxic in the amounts that are permitted in food. By the way, both examples — cyanide and vitamin C — are *natural* chemicals, one benefi-cial, one not so much.

Explaining carcinogens

A *carcinogen* is a substance that causes cancer. Some natural chemicals, such as *aflatoxins,* which are poisons produced by molds that grow on peanuts, are carcinogens. Some synthetic chemicals, such as specific dyes, are also potentially carcinogenic.

The nitrate/nitrite conundrum

Some preservatives are double-edged — good and not-so-good at the same time. For example, nitrates and nitrites are effective preservatives that prevent the growth of disease-bearing organisms in cured meat. But when they reach your stomach, nitrates and nitrites react with natural ammonia compounds called *amines* to form *nitrosamines,* substances known to cause cancer in animals fed amounts of nitrosamines much higher than found in any human food.

But avoiding foods with added nitrates and nitrites won't prevent your having to cope with nitrosamines. Beets, celery, eggplant, lettuce, radishes, spinach, and turnip greens all contain naturally occurring nitrates and nitrites,

sometimes at higher levels than in cured meat products. When their nitrates and nitrates shake hands in your stomach, they make — you got it! — nitrosamines.

To take the sting out of added nitrates and nitrites in foods such as cured meats, the USDA, which regulates meat, fish, and poultry, sensibly requires manufacturers to add an antioxidant vitamin C compound such as sodium ascorbate or an antioxidant vitamin E compound (a tocopherol). The antioxidant vitamins prevent the formation of nitrosamines while boosting the antimicrobial powers of the nitrates and nitrites.

In 1958, driven by a fear of potentially carcinogenic pesticide residues in food, New York Congressman James Delaney proposed and Congress enacted into law an amendment to the Food, Drug, and Cosmetic Act that banned from food any synthetic chemical known to cause cancer (in animals or human beings) when ingested in *any* amount, no matter how small. (The Delaney clause did not apply to natural chemicals, even those known to cause cancer.)

For a time, the only exception to the Delaney clause was saccharin, which was exempted in 1970. Although ingesting very large amounts of the artificial sweetener is known to cause bladder cancer in animals, no similar link was ever found to human cancers. Nonetheless, in 1977, Congress required all products containing saccharin to carry a warning statement: *Use of this product may be hazardous to your health. This product contains saccharin, which has been determined to cause cancer in laboratory animals.*

When the Delaney clause was introduced, ingredients such as additives were measured in parts (of the additive) per thousand parts (of the product). Today, scientists have the ability to measure an ingredient in parts per trillionths. As a result, the zero-risk standard of the Delaney clause in regard to pesticide residue in food was repealed and replaced with a standard of "reasonable risk." The zero risk standard still applies to food additives; the saccharin warning was lifted in 2000.

Listing allergens

Allergens are substances that trigger allergic reactions. Some foods, such as peanuts, contain natural allergens that can provoke fatal allergic reactions.

The best-known example of an allergenic food additive is sulfites, a group of preservatives that

- ✔ Keep light-colored fruits and vegetables (apples, potatoes) from browning when exposed to air
- ✔ Prevent shellfish (shrimp and lobster) from developing black spots
- ✔ Reduce the growth of bacteria in fermenting wine and beer
- ✔ Bleach food starches
- ✔ Make dough easier to handle

Sulfites are safe for most people but not for all. In fact, the FDA estimates that 1 out of every 100 people is sensitive to these chemicals; among people with asthma, the number rises to 5 out of every 100. For people sensitive to sulfites, even infinitesimally small amounts may trigger a serious allergic reaction, and asthmatics may develop breathing problems by simply inhaling fumes from sulfite-treated foods.

The FDA tried banning sulfites from food but lost in a court case brought by food manufacturers who wanted to use the additive. To protect sulfite-sensitive people, the FDA created rules for safe use of the preservatives. The rules called for a total ban on sulfites in food at salad bars and a requirement that sulfites be listed on the label of any food or beverage product with more than ten parts sulfites to every million parts food (10 ppm). These rules, plus plenty of press information about the risks of sulfites, have led to a dramatic decrease in the number of sulfite reactions.

Looking Beyond Additives: Foods Nature Never Made

Genetically engineered foods, also known as bioengineered foods, are foods with extra genes added artificially through special laboratory processes. Like preservatives, flavor enhancers, and other chemical boosters used in food, the genes — which may come from plants, animals, or microorganisms such as bacteria — are used to make foods

✔ More resistant to disease and insects

✔ More nutritious

✔ Better tasting

Genetic engineering may also help plants and animals grow faster and larger, thus increasing the food supply. And it may enable us to produce foods with medicines bred right into the food itself. (Check out Chapter 26.)

The Big Question is "Are genetically engineered foods safe?" The best answer may be that only time can tell. As you can imagine, many people don't want to wait to find out.

To permit consumers to make a clear choice — "Yes, I'll take that biotech food" or "No, I won't" — the European Union requires food labels to specifically state the presence of any genetically altered ingredients. In the United States, the FDA currently requires wording on labels to alert consumers to genetic engineering only when it results in an unexpected allergen, such as corn genes in tomatoes, or changes the nutritional content of a food.

Whether the wording on the label matters to most consumers or whether most consumers are willing to accept genetically altered foods seems to depend on whom you ask and how you ask.

The International Food Information Council (IFIC), a trade group for the food industry, accepts the current label-wording rules. The Center for Science in the Public Interest (CSPI), a Washington-based consumer advocacy group, wants to see the words "genetically altered" on all foods that have been, well, genetically altered. CSPI also wants the FDA to finalize a rule requiring food marketers to notify the agency in advance when introducing a new altered food or plant, a policy that's already in place for foods from genetically altered animals.

Naturally, each organization has conducted a survey to bolster its point of view. For example, IFIC's survey says that nearly two-thirds (61 percent) of Americans expect food technology to serve up better-quality, better-tasting food. CSPI's competing survey says, "Not so fast." The difference lies in the questions. The IFIC's survey questions emphasize the benefits of biotech; CSPI's survey questions lean more heavily on the drawbacks. Here are a couple of comparable questions from the CSPI and IFIC surveys:

1. **Question**

    CSPI Version: Should food labels tell you if a food has been genetically altered in any way? 70 percent (Yes)

    IFIC Version: Would you say you support or oppose FDA's [current labeling] policy? 59 percent (Support)

2. Question

CSPI Version: Would you buy food labeled "genetically engineered"? 43 percent (Yes)

IFIC Version: Would you buy a food if it had been modified by biotechnology to taste better or fresher? Or stay fresher? 54 percent (Yes)

In other words, despite a slight wariness about exploring new nutritional ground, Americans seem intrigued by the promise of food innovations and are willing to give the whole idea a try. After that, the proof will be in the — genetically engineered — pudding.

To read the CSPI survey, go to www.cspinet.org, choose Reports, and scroll down to National Opinion Poll on Labeling of Genetically Engineered Foods. To read the IFIC survey, type this into your search bar: ific.nisgroup. com/research/upload/2005BiotechSurvey.pdf.

Part V
Food and Medicine

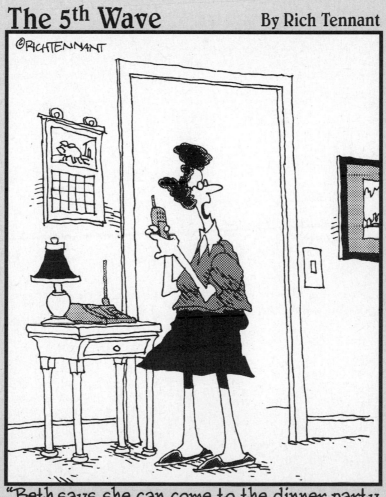

"Beth says she can come to the dinner party, but she's allergic to cow's milk. Does that mean we can't invite your mother?"

In this part . . .

How come a civilization (yours) that has antibiotics, analgesics, and decongestants still serves up chicken soup for a cold, coffee for a headache, and chocolate for a broken heart? Because they work.

Food and medicine are natural partners. Sometimes they fight (the technical term is *food/drug interactions*), but more often, as this part explains, they march together to keep your body in tip-top shape.

Chapter 23

When Food Gives You Hives

According to the Food Allergy & Anaphylaxis Network (FAAN), at least 11.4 million Americans have true *food allergies* (also known as *food hypersensitivity*).

This number includes more children than adults because many childhood allergies seem to fade with age. But food allergies that don't disappear can trigger reactions ranging from the trivial (a stuffy nose the day after you eat the food) to the truly dangerous (immediate respiratory failure). And, a person with food allergies is likely to be allergic to other things, such as dust, pollen, or the family cat. So, forewarned (about food allergies) is forearmed (against the rest).

A word to the allergy-wise: You can stay current with allergy news via these two Web sites:

✔ The American Academy of Allergy, Asthma, & Immunology (www.aaaai.org)

✔ The Food Allergy & Anaphylaxis Network (www.foodallergy.org)

Finding Out More About Food Allergies

Your immune system is designed to protect your body from harmful invaders, such as bacteria. Sometimes, however, the system responds to substances normally considered harmless. The substance that provokes the attack is called an *allergen;* the substances that attack the allergen are called *antibodies.*

A food allergy can provoke such a response as your body releases antibodies to attack specific proteins in food. When this happens, some of the physical reactions include

- ✔ Hives

- ✔ Itching

- ✔ Swelling of the face, tongue, lips, eyelids, hands, and feet

- ✔ Rashes

- ✔ Headaches, migraines

- ✔ Nausea and/or vomiting

- ✔ Diarrhea, sometimes bloody

- ✔ Sneezing, coughing

- ✔ Asthma

- ✔ Breathing difficulties caused by *tightening* (swelling) of tissues in the throat

- ✔ Loss of consciousness (from anaphylactic shock)

If you're sensitive to a specific food, you may not have to eat the food to have the reaction. For example, people sensitive to peanuts may break out in hives just from touching a peanut or peanut butter and may suffer a potentially fatal reaction after tasting chocolate that has touched factory machinery that previously touched peanuts. People sensitive to seafood — fin fish and shellfish — have been known to develop breathing problems after simply inhaling the vapors or steam produced by cooking the fish.

Understanding how an allergic reaction occurs

When you eat a food containing a protein to which you're sensitive, the protein reaches antibodies on the surface of white blood cells called *basophils* and immune system cells called mast cells either in your gastro-intestinal tract or by circulating through the blood stream.

The basophils and mast cells produce, store, and release *histamine,* a natural body chemical that causes the symptoms — itching, swelling, hives — associated with allergic reactions (some allergy pills designed to counter this are called *antihistamines*). When the antibodies on the surface of the basophils and mast cells come in contact with food allergens, the cells release histamine, and the result is an *allergic reaction.*

Allergy glossary

allergen: Any substance that sets off an allergic reaction (see "antigen" in this sidebar).

anaphylaxis: A potentially life-threatening allergic reaction that involves many body systems, creating a cascade of adverse effects beginning with sudden, severe itching and moving on to tissue swelling in the air passages that can lead to breathing difficulties, falling blood pressure, unconsciousness, and death.

antibody: A protein in your blood that reacts to an antigen and tries to render it harmless.

antigen: A substance that stimulates a response from the immune system; an allergen is a specific type of antigen.

basophil: A white blood cell that carries IgE and releases histamine.

ELISA: Short for *enzyme-linked immunosorbent assay,* a test used to determine the presence of antibodies in your blood, including antibodies to specific allergens.

epinephrine: Adrenaline, the medicine used to treat severe allergic reactions.

histamine: The substance released by the immune system (specifically by basophils and mast cells) that produces the symptoms of an allergic reaction, such as itching and swelling.

IgE: An abbreviation for *immunoglobulin E,* the antibody that reacts to allergens.

intolerance: A nonallergic adverse reaction to food.

mast cell: A cell in body tissue that releases histamine.

RAST: An abbreviation for *radioallergosorbent test,* a blood test used to determine whether you're allergic to certain foods.

urticaria: The medical name for hives.

Investigating two kinds of allergic reactions

Your body may react to an allergen in one of two ways — immediately or later on:

- ✔ **Immediate reactions** are more dangerous because they involve a fast swelling of tissue, sometimes within seconds after contact with the offending food.

- ✔ **Delayed reactions,** which may occur as long as 24 to 48 hours after you've been exposed to the offending food, are usually much milder, perhaps a slight cough or nasal congestion caused by swollen tissues.

Most allergic reactions to food are unpleasant but essentially mild. However, as many as 150 to 200 people die every year in the United States from a severe reaction to a food allergen.

Call 911 immediately if you or a friend or relative show any signs of an allergic reaction — including an allergic reaction to food — that affects breathing.

Identifying food allergies

A tendency toward allergies (although not necessarily the specific allergy itself) is inherited. If one of your parents has an allergy, your risk of having one is two times higher than it would be if neither of your parents had a history of allergic disease. If both your mother and your father have allergies, your risk is four times higher.

To identify the culprit causing your food allergy, your doctor may suggest an *elimination diet.* This regimen removes from your diet foods — most commonly milk, egg, soy, wheat, peanuts — known to cause allergic reactions in many people. Then, one at a time, the foods are added back. If you react to one, bingo! That's a clue to what triggers your immune response.

To be absolutely certain, your doctor may challenge your immune system by introducing foods in a form (maybe a capsule) that neither you nor he can identify as a specific food. Doing so rules out any possibility that your reaction has been triggered by emotional stimuli — that is, seeing, tasting, or smelling the food.

Other tests that can identify allergens to specific foods include skin tests and two types of blood tests — *ELISA* (enzyme-linked immunosorbent assay) and *RAST* (radioallergosorbent test) — that can identify antibodies to specific allergens in your blood. But these two tests are rarely required.

Coping with Food Allergies

To keep yourself or your allergic friends and family safe in a world practically teeming with allergens, know what's in your food, check out unusual allergenic couplings, work with others to make rules that work, and practice simple protection.

Reading the food ingredient label

According to the Food Allergy and Anaphylaxis Network, more than 90 percent of all allergic reactions to foods are caused by just eight foods: Eggs, fish, milk, peanuts, shellfish, soy, tree nuts, and wheat.

If you're sensitive to one of these foods, the best way to avoid an allergic reaction is to avoid the food. And you can do that by reading the label to ferret out hidden ingredients — peanuts in the chili or caviar (fish eggs) in the dip.

In the past, a hidden allergen might be hidden in plain sight on a food label that used alternative or chemical code names, such as whey or casein or lactoglobulin for milk. But in 2004, Congress passed and the president signed into law the Food Allergen Labeling and Consumer Protection Act. As of January 1, 2006, all food labels must use plain English words for the eight most-common food allergens.

Table 23-1 lists and describes The Allergy Eight, with special attention to those unexpected appearances on the menu (also see Figure 23-1).

Table 23-1	The Allergy Eight	
Food	*People Affected[1]*	*Where This Food May Hide in Commercial Products*
Eggs	1–2% of young children; most outgrow this allergy	Foam/topping on coffee drinks; egg substitutes; pasta in prepared foods (like soups); pretzels/bread (egg wash on crust)
Fish	2.3% of all Americans (children and adults)	Dressings and sauces (Worcestershire sauce); Asian and Mexican dishes; prepared meat products (like meatloaf)
Milk	2.3% of children under 3; most outgrow this allergy	Canned tuna, meat, and nondairy products (as casein, the protein in milk)
Peanuts[2]	1% of American children and adults; recent studies suggest that up to 20% of allergic children may outgrow this allergy	Dressings and sauces; marinades; pizza; Asian and Mexican dishes; meat substitutes
Shellfish	2.3% of all Americans	Sauces (like fish sauce); Asian dishes
Soy	NA[3]; many children outgrow this allergy	Baked products including cereals and snacks; margarines; meat substitutes (textured vegetable protein); nut butters; sauces; prepared soups

(continued)

Table 23-1 *(continued)*

Food	People Affected[1]	Where This Food May Hide in Commercial Products
Tree nuts[4]	0.5% of American children and adults	Salad dressings; sauces (barbecue sauce); breaded foods; meat substitutes (vegetarian burgers); pastas
Wheat[5]	>1% of children younger than 3; most outgrow this allergy	Various foods including ice cream; chips; meat, fish, and poultry products (prepared burgers, hot dogs, imitation crab meat [surimi])

(1) *Estimates.*
(2) *Peanuts, sometimes known as ground nuts, are legumes, a vegetable class that includes peas and beans.*
(3) *Depending on the source, estimates range from a low of 0.3% of young children to a high of 20% of all children and adults.*
(4) *Including, among others, almonds, Brazil nuts, cashews, chestnuts, coconuts, hazelnuts, Macadamia nuts, pecans, pistachios, walnuts.*
(5) *Wheat allergy has no relationship with celiac disease, a genetic malabsorption disorder in which the body reacts to gluten, a protein in some grains (primarily wheat, barley, oats, and rye). Celiac disease is a lifelong condition.*
Sources: About.com, http://foodallergies.about.com/od/soyallergies/p/soyallergy.htm, Food Allergy and Anaphylaxis Network, www.foodallergy.org; Mayo Clinic, www.mayoclinic.com/health/soy-allergy/DS00970; "Is Soy Allergy Overestimated?," Luisa Businco. Pediatric Asthma, Allergy & Immunology, Summer 1993, 7(2): 73-76.

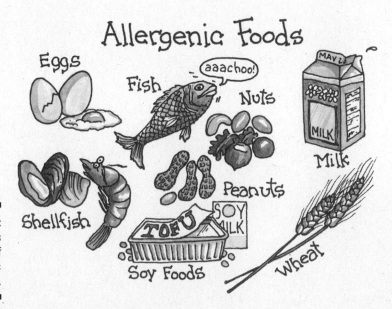

Figure 23-1: These foods can set off an allergic reaction.

Avoiding unusual interactions

Sometimes a food label doesn't list an allergen because the allergen is simply (surprise!) a natural component of the food.

Salicylates are a perfect example. These natural chemicals occur in many plants, including some plants that end up on the dinner table. The salicylates protect the plants by destroying mold and other microorganisms. For human beings, salicylates act as analgesics (pain killers), the most famous of which is *acetylsalicylic acid,* better known as *aspirin.* People who are sensitive to salicylates may experience an allergic reaction (asthmalike breathing difficulty, headache, hives, rash or itchy skin, and swollen hands, feet, or face) when exposed even to very small amounts, including the salicylates in otherwise highly nutritious plant foods such as fruits and vegetables.

If you or someone you know is sensitive to salicylates, you'll be pleased to know that the allergy experts at the Wegeningen University in The Netherlands have put together a nifty little list of foods grouped into five categories according to the amount of salicylates they contain. (One regular aspirin contains 365 mg acetylsalicylic acid; one low-dose aspirin, the medicine prescribed to reduce the risk of heart disease, has 81 mg.)

The following list is a basic guide to the salicylate content of common foods:

- **Foods with negligible amounts of salicylates:** Bananas, cabbage, cashews, celery, chives, garlic, green beans, pears, peas, lentils

- **Foods low in salicylates (0.1–0.25 mg per 3.5 oz/100 g):** Apples (golden, red delicious), asparagus (fresh), cauliflower, cherries (sour), grapes (green), hazel nuts, lemon, mango, mushrooms (fresh), onions, passion fruit, pecans peanut butter, tamarillo, saffron, sesame seeds, soy sauce, vinegar

- **Foods moderate in salicylates (0.25–0.49 mg per 3.5 z/100g):** Asparagus (canned), Brazil nuts, Chinese vegetables, coconut, fennel, grapefruit juice, loquat, lychee, marrow (the British/European term for zucchini), nectarines, olives (black), plum, pumpkin, snow peas, watermelon

- **Foods high in salicylates (0.5–1.0 mg per 3.5 oz/100 g):** Alfalfa, apples (Granny Smith), avocado, broccoli, cherries (red), cucumber, fava beans, Macadamia nuts, mandarin oranges, pine nuts, pistachios, spinach, sweet potato, tangelo (tangerine/grapefruit, a.k.a. honeybell), vegemite (a salty food paste made from yeast)

- **Foods very high in salicylates (>1 mg per 3.5 oz/100g):** Almonds, apricots, blackberries, blueberries, canella (a cinnamon-like seasoning), cantaloupe, chicory, cumin, curry powder, dates, dill (dried), green pepper, guava, mushrooms (canned), mustard, olive, oregano, paprika (hot), peanuts, radish, raisins, rosemary, thyme, tomatoes, turmeric

Working to change an allergenic environment

In the real world, having a peanut allergy may affect your ability to enjoy simple pleasures, such as a baseball game where peanuts are sold. So imagine the delight of parents in New Britain, Connecticut, when the local Eastern League team (the Rock Cats) decided to set aside a special 138-seat food-free section during its 2002 season for baseball-crazy but peanut-allergic kids and their families at a game between the Rock Cats and the New Haven Ravens.

The Rock Cats and the Food Allergy & Anaphylaxis Network, a national consumer advocacy group with 250 members in the Hartford area, cooked up the idea because, as Rock Cats general manager John Willi has said, "No child should be deprived of the Rock Cats experience."

By 2010, the peanut-free theme had moved well into the majors, with more than one-third of the major-league baseball teams designating games with peanut-free areas. And some people take peanut-free very seriously indeed: The Washington Nationals wash the sections down twice before each peanut-free game.

But as Robert Wood, MD, director of pediatric allergy and immunology at the Johns Hopkins Children's Center in Baltimore, author of *Food Allergies For Dummies* (Wiley), and a person with a peanut allergy himself, has noted, watching a game in an outdoor ballpark is less hazardous than, say, sitting in the cabin in an airplane where the air carries peanut particles and scattered crumbs on the floor or seats.

Funny he should mention that. In the spring of 2010, the U.S. Department of Transportation once again considered imposing a ban on peanuts on U.S. carriers. (They had tried this once before, in 1998, only to be stymied by representatives from peanut-growing states.)

The DOT's current proposals include the following options:

✔ An outright ban on airlines serving peanuts and peanut products

✔ Banning service of peanuts and peanut products only on a flight where a passenger with a peanut allergy requests a peanut-free flight in advance

✔ Requiring the airline to provide a peanut-free buffer zone around a passenger with a medically documented severe peanut allergy if the passenger makes a request in advance

While you're waiting to see whether these proposals fly, remember to check with the airline when making reservations. Some carriers are already piloting peanut-free planes.

Practicing pragmatic protection

If you're someone with a known potentially life-threatening allergy to food (or another allergen, such as wasp venom), your doctor may suggest that you carry a syringe prefilled with *epinephrine*, a drug that counteracts the reactions.

You may also decide to wear a tag that identifies you as a person with a serious allergic problem. One company that provides these tags is Medic-Alert Foundation International, a 40+-year-old firm located in Turlock, California. The 24/7 telephone number for Medic-Alert is 888-633-4298;Web site: www. medicalert.org.

Recognizing Other Body Reactions to Food

Allergic reactions aren't the only way your body registers a protest against certain foods. Other reactions to foods include

✔ **A metabolic reaction:** Food intolerance, also known as a non-allergic food hypersensitivity, is an inherited inability to metabolize (digest) certain foods, such as fat or lactose (the naturally occurring sugar in milk). The reaction may include intestinal gas, diarrhea, or other signs of gastric revolt.

✔ **A physical reaction to a specific chemical:** Your body may react to things such as the laxative substance in prunes or monosodium glutamate (MSG), the flavor enhancer commonly found in Asian food. Although some people are more sensitive than others to these chemicals, their reaction is a physical one. It does not involve the immune system.

✔ **A body response to psychological triggers:** When you're very fearful or very anxious or very excited, your body moves into hyper drive, secreting hormones that pump up your heartbeat and respiration, speed the passage of food through your gut, and cause you to empty your bowels and bladder. The entire process, called the *fight-or-flight response,* prepares your body to defend itself by either fighting or running. On a more prosaic level, a strong reaction to your food may cause diarrhea. It isn't an allergy; it's your hormones.

✔ **A change in mood and/or behavior.** Some foods, such as coffee, contain chemicals, such as caffeine, may cause hyperactivity, as well as having a real effect on mood and behavior, the subject of Chapter 24.

Chapter 24

Brain Food

. . . .

In This Chapter

▶ Identifying food's effects on the brain

▶ Explaining thought and memory

▶ Matching your diet to your brain's age

▶ Choosing food to change your mood

. . . .

Are you an average adult? Then your average brain weighs an average 3 pounds, about 2 percent of your average (150 pounds) body weight. But that 2 percent uses nearly 20 percent of the calories you consume each day to power more than 100 billion neurons (nerve cells) that, working at top speed, convert those calories into enough energy to turn on a 25-watt incandescent light bulb.

Calories aren't the whole story, of course. *What* you eat and *when* you eat it also matter. This chapter tells you *why* and introduces you to a new and exciting field of investigative science: Food and your brain.

Nourishing the Developing Brain

In 1987, pediatricians at North Shore University Hospital in Manhasset, New York, faced an unusual situation. In a thriving middle class community, they were suddenly called to treat seven infants who were definitely *not* thriving, meaning that the babies' bodies and, more disturbing, their brains, were not developing as expected.

Failure to thrive is commonly linked to malnutrition. And, in an unusual way, this failure turned out to be the case. After a series of diagnostic exams and questions, the Long Island doctors discovered that seven sets of nutrition-conscious parents had been feeding their children a lowfat, low cholesterol diet meant to protect adults at risk of heart disease.

Happily, the doctors changed the diet, the infants recovered, and everybody got the point: Not only does a developing brain need plenty of calories; a lot of those calories should come from fats, particularly the polyunsaturated omaga-3 fatty acid docosahexaenoic acid, better known as DHA.

Fats and the fetal brain

The human body is about 60 percent water. The human brain is about 60 percent fat, and most of that is DHA. This fatty acid is vital for the proper functioning of the adult brain but even more important for the development of the fetal brain and spinal cord. (Consuming foods with DHA also helps reduce the risk of cardiovascular disease, but that's a story for another chapter or another book, perhaps *Controlling Cholesterol For Dummies*.)

More than 20 years after the seven fat-deprived babies showed up at North Shore, an entire catalogue of well-designed studies has documented the advantages conferred on infants whose mothers get plenty of DHA — the best source is fish oils, fish, and seafood (see Table 24-2) while pregnant — along with all the normal vitamins, minerals, and other essential components of a healthful diet, of course.

Right from the start, babies delivered by women with higher blood levels of DHA are more attentive to new stimuli. For the next six months, they score higher on tests of cognition (thinking processes) than babies born to women with lower levels of DHA. According to Emily Oken of Harvard Medical School, by the time the DHA-enriched babies are three years old, they may also score several points higher on the Peabody Picture Vocabulary Test, a quiz that is to babies what a spoken or written vocabulary test is to older children and adults.

But DHA's brain benefit doesn't end with babies.

Fish and the teenage brain

The next time your teen brother, nephew, son, or friend tells you he's a grown-up, smile pleasantly and hand him a tuna sandwich. In fact, the brain of an older teen — think 15, 16, 17, 18 — is particularly "plastic," meaning particularly able to build the new connections required to learn new things like high school math, science, history, and literature.

Data from a 2009 study at Sweden's Goteborg University showed that 15-year-old boys who eat fish more than once a week score higher than their non-fish-eating friends on intelligence tests.

Unless they're totally chauvinistic, sometime soon the Goteberg researchers are likely to file another report, this one on the plastic female brain. While we're waiting, make sure your teen brother, nephew, son, or friend shares that tuna sandwich with his sister, niece, daughter, or girlfriend.

How much DHA does a body need?

In 2002, the National Academy of Science's Food and Nutrition Board set recommendations for daily consumption of omega-3 fatty acids as shown in Table 24-1. By the way, as explained in Chapter 5, the Adequate Intake (AI) is a recommendation for nutrients for which there is no RDA.

Table 24-1	Daily Adequate Intake (AI) for Omega-3s	
Infants	0–12 months	0.6 g/600 mg
Children	1–3 years	0.7 g/700 mg
	4–8 years	0.9h/900 mg
	9–13 years	1.2 g/1,200 mg
	14–18 years	1.6 g/1,600 mg (boys)
		1.1 g/1,100 mg (girls)
Pregnant women		1.4 g/1,400 mg
Breastfeeding women		1.3 g/1,300mg
Adults	19+	1.6 g/1,600 mg (men)
		1.1 g/1,100 mg (women)

Source: Food and Nutrition Board, National Academy of Sciences, "Dietary Reference Intakes for Energy, Carbohydrate, Fiber, Fat, Fatty Acids, Cholesterol, Protein, and Amino Acids," September 5, 2002

Avoiding malicious mercury

Naturally, there is a catch in the day's catch. Some fish contain an unhealthful amount of methylmercury, a compound produced by bacteria that chemically alter the naturally occurring mercury in rock and soil or the mercury released into water through industrial pollution.

Little fish eat mercury-contaminated algae, bigger fish eat the smaller fish, we eat the bigger fish, and the mercury ends up in us. The larger the fish and the longer it lives, the higher its mercury content is likely to be. To reduce the risk to fetal development, the 2010 Dietary Guidelines for Americans advisory committee advises pregnant woman to avoid the Mercury Big Four (shark, swordfish, king mackerel, tilefish) and limit their weekly consumption of seafood to two or less 4-ounce servings of seafood high in omega-3s and low in mercury.

Luckily, you can also get DHA from nonfish sources. For example, many infant formulas now contain DHA derived from fermented algae, and health-food stores sell algae-based DHA supplements for adults. One plain egg yolk contains 20 mg/0.02 g DHA; an egg yolk from an egg laid by a hen fed a DHA-enriched diet may contain up to 200 mg/0.2 g DHA. Some nuts and seeds (think walnuts and flax seed) contain alpha linolenic acid, a precursor converted by our bodies to DHA.

Table 24-2 shows the DHA and mercury content of some popular fish and shellfish.

Table 24-2	DHA & Mercury Content of Popular Fish & Seafood	
Fish	*DHA per 100g/3.5 oz*	*Mercury Content**
Anchovy	1.3	Low
Catfish	0.13	Low
Clams	0.15	Not detectible
King Mackeral	0.23	High
Salmon, Atlantic, wild	1.43	Low
Sardine,#	0.51	Low
Scallop	0.10	Low
Shark, raw	0.53	High
Swordfish	0.68	High
Tilefish	0.73	High
Trout, mixed species	0.68	Low

* Low = less than 0.12 ppm; high = more than 0.730 ppm.
 # canned, drained.
Source: USDA, Appendix G2: Original Food Guide Pyramid Patterns and Descriptions of USDA Analyses, Addition A: EPA and DHA Content of Fish Species, 2005, www.health.gov/dietaryguidelines/ dga2005/report/html/table_g2_adda2.htm; FDA, Mercury Levels in Commercial Fish and Shellfish, 2006, www.fda.gov/food/foodsafety/product-specificinformation/seafood/foodbornepathogens contaminants/methylmercury/ucm115644.htm.

Protecting the Adult Brain

Once you and your brain make it past the teen years and into your 20s, the support system that once mentored the birth and maturity of as many as several hundred thousand new neurons a day apparently goes to sleep. Currently, some researchers are working on ways to wake it up, but that's a story for the future. Right now, barring illness or injury, what you have — structurally speaking — is pretty much what you will have until The End.

Of course, you can and certainly should use your full-grown brain to learn new things, creating new connections among brain cells and assimilating new information about the world around you.

But whether you are 30 or 70, from now on your primary task is to protect and preserve your intellectual brain functions: *cognition* (the processes of learning, thinking, and reasoning) and *memory* (the ability to retain and recall past experiences).

The natural enemies of thought and memory

The old news was that after a certain age, say, 30, your brain begins to shrink until it simply shrivels into nothing. The new news is that scientists who have actually taken the time to sit down and count brain cells find practically no age-related loss of cells responsible for cognition and memory.

Remember this

Short-term memory lasts a few minutes. If you are reading a book, and you put it down to answer the phone, short-term memory enables you to go back and recognize where you left off. Or to remember a strange phone number long enough to dial it.

Long-term memory lasts for years. If what you were reading strikes a chord, you may store it in your brain and pull it out from time to time. For example, few people who read Charles Dickens' *A Tale of Two Cities* ever forget the first line: "It was the best of times. It was the worst of times." Or, on a more practical level, their own phone numbers.

Amnesia is loss of memory related to an illness or an injury. *Retrograde amnesia* is the inability to remember things that happened before the illness or injury; *anterograde amnesia* is the inability to form new memories afterwards. With the former, you can't remember the phone number you had in high school. With the latter, you won't be able to remember the new phone number you might get tomorrow.

Are vitamins vital?

Using nutritional supplements to boost brain power is an iffy proposition, long on theory and short on proof.

True, deficiencies of specific nutrients, such as iron, can adversely affect brain development and function. For example, in 1996, researchers at Johns Hopkins Children's Center recruited iron-deficient but not-yet-anemic high school girls from four Baltimore high schools, gave them iron supplements, and watched their test scores rise.

But do supplements increase brain health for healthy people? Yes. No. And maybe — the evidence is far from conclusive. As for herbs. Ginko biloba, ginseng, gotu kola — is there something special in plants beginning with the letter "g"? — come into vogue and then slide out again as scientific studies show a lack of effect.

The best advice on nutrients for your brain? As always, stick to that boring but effective varied diet.

However, the cells in your adult brain — like other body cells — face two natural enemies: oxidative stress and inflammation.

- *Oxidative stress* is damage done by particles called *free radicals* that form during chemical reactions occurring in the body. As you grow older, your cells' sensitivity to this kind of injury goes up while your ability to heal afterwards goes down.

- *Inflammation* is your immune system's natural response to injury: swelling, heat, and pain. The American Heart Association regards *C-reactive protein* (CRP), a protein whose presence increases during inflammation, as a risk factor for heart disease and stroke. A natural increase in the level of *tumor necrosis factor alpha* and *interleukin-6,* two inflammatory agents in your brain and spinal cord, appears to play a role in the age-related loss of both cognition and memory.

How to counter these two enemies? One possible answer: Food. Maybe.

Dieting to keep your brain in shape

Some people say that whatever you eat goes straight to your hips. Two nutrition researchers suggest that's just a short stop on the way to your brain, and that as you age, expanding hips may mean shrinking brainpower.

Although there is no evidence that cutting back on calories extends human life or preserves human cognition, more than 20 years' worth of studies show that it works for lab rats. In 2001, Christiaan Leeuwenburgh, director of the Biochemistry of Aging Laboratory at the University of Florida College of Health and Human Performance, suggested one reason why.

As a body ages, it churns out higher levels of certain proteins, such as *cytochrome C,* which trigger *apoptosis,* science-speak for cell death. In Leeuwenburgh's studies, rats given food with plenty of nutrients but 40 percent fewer calories than the normal rat diet had lower levels of cytochrome C in their brains. They also had higher brain levels of *apoptosis receptor caspase (aka ARC),* a protein that slows production of cytochrome C, thus preserving brain cells.

Leeuwenburgh wasn't the only one to see a link between weight and brain health. In 2004, Miia Kivipelto of the Karolinska Institute in Stockholm told the 4,500 scientists at the Ninth International Conference on Alzheimer's Disease and Related Disorders that chubby middle-agers are at a higher risk of developing dementia later in life. Kivipelto based her assumption on data of 1,499 Finnish men and women showing a BMI (body mass index) higher than 30 at age 50 — about 197 pounds for a 5'8" man or woman — doubles the risk. Add in a total cholesterol level higher than 250 and a blood pressure reading with one number higher than 140, and the Kivipelto says the risk is six times higher.

For more on Body Mass Index, turn to Chapter 4.

And maintain your healthful weight.

Choosing foods that boost the brain

Plants are deceptive. On the outside, they are mostly green and calm. On the inside, they are busy little chemical factories churning out multitudinous compounds, many of which have properties that protect the plant — and various parts of your body, including, of course, your brain.

One class of these natural chemicals is the *polyphenols,* so-named because their molecules are built of many *(poly-)* phenol- (ringlike) components.

Polyphenols are widely distributed in fruits and vegetables, as well as in nuts, seeds, and grains. Some have antioxidant, anti-allergic, anti-inflammatory, antiviral, antiproliferative (prevents cell from irregular reproduction, an anticancer trait), or anticarcinogenic effects.

One group of important antioxidant and anti-inflammatory polyphenols are the *flavonoids* (sometimes spelled flavanoids), the pigments that color plants yellow, red, orange, green, or white. Some flavonoids may also be antiviral and antiproliferative. Altogether, flavonoids protect plants from oxidative stress, including stress triggered by attacks from insects, fungi, and microbes.

Flavonoids may protect us, as well. Tests performed on living animals are called *in vivo,* from the Latin word for *life;* those done in test tubes are called *in vitro,* from the Latin word for *glass.* During *in vitro* experiments, some flavonoids have shown even more powerful antioxidant effects than the antioxidant vitamins C and E, thus providing a scientific rationale for the relatively new advice to choose your diet by color, opting always for the most brilliant fruits and vegetables.

Or memorize the ORAC ratings.

ORAC rules

One way to rank the antioxidant potential of a food is to evaluate its Oxygen Radical Absorbance Capacity (ORAC).

The original ORAC evaluations were done in test tubes using a procedure created in 1994 by Guohua Cao and Richard Cutler of the Jean Mayer USDA Human Nutrition Research Center on Aging at Tufts University in Boston. Eventually, another USDA/Mayer scientist, Ronald Prior, automated the test, thus saving everyone much time and effort.

The brain power of chocolate and berries

Dark chocolate scores high on the ORAC scale, so it, along with blueberries (another ORAC champion), hit the headlines in virtually every news story on the virtues of antioxidant foods for the adult brain. Actually, while chocolate is sexier (see the section "Altering the Emotional Brain," later in this chapter), berries, including blue ones, have the better science backup.

In January 2010, a team of researchers from the University of Cincinnati, the USDA, and the Canadian Department of Agriculture released data from a study in which volunteers in their 70s exhibiting early symptoms of memory loss were given either the equivalent of 2 to 2½ cups of blueberry juice or a lookalike substitute every day for two months. When the testing ended, the blueberry people had improved their performance on memory tests; the lookalike group had not.

Eight months later, in the summer of 2010, another group of blueberry fans told attendees at the 240th National Meeting of the American Chemical Society (ACS) that eating blueberries, strawberries, and acai berries — and maybe walnuts — might protect an older brain by powering up its natural mechanisms for eliminating toxins linked to age-related memory loss and other mental deficits.

Quantifying ORAC consumption

Right now, and probably subject to change, the USDA recommends that each of us consume foods providing at least 3,000 to 5,000 ORAC units every day. To simplify the task, in 2007 the agency put together a database listing the ORAC numbers for more than 300 foods.

You can access the report describing this database by going to the USDA Web site at `www.ars.usda.gov/Services/docs.htm?docid=15866` and clicking ORAC Report to pull up a PDF with a sampling of the foods already evaluated. For the complete, 300-plus foods list, click ORAC R2.mdb. *Caveat emptor:* To open this file you must have Microsoft Access.

Table 24-3 is a representative list of high-ORAC foods.

Table 24-3 ORAC Scores for Selected Foods	
Food	*ORAC Value* (per 100 g/3.5 oz)*
Almonds	4454
Apple, red delicious	4275
Black beans (boiled)	2249
Blackberries	5908
Blueberries	4669
Bread, pumpernickel	1963
Cabbage, red	2496
Cauliflower, purple	2210
Grapefruit, pink, white	1640
Hazelnuts	9645
Lettuce, Boston, Bibb	1423
Lettuce, red leaf	2426
Oats, old fashioned	1708
Oats, quick cook	2169
Onions, red	1521
Peanut butter, smooth	3432
Pecans	17940
Popcorn, air-popped	1743
Potatoes w/skin baked, Russet	1680
Potatoes w/skin baked, white	1138
Spinach	1573
Sweet potato, baked w/skin	2115
Walnuts	13541
Wine, red	3607

*Unless otherwise noted, values are for raw foods.
Source: USDA Agricultural Research Service, Oxygen Radical Absorbance Capacity (ORAC) of Selected Foods, Release 2 (2010), www.ars.usda.gov/Services/docs.htm?docid=15866.

Measuring the male mind

Mild cognitive impairment (Where did I leave my keys?) may be a precursor to various forms of age-related dementia (What are keys used for?), so the Mayo Alzheimer's Disease Research Center recently decided to calculate the incidence of cognitive problems with a survey of 1,969 randomly selected volunteers age 70 to 80.

The results, published in the journal *Neurology* in 2010, were interesting. Although Alzheimer's is more prevalent among women, mild cognitive dysfunction — those missing keys — showed up in 19 percent of the Mayo men but only 14 percent of the women. Statistically, that means it was 1.5 times more common among men than among women.

"The finding was unexpected, since the frequency of Alzheimer's disease is actually greater in women," says Ronald Petersen, MD, PhD, neurologist and director of the Mayo Clinic Alzheimer's Disease Research Center.

Do you see another study looming in the near future?

Altering the Emotional Brain

A *mood* is a feeling, an internal emotional state that can affect how you see the world. If your team wins the World Series, your happiness may last for days, making you feel so mellow that you simply shrug off minor annoyances such as finding a ticket on your windshield because your parking meter expired while you were having lunch. If you're sad because the project you spent six months setting up didn't work out, your disappointment can linger long enough to make your work seem temporarily unrewarding or your favorite television sitcom totally unfunny.

Most of the time, after shifting one way or the other, your mood swings back to center fairly soon. You come down from your high or recover from your disappointment, and life resumes its normal pace — some good news here, some bad news there, but all in all, a relatively level field.

Occasionally, however, your mood may go haywire. Your happiness over your team's victory escalates to the point where you find yourself rushing from store to store buying things you can't afford, or your sadness over your failure at work deepens into a gloom that steals joy from everything else. This unpleasant state of affairs — a mood out of control — is called a *mood disorder*.

Mood malfunctions

Approximately one in every four human beings (more frequently a woman than a man) experiences some form of mood disturbance during his or her lifetime. Eight or nine out of every 100 people will experience a *clinical mood disorder,* a mood disorder serious enough to be diagnosed as a disease.

The two most common moods are happiness and sadness. The two most common mood disorders are *clinical depression,* an elongated period of overly intense sadness, and *clinical mania,* an elongated period of overly intense elation. Clinical depression alone is called a *unipolar* (one-part) *disorder;* clinical depression plus clinical mania is a *bipolar* (two-part) *disorder.*

Natural chemicals that affect mood

Your body makes a group of substances called *neurotransmitters,* which are chemicals that enable brain cells to send messages back and forth. Three important neurotransmitters are

- Dopamine *(DOE-pa-meen)*
- Norepinephrine *(NOR-e-pe-NEF-rin)*
- Serotonin *(ser-a-TOE-nin)*

Dopamine and *norepinephrine* are chemicals that make you feel alert and energized. *Serotonin* is a chemical that can make you feel smooth and calm. Some forms of clinical depression appear to be a malfunction of the body's ability to handle these neurotransmitters effectively.

Mood meds

Several medical drugs are useful in making neurotransmitters more available to your brain or enabling your brain to use them more efficiently. These medications include

- **Tricyclic antidepressants:** These drugs were the first truly effective antidepressants. They are named for their chemical structure: three ring-shaped groups of atoms (*tri* = three; *cyclic* = ring). They relieve symptoms by increasing the availability of serotonin. One well-known tricyclic is amitriptyline (Elavil).

- **Monoamine oxidase inhibitors (MAO inhibitors):** These drugs interrupt the actions of an enzyme that triggers the natural elimination of dopamine and other neurotransmitters so that they remain available for your brain. Phenelzine (Nardil) and tranylcypromine (Parnate) are MAO inhibitors.

- **Selective serotonin reuptake inhibitors (SSRIs):** These medicines slow the body's natural re-absorption of serotonin, leaving more serotonin available to your brain. Celexa (citalopram), Lexapro (escitalopram oxalate), Luvox (fluoxamine), Paxil (paroxetie), Prozac (fluoxetine), and Zoloft (sertraline) are SSRIs.

> ✔ **Selective serotonin-norepinephrine reuptake inhibitors (SNRIs):** These medicines slow the body's natural re-absorption of both serotonin and norepinephrine. Cymbalta (duloxetine), Effexor (venlafaxine), and Priztiq (desvenlafaxine) are SNRIs.
>
> ✔ **Norepinephrine and dopamine reuptake inhibitor (NDRI):** This medicine slows the body's natural re-absorption of norepinephrine and dopamine. Wellbutrin (buproprion) is an NDRI. *Note:* Buproprion is also marketed as an antismoking drug under the brand name Zyban.

How food affects mood

Good morning: Time to wake up, roll out of bed, and sleepwalk into the kitchen for a cup of coffee.

Good afternoon: Time for a moderate glass of whiskey or wine to soothe away the tensions of the day.

Good grief: Your lover has left. Time for chocolate, *lots* of chocolate, to soothe the pain.

Good night: Time for milk and cookies to ease your way to Dreamland.

For centuries, millions of people have used these foods in these situations, secure in the knowledge that each food will work its mood magic. Today, modern science knows why. Having discovered that your emotions are linked to your production or use of neurotransmitters, nutrition scientists have been able to identify the natural chemicals in food that change the way you feel by

> ✔ Influencing the production of neurotransmitters
>
> ✔ Hooking onto brain cells and changing the way the cells behave
>
> ✔ Opening pathways to brain cells so that other mood-altering chemicals can come on board

The following sections describe chemicals in food commonly known to affect mood.

Alcohol

Alcohol is man's (and woman's) most widely used natural relaxant. Contrary to common belief, alcohol is a depressant, not a mood elevator. If you feel relaxed or, conversely, exuberant after one drink, the reason isn't that the alcohol is speeding up your brain; it's that alcohol loosens your *controls,* the brain signals that normally tell you not to put a lampshade on your head or take off your clothes in public.

For more about alcohol's effects on virtually every body organ and system, turn to Chapter 10. In this chapter, it's enough to say that many people find that, taken with food and in moderation — defined as one drink a day for a woman and two for a man — alcohol can comfortably change a mood from tense to mellow.

Anandamide

Anandamide is a *cannabinoid,* a chemical that hooks up to the same brain receptors that catch similar ingredients in marijuana smoke. Your brain produces some anandamide naturally, but you also get very small amounts of the chemical from cocoa bean products — chocolate. In addition, chocolate contains two chemicals similar to anandamide that slow the breakdown of the anandamide produced in your brain, thus intensifying its effects.

Maybe that's why eating chocolate makes you feel so good. And that really does mean *mildly:* You'd have to eat at least 25 pounds of chocolate at one time to get any marijuana-like effect. In 2009, a team of nutrition scientists at the Nestle Research Center in Lausanne (Switzerland) put the beneficial calming effects and reduction in the body's production of stress hormones dose at 40 grams (about 1.5 ounces) of dark chocolate a day. The chocolate used in the study was 74 percent cocoa, served in two daily doses, 20 grams in the morning and 20 grams in the afternoon, after which the researchers tested the volunteers' blood to measure levels of stress hormones. They discovered the levels of stress hormones went down among the chocolate eaters, thus making chocoholics everywhere even happier than usual.

Caffeine

Caffeine is a mild stimulant that

- ✔ Raises your blood pressure
- ✔ Speeds up your heartbeat
- ✔ Makes you burn calories faster
- ✔ Makes you urinate more frequently
- ✔ Causes your intestinal tract to move food more quickly through your body

Although it increases the level of serotonin, the calming neurotransmitter, caffeine also hooks up at specific receptors (sites on the surface of brain cells) normally reserved for another naturally occurring tranquilizer, *adenosine (a-DEN-o-seen).* When caffeine latches on in place of adenosine, brain cells become more reactive to stimulants such as noise and light, making you talk faster and think faster.

But caffeine can be confusing. People react to it in highly individual ways. Some can drink seven cups of regular ("with caffeine") coffee and still stay calm all day and sleep like a baby at night. Others tend to hop about on decaf. Perhaps those who stay calm have enough brain receptors to accommodate both adenosine and caffeine, or perhaps they're more sensitive to the adenosine that manages to hook up to brain cells. Nobody really knows. Either way, caffeine's bouncy effects may last anywhere from one to seven hours.

Table 24-4 lists some common food sources of caffeine. The caffeine content listed here is an average for the generic versions of the food or drink — in other words, plain, no-brand products. You can check out the caffeine content of brand-name products such as a Starbucks Espresso Solo (75 mg/oz) or Ben and Jerry's coffee flavored ice cream (34 mg/4 oz) at the Center for Science In the Public Interest Web site at `www.cspinet.org/new/cafchart.htm`.

Table 24-4	Foods That Give You Caffeine
Food	*Average Amount of Caffeine (mg)*
6-ounce cups	
Coffee, regular, drip	71
Coffee, regular, instant	47
Coffee, decaffeinated	1
Tea	36
Tea, instant	20
Cocoa (mix + water)	4
12-ounce can	
Soft drinks, cola	29
8-ounce container	
Chocolate milk (commercial, lowfat)	5
1-ounce serving	
Milk chocolate	6
Semisweet chocolate	24
Bitter (baker's) chocolate	23

USDA National Nutrient Database for Standard Reference, www.nal.usda.gov/fnic/foodcomp/search.

Tryptophan and glucose

Tryptophan is an amino acid, another one of those "building blocks of protein" (see Chapter 7). Glucose, the end product of carbohydrate metabolism, is the sugar that circulates in your blood, the basic fuel on which your body runs (see Chapter 9). Milk and cookies, a classic calming combo, owe their power to the tryptophan/glucose team.

Start with the fact that the neurotransmitters dopamine, norepinephrine, and serotonin are made from the amino acids tyrosine and tryptophan, which are found in protein foods (like milk). *Tyrosine* is the most important ingredient in dopamine and norepinephrine, the alertness neurotransmitters. *Tryptophan* is the most important ingredient in serotonin, the calming neurotransmitter.

All amino acids ride into your brain on chemical pathways, but your brain makes way for the bouncy tyrosine first and the soothing tryptophan last. That's why a high-protein meal heightens your alertness.

To move the tryptophan along faster, you need glucose, and that means carbohydrate foods (like those cookies). When you eat carbs, your pancreas releases *insulin,* a hormone that enables you to metabolize the carbs and produce glucose. The insulin also keeps tyrosine and other amino acids circulating in your blood so that tryptophan travels on plenty of open paths to the brain. With more tryptophan coming in, your brain can increase its production of soothing serotonin. That's why a meal of starchy pasta (starch is composed of chains of glucose molecules, as explained in Chapter 9) makes you feel calm and cool.

The effects of simple sugars, such as sucrose (table sugar), are more complicated. If you eat simple sugars on an empty stomach, the sugars are absorbed rapidly, triggering an equally rapid increase in the secretion of insulin, a hormone needed to digest carbohydrates. The result is a rapid decrease in the amount of sugar circulating in your blood, a condition known as *hypoglycemia* (*hypo* = low; *glycemia* = sugar in the blood) that can make you feel temporarily jumpy rather than calm. However, when eaten on a full stomach — dessert after a full meal — simple sugars are absorbed more slowly and may exert the calming effect usually linked to complex carbohydrates (starchy foods).

Obvious conclusion: Some foods, such as meat, fish, and poultry, make you more alert. Others, such as pasta, bread, potatoes, rice, and other grains, calm you down. The effect of the food depends on its ability to alter the amount of serotonin available to your brain (see Figure 24-1).

Fascinating factoid: Even though turkey is high in protein, it's also high in tryptophan, the precursor of (chemical that leads to the creation of) serotonin, which may explain why so many people nod off after Thanksgiving dinner.

Caution! Medicine at work

Some of the mood-altering chemicals in food interact with medicines. As you may have guessed, the two most notable examples are caffeine and alcohol.

✔ Caffeine makes painkillers such as aspirin and acetaminophen more effective. On the other hand, many over-the-counter (OTC) painkillers and cold medicines already contain caffeine. If you take the pill with a cup of java, you may increase your caffeine intake past the jitters stage.

✔ Alcohol is a no-no with most medicines because it increases the sedative or depressant effects of some drugs, such as antihistamines and painkillers, and alters the rate at which you absorb or excrete others.

Always ask your pharmacist about food/drug interactions (you can read more about this in Chapter 25) when you fill a prescription or purchase an OTC product.

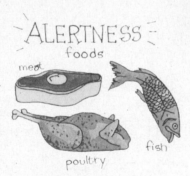 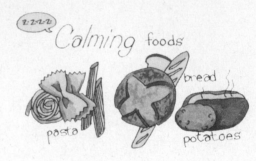

Figure 24-1:
Some foods may calm you, and some foods may make you more alert.

Phenylethylamine (PEA)

Phenylethylamine — sometimes abbreviated PEA — is a natural chemical that your body releases when you're in love, making you feel, well, good all over. A big splash occurred in the late 1980s when researchers discovered that chocolate, the food of lovers, is a fine source of PEA.

In fact, many people think that PEA has a lot to do with chocolate's reputation as the food of love and consolation. Of course, to be fair about it, chocolate also contains the mood-elevator caffeine, the muscle stimulant theobromine, and the cannabinoid anandamide (see the earlier section on anandamide).

Using food to manage mood

No food will change your personality or alter the course of a mood disorder. But some may add a little lift or a small moment of calm to your day, increase your effectiveness at certain tasks, make you more alert, or give you a neat little push over the finish line.

The watchword is balance:

- ✔ One cup of coffee in the a.m. is a pleasant push into alertness. Seven cups of coffee a day can make your hands shake.

- ✔ One alcohol drink is generally a safe way to relax. Three may be a disaster.

- ✔ A grilled chicken breast (white meat, no skin) for breakfast on a day when you have to be on your toes before lunch can help make you sharp as a tack.

- ✔ Got an important lunch meeting? Order starches without fats or oils: pasta with fresh tomatoes and basil, no oil, no cheese; rice with veggies; rice with fruit. Your aim is to get the calming carbs without the high-fat food that slows thinking and makes you feel sleepy.

In this, as in other aspects of a healthy life, the point is to make sure that you use the tool (in this case, food), not the other way around.

Healing the Injured Brain

Slice off your finger while chopping wood, and as you're on the way to the emergency room, some helpful passerby can pick up the finger, hopefully stick it into a cup of ice to chill and preserve the tissues, and dawdle his way over to the hospital to meet you. If the finger arrives within a couple of hours, it likely can be successfully re-implanted. New cells will grow to heal the damage. Blood will flow through reattached vessels. Newly stitched nerves and muscles will signal and move. Bones will knit together. And you may well enjoy a working five-fingered hand.

But hit your head hard enough to injure brain cells, suffer a stroke, or have a heart attack that interrupts the flow of oxygenated blood to the brain, and your brain cells begin to die within minutes. They won't grow back, either (see the earlier section, "Protecting the Adult Brain"). Recovery after brain injury pretty much depends not on creating new cells but on the brain's ability to efficiently switch tasks from one area to another.

To reduce the loss of brain cells and limit damage to an injured brain, doctors concentrate on ensuring an adequate supply of oxygen and controlling swelling that pushes the soft brain against the inside of the hard skull.

But there may be another weapon in the arsenal: Food.

The 5, 7, 2, 4, 100, 200 solution

After any injury, your body goes into a *hypermetabolic state* (*hyper* = the Greek word for "over"), meaning that it suddenly requires more calories than normal to provide the energy and material to rebuild damaged tissues. True, an injured brain won't be producing new cells, but this 2 percent of your weight that consumes 20 percent of your calorie intake will need extra energy to establish the new connections that can enable you to function.

In fact, feeding patients with brain injuries is so important that neurologists at Presbyterian Hospital/Weill Cornell Medical Center in New York have actually put some hard numbers to it: 5, 7, 2, 4, 100, 200.

Translation: Patients with brain injury who are not fed either intravenously or through a tube into the stomach within *5* days after the injury occurs are *2* times more likely to die than are patients who get fed. Patients not fed within *7* days are *4* times more likely to die. And the best menu provides *100* percent of the normal recommended daily calories for that particular patient (see Chapter 3); up to *200* percent is even better.

"There is no miracle drug for patients with severe traumatic brain injury," says Roger Hartl, director of neurotrauma at the Brain and Spine Center of Weill Cornell Medical College. "But we have been able to reduce the mortality and improve outcome in these patients dramatically over the past 15 years by maintaining their blood pressure and supplying the brain early on with oxygen and nutrients. We now start feeding patients with severe brain injuries very aggressively from the moment they first hit the intensive care unit, and early nutrition is now recognized as one of the most important factors improving outcome in these patients." So important, in fact, that the regimen has now been incorporated in the international Guidelines for Management of Severe Traumatic Brain injury.

Protein possibilities

Leucine, isoleucine, and valine are amino acids, the building blocks of protein described in Chapter 7. Because these three particular amino acids share a distinct chemical structure — a long central chain with smaller side chains branching off — they are called *branched chain amino acids* (BCAA, for short).

The body uses BCAA to build neurotransmitters, the naturally occurring chemicals that enable cells to exchange messages: Think! Move! Feel! Unfortunately, an injury to the brain that damages the hippocampus, a part of the brain that helps direct memory and cognition, may reduce brain levels of leucine, isoleucine, and valine.

As long ago as 1983, studies suggested that intravenous doses of BCAA would benefit patients with liver disease by forcing additional amino acids into their brain. Some sports nutritionists think that BCAA supplements can improve muscle performance.

Neuroscientist Akiva Cohen and his team at The Children's Hospital of Philadelphia see a more direct application. When they added BCAA to the drinking water of brain-injured mice, Cohen's team observed improvements in both mouse memory and cognition. If future studies with human beings demonstrate the same effect, patients with traumatic brain injuries might be able to avoid the feeding tubes and intravenous needles to improve their thinking and remembering simply by sipping a glass of branched-chain-amino-acid-enriched (building blocks of protein) water.

The (eventual) official word

The National Academy of Sciences is a private group in Washington that serves as an official adviser to the federal government on science and technology.

The Institute of Medicine (IOM) is the division of the Academy that sets and publishes the RDAs, RDIs, and other nutritional recommendations listed in Chapter 5. In 2009, IOM set up a *Consensus Study on Nutrition, Trauma, and the Brain* to determine (and I quote), ". . . the potential role for nutrition in providing resilience (i.e., protecting), mitigating or treating of primary (i.e., within minutes of insult), secondary (i.e., within 24 hours of insult), and long-term (i.e., more than 24 hours after insult) associated effects of neurotrauma, with a focus on traumatic brain injury."

The first part of the study will consider how the body's responses to a brain injury affect a patient's need for and ability to handle nutrients. The second will concentrate on how a patient's nutritional status affects his long-term prognosis. Sooner or later — most likely the latter — there will be a final report.

The (Current) (Nutritious) Last Word

While you're waiting for nutrition science to catch up with your brain, make your own medicine with these four simple rules for a diet that benefits your brain and your body, too:

✔ **Eat enough food.** Sounds foolish in a country where obesity is a problem, doesn't it? But constant on-and-off dieting or even occasional crash dieting can rob your brain of energy without producing lasting weight control. Get the calories you need. And not a smidgen more. (For your calorie requirements, see Chapter 3.)

✔ **Eat smaller portions, but more often.** Who says three scheduled large meals a day are right for every body? Frequent smaller meals provide a continuous flow of energy to your brain. And by allowing them to eat before they are ravenously hungry, these grazing moments may enable some people to keep from overeating. (Want to know why you eat, when you eat? See Chapter 14.)

✔ **Choose foods that turn to energy slower rather than faster.** Simple carbs, such as table sugar, pep you up fast and then let you down just as quickly. Your body metabolizes complex carbs such as fruits and vegetables and whole grains more slowly, so their effect on your brain's energy bank is smoother and lasts longer. (For more about which carbs are which, see Chapter 9.)

✔ **Pick the perfect fats.** Protect your brain as well as your heart by emphasizing fats that build you up without blocking arteries, including those in your brain. (What you need to know is in Chapter 8.)

Chapter 25

Food and Drug Interactions

Foods nourish your body. Medicines cure (or relieve) what ails you. The two should work together in perfect harmony to protect your body. Sometimes they do. Occasionally, however, foods and drugs fight: The drug keeps your body from absorbing or using the nutrients in food, or the food (or nutrient) prevents you from getting the benefits of certain medicines.

The medical phrase for this is *adverse interaction*. This chapter describes several adverse interactions and lays out some simple strategies that enable you to short-circuit them.

How a Food and Drug Interaction Happens

When you eat, food moves from your mouth to your stomach to your small intestine, where the nutrients that keep you strong and healthy are absorbed into your bloodstream and distributed throughout your body. Take medicine by mouth, and it follows pretty much the same path from your mouth to your stomach, where it's dissolved and passed along to the small intestine for absorption. Nothing is unusual about that.

A problem may arise when a food or drug brings the process to a halt by behaving in a way that stops your body from using either the drug or the food (see Figure 25-1). For example:

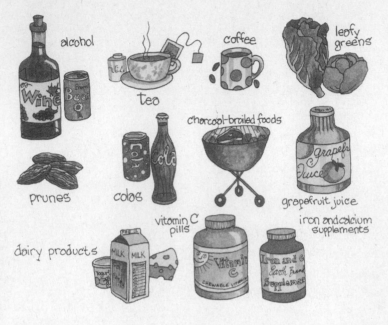

Figure 25-1:
Some foods
may affect
the way
your body
interacts
with drugs.

✔ Some drugs or foods change the natural acidity of your digestive tract so that you absorb nutrients less efficiently. For example, your body absorbs iron best when your stomach is acidic. Taking antacids reduces stomach acidity — and iron absorption.

✔ Some drugs or foods change the rate at which food moves through your digestive tract, which means that you absorb more (or less) of a particular nutrient or drug. For example, eating prunes (a laxative food) or taking a laxative drug speeds things up so that foods (and drugs) move more quickly through your body, giving you less time to absorb medicine or nutrients.

✔ Some drugs and nutrients *bond* (link up with each other) to form insoluble compounds that your body can't break apart. As a result, you get less of the drug and less of the nutrient. The best-known example: Calcium (in dairy foods) bonds to the antibiotic tetracycline so that both move swiftly out of your body.

✔ Some drugs and nutrients have similar chemical structures. Taking them at the same time fools your body into absorbing or using the nutrient rather than the drug. One good example is coumadin (the generic version of Warfarin, a drug that keeps blood from clotting) and vitamin K (a nutrient that makes blood clot). Eating lots of vitamin K–rich leafy greens counteracts the intended effect of taking warfarin.

✔ Some foods contain chemicals that either lessen or intensify the natural side effects of certain drugs. For example, the caffeine in coffee, tea, and cola drinks reduces the sedative effects of antihistamines and some anti-depressant drugs but increases the nervousness, insomnia, and shakiness common with some diet pills and cold medications containing caffeine or a *decongestant* (an ingredient that temporarily clears a stuffy nose).

Food Fights: Drugs versus Foods

Sometimes the combinations of interacting foods and drugs are surprising. Astounding. Or breathtaking.

Everyone knows that people with asthma may find it hard to take a deep breath around the barbecue. The culprit's the smoke, right? Yes. And no. Breathing in smoke does irritate air passages, but — the surprise — eating charcoal-broiled food speeds the body's elimination of *theophylline,* a widely used asthma drug, reducing the drug's ability to protect against wheezing. Take the drug, eat the food, and maybe end up wheezing.

Another potential troublemaker is an acidic beverage, such as fruit juice or soft drinks, which may inactivate the antibiotics erythromycin, ampicillin, and penicillin. Grapefruit juice is a particularly potent offender.

In the mid-1990s, researchers tracking the effects of alcohol beverages on the blood pressure drug felodipine (Plendil) tripped across the *Grapefruit Effect,* a dramatic reduction in the ability to metabolize and eliminate certain drugs. The explanation: Grapefruit juice contains substances that suppress the effectiveness of CYP 3A4, an intestinal enzyme required to convert many drugs to water-soluble substances you can flush out of your body; without the enzyme, you can't get rid of the drug. The result may be an equally dramatic rise in the amount of medication in your body, leading to unpleasant side effects. Table 25-1 lists the medicines known to be affected by grapefruit juice.

Caveat #1: Taking a slow-release medicine along with grapefruit juice may cause the entire dose of medicine in the pill or capsule to be released and metabolized at once. *Caveat #2:* Table 25-1 is not a complete list of medicines subject to the grapefruit effect. Check with your doctor or pharmacist whenever a new medicine is prescribed.

Table 25-1	Grapefruit Juice versus Meds	
Condition	**Drug Class**	**Drug (Brand Name)**
Allergy	Antihistamine	fexofenadine (Allegra)
Cough	Cough suppressant	dextromethorphan (DXM)
Depression	Antidepressant	fluvoxamine (Luvox, Faverin)
Diabetes, Type 2	Meglitinide (lowers blood sugar)	repaglinide (Prandin)
Erectile dysfunction	Enzyme inhibitor (increases blood flow)	sildenafil (Viagra), tadalafil (Cialis), vardenafil (Levitra)
High cholesterol	Statins	atorvastatin (Lipitor), lovastatin (Mevacor), simvastatin Zocor. **Note:** pravastatin (Pravachol) is not affected
HIV	Antiretoviral	ritonavir (Novir), saquinavir (Invirase, Fortovase)
Hypertension	Calcium channel blocker	felodipine (Nitrendipine, Plendil), losartan (Cozaar), nicardipine (Cardene), nimodipine (Nimotop), nisoldipine (Sular), verapamil (Verelan)
Insomnia	Sleep aid	zolpidem (Ambien)
Irregular heartbeat	Antiarrhythmic	amiodarone (Cordarone), carvedilol/verapamil (Calan SR, Covera HS, Isoptin SR, Verelan), dronedarone (Multaq), disopyramide (Norpace), quinidine (Quinidex, Cardioquin, Quinora)
Migraine	Ergot alkaloid	ergotamine, ergotamine & caffeine (Cafergot, Ergomar), OCD
Pain	Narcotics	codeine, methadone, morphine, oxycodone
Psychosis	Anti psychotic	quetiapine (Seroquel)
Seizures	Antiseizure	carbamazepine (Tegretol)
Transplants, severe	Immunosuppressant	cyclosporine (Neoral, Sandimmune), rheumatoid arthritis tacrolimus (Prograf) psoriasis

Source: MedicineNet.com, www.medicinenet.com/script/main/art.asp?articlekey=14760#; Rolfes, Sharon Rady, Kathryn Pinna, and Elie Whitney, Understanding Normal and Clinical Nutrition, Seventh edition (Belmont, CA: Thomason Higher Education, 2006).

Drugs versus Nutrients

Like food, individual nutrients — vitamins and minerals — may also interact with medicines.

Water pills, more properly known as *diuretics,* make you urinate more often and more copiously, thus increasing your elimination of the mineral potassium. To make up what you lose, experts suggest adding potatoes, bananas, oranges, spinach, corn, and tomatoes to your diet. Consuming less sodium (salt) while you're using water pills makes the water pills more effective and decreases your loss of potassium.

Oral contraceptives seem to reduce the ability to absorb B vitamins, including folate. Taking lots of aspirin or other NSAIDs (nonsteroidal anti-inflammatory drugs) such as ibuprofen can trigger a painless, slow but steady loss of small amounts of blood from the lining of your stomach that may lead to iron-deficiency anemia.

Persistent use of antacids made with aluminum compounds may lead to loss of the bone-building mineral phosphorus, which binds to aluminum and rides right out of the body. Laxatives increase the loss of minerals (calcium and others) in feces.

The antiulcer drugs cimetidine (Tagamet) and ranitidine (Zantac) can make you positively giddy. These drugs reduce stomach acidity, which means the body absorbs alcohol more efficiently. According to experts at the Mayo Clinic, taking ulcer medication with alcohol leads to twice the wallop, similar to drinking one beer and feeling the effects of two.

The point, of course, is to read the label and definitely check with your doctor or pharmacist for any potential food and drug interactions whenever you take medication.

Finally, consider nutritional supplements. The vitamins and minerals in nutritional supplements are simply food reduced to its basic nutrients, so interactions between drugs and supplements aren't a surprise. Table 25-2 lists some common vitamin/mineral and drug interactions. (For more information on supplements, see Chapter 6.)

Table 25-2	Battling Nutrients and Medications
You Absorb Less . . .	*When You Take . . .*
Vitamin A	Aluminum antacids Bisacodyl (laxative) Cholestyramine (lower cholesterol) Fenfluramine (diet pill) Mineral oil (laxative) Neomycin (antibiotic)
Vitamin D	Bisacodyl (laxative) Cholestyramine (lowers cholesterol) Mineral oil (laxative) Neomycin (antibiotic)
Vitamin K	Bisacodyl (laxative) Cholestyramine (lowers cholesterol) Mineral oil (laxative) Neomycin (antibiotic)
Vitamin C	Aspirin Barbiturates (sleeping pills) Cortisone and related steroid drugs
Thiamin	Antacids (calcium) Aspirin Cortisone and related steroid drugs
Riboflavin	Birth control pills
Folate	Aspirin Cholestyramine (lowers cholesterol) Penicillin Phenobarbital, primidone, phenothiazines (antiseizure drugs) Sulfa drugs
Vitamin B12	Cholestyramine (lowers cholesterol) Neomycin (antibiotic)
Calcium	Cortisone and related steroid drugs Diuretics (water pills) Magnesium antacids Neomycin (antibiotic) Phosphorus laxatives Tetracycline (antibiotic)
Phosphorus	Aluminum antacids
Magnesium	Amphotericin B (antibiotic) Diuretics (water pills) Tetracycline (antibiotic)

You Absorb Less . . .	When You Take . . .
Iron	Aspirin and other nonsteroidal anti-inflammatory drugs
	Calcium antacids
	Calcium supplements (with meals)
	Cholestyramine (lowers cholesterol)
	Neomycin (antibiotic)
	Penicillin (antibiotic)
	Tetracycline (antibiotic)
Zinc	Diuretics (water pills)

James J. Rybacki, The Essential Guide to Prescription Drugs 2002 (New York: Harper Collins, 2001); Brian L. G. Morgan, The Food and Drug Interaction Guide (New York: Simon and Schuster, 1986); Eleanor Noss Whitney, Corinne Balog Cataldo, and Sharon Rady Rolfes, Understanding Normal and Clinical Nutrition, 4th ed. (Minneapolis/St. Paul: West Publishing, 1994)

Using Food to Improve a Drug's Performance

Not every food and drug interaction is an adverse one. Sometimes a drug works better or is less likely to cause side effects when you take it on a full stomach. For example, aspirin is less likely to upset your stomach if you take the painkiller with food, and eating stimulates the release of stomach juices that improve your ability to absorb griseofulvin, an antifungus drug.

Table 25-3 lists some drugs that may work better when your stomach is full.

Table 25-3	Drugs That Work Better on a Full Stomach
Purpose	**Drug**
Analgesics (painkillers)	Acetaminophen
	Aspirin
	Codeine
	Ibuprofen
	Indomethacin
	Mefenamic acid
	Metronidazole
	Naproxen/naproxen sodium

(continued)

Table 25-3 *(continued)*

Purpose	Drug
Antibiotics, Antivirals, Antifungals	Ethambutol
	Griseofulvin
	Isoniazid
	Ketoconazole
	Pyrimethamine
Antidiabetic Agents	Glipizide
	Glyburide
	Tolazamide
	Tolbutamide
Cholesterol-Lowering Agents	Cholestyramine
	Colestipol
	Lovastatin
	Probucol
Gastric Medications	Cimetidine
	Ranitidine

James J. Rybacki, The Essential Guide to Prescription Drugs 2002 (New York: Harper Collins, 2001).

With this medicine, who can eat?

Interactions aren't the only drug reactions that keep you from getting nutrients from food. Some drugs have side effects that also reduce the value of food. For example, a drug may

✔ Sharply reduce your appetite so that you simply don't eat much. The best-known example may be the amphetamine and amphetamine-like drugs such as fenfluramine used (surprise!) as diet pills.

✔ Make food taste or smell bad or steal away your senses of taste or smell so that eating isn't pleasurable. One example is the anti-depressant drug amitriptyline (Elavil), which can leave a peculiar taste in your mouth.

✔ Cause nausea, vomiting, or diarrhea so that you either can't eat or do not retain nutrients from the food you do eat. Examples include the antibiotic erythromycin and many drugs used to treat cancer.

✔ Irritate the lining of your intestinal tract so that even if you do eat, your body has a hard time absorbing nutrients from food. The most common examples of this kind of interaction occur with drugs used in cancer chemotherapy.

The moderately good news is that new medications appear to make some drugs (including anticancer drugs) less likely to cause nausea and vomiting. The best news is that many drugs are less likely to upset your stomach or irritate your gut if you take them with food (refer to Table 25-3). For example, taking aspirin and other non-prescription painkillers such as ibuprofen with food or a full glass of water may reduce their natural tendency to irritate the lining of your stomach.

Chapter 26

Using Food as Medicine

A healthful diet gives you the nutrients you need to keep your body in top-flight condition. In addition, evidence suggests that eating well may prevent or minimize the risk of a long list of serious medical conditions, including heart disease, high blood pressure, and cancer.

This chapter describes what nutritionists know right now about how to use food to prevent, alleviate, or cure what ails you — with a couple of hints about what's to come in the evolving world of medical nutrition.

Defining Food as Medicine

Start with a definition. A food that acts like a medicine is one that increases or reduces your risk of a specific medical condition or cures or alleviates the effects of a medical condition. For example:

✔ Eating foods, such as wheat bran, that are high in *insoluble dietary fiber* (the kind of fiber that doesn't dissolve in your gut) moves food more quickly through your intestinal tract and produces soft, bulky stool that reduces your risk of constipation.

✔ Eating foods such as beans that are rich in *soluble dietary fiber* (fiber that dissolves in your intestinal tract) seems to help your body mop up the cholesterol circulating in your bloodstream, preventing it from sticking to the walls of your arteries. This reduces your risk of heart disease.

✔ Eating sufficient amounts of calcium-rich foods (accompanied by vitamin D, as noted in Chapter 11) ensures the growth of strong bones early in life and protects bone density later on.

✔ Eating very spicy foods, such as chili, makes the membrane lining your nose and throat weep a watery fluid that makes blowing your nose or coughing up mucus easier when you have a cold.

✔ Eating (or drinking) foods (or beverages) with mood-altering substances such as caffeine, alcohol, and phenylethylamine (PEA) may lend a lift when you're feeling down or help you chill when you're tense. (For more on food and mood, see Chapter 24.)

The joy of food-as-medicine is that it's cheaper and much more pleasant than managing illness with drugs. Given the choice, who wouldn't opt to control cholesterol levels with oats or chili (all those yummy beans packed with soluble dietary fiber) than with a list of medicines whose possible side effects include kidney failure and liver damage? Right.

Examining Diets with Absolutely, Positively Beneficial Medical Effects

Some foods and some diet plans are so obviously good for your body that no one questions their ability to keep you healthy or make you feel better when you're ill. For example, if you've ever had abdominal surgery, you know all about liquid diets — the water–gelatin–clear broth regimen your doctor prescribed right after the operation to enable you to take some nourishment by mouth without upsetting your intestines.

Or if you have *type 1 diabetes* (an inherited inability to produce the insulin needed to process carbohydrates), you know that your ability to balance the carbohydrates, fats, and proteins in your daily diet is important to stabilizing your illness.

Other proven diet regimens include

✔ **The low-cholesterol, low-saturated-fat diet:** The basic version, known as the *Stage 1 Diet,* is used as a first step in lowering a person's cholesterol level. The diet limits cholesterol consumption to no more than 300 milligrams a day and total fat intake to no more than 30 percent of your total daily calories (see Chapter 16).

A nifty bonus to this diet is that it's a relatively painless way of losing weight.

✔ **The high-fiber diet:** A high-fiber diet quickens the passage of food through the digestive tract. This diet is used to prevent constipation. If you have *diverticula* (outpouchings) in the wall of your colon, a high-fiber diet may reduce the possibility of an infection. It can also alleviate the discomfort of irritable bowel syndrome (sometimes called a nervous stomach). Extra bonus: A diet high in soluble fiber also lowers cholesterol (see the preceding section, "Defining Food as Medicine"). A word to the wise: When increasing your dietary fiber intake, be sure to drink enough fluid (see Chapter 13) to prevent the fiber from clumping in and maybe even blocking your digestive tract.

✔ **The sodium-restricted diet:** Sodium is hydrophilic (hydro = water; philic = loving). It increases the amount of water held in body tissues. A diet low in salt often lowers water retention, which can be useful in treating high blood pressure, congestive heart failure, and long-term liver disease. By the way, not all the sodium in your diet comes from table salt. Check out Chapter 16 for a list of the sodium compounds used in food.

✔ **The extra-potassium diet:** People use this diet to counteract the loss of potassium caused by *diuretics* (drugs that make you urinate more frequently and more copiously, causing you to lose excess amounts of potassium in urine). Some evidence also suggests that the high-potassium diet may lower blood pressure a bit.

✔ **The low-protein diet:** This diet is prescribed for people with chronic liver or kidney disease or an inherited inability to metabolize amino acids, the building blocks of proteins. The low-protein regimen reduces the amount of protein waste products in body tissues, thus reducing the possibility of tissue damage.

Using Food to Prevent Disease

Using food as a general preventive is an intriguing subject. True, much anecdotal evidence ("I did this, and that happened") suggests that eating some foods and avoiding others can raise or lower your risk of some serious diseases. But anecdotes aren't science. The more important indicator is the evidence from scientific studies tracking groups of people on different diets to see how things such as eating or avoiding fat, fiber, meat, dairy foods, salt, and other foods affects their risk of specific diseases.

The general name for foods that deliver a health benefit is *functional foods.* One example of a group of natural functional foods that prevent illness is the vitamin A-rich collection of dark green, yellow, red, and orange fruits and vegetables that protect the ability to see in dim light. An example of a manufactured functional food is margarines made with heart-and-brain protective omega-3 fatty acids, whipped up by food technologists. (See Chapters 4 and 24 for more on these nutritious fats.)

Battling deficiency diseases

The simplest example of food's ability to act as preventive medicine is its ability to ward off a *deficiency disease,* a condition that occurs when you don't get sufficient amounts of a specific nutrient. For example, people deprived of vitamin C develop scurvy, the vitamin C–deficiency disease.

The identifying characteristic of a deficiency disease is that simply adding the missing nutrient to your diet can cure it; scurvy disappears when people eat foods, such as citrus fruits, that are high in vitamin C.

Fighting off cancer with food

Is there really an anticancer diet? Right now, the answer seems to be a definite *maybe.* The problem is that cancer isn't one disease; it's many diseases with many causes. Some foods seem to protect against some specific cancers, but none seem to protect against all. For example:

✔ **Fruits and vegetables:** Plants contain some potential anticancer substances, such as *antioxidants* (chemicals that prevent molecular fragments called *free radicals* from hooking up to form cancer-causing compounds); hormone-like compounds that displace natural and synthetic estrogens; and sulfur compounds that interfere with biochemical reactions leading to the birth and growth of cancer cells. (For more about these protective substances in plant foods, see Chapter 12.)

Despite early predictions that antioxidant-rich plant foods would reduce the risk of cancer overall, to date, no seriously controlled study has ever shown that belief to be true. However, several such studies do demonstrate a relationship between eating lots of fruits and vegetables and having a lower risk of a specific type of cancer. For example, in 2010, data from a study conducted by The National Institute for Public Health and the Environment in the Netherlands and published in *Cancer Epidemiology, Biomarkers & Prevention,* a journal of the American Association for Cancer Research, did suggest that this kind of diet would decrease the risk of one type of lung cancer in current smokers.

✔ **Foods high in dietary fiber:** Human beings can't digest dietary fiber, but friendly bacteria living in your gut can. Chomping away on the fiber, the bacteria excrete fatty acids that appear to keep cells from turning cancerous. In addition, insoluble dietary fiber helps speed food through your body, reducing the formation of carcinogenic compounds.

For more than 30 years, doctors have assumed that eating lots of dietary fiber reduces the risk of colon cancer, but in 1999, data from the long-running Nurses' Health Study at Boston's Brigham and Women's Hospital and Harvard's School of Public Health threw this assumption into question. By 2005, several very large studies — one with more than

350,000 people! — confirmed that dietary fiber has no protective effect against colon cancer. But even if dietary fiber doesn't fight cancer, it does prevent constipation. One out of two ain't bad.

✔ **Lowfat foods:** Dietary fat appears to increase the proliferation of various types of body cells, a situation that may lead to the out-of-control reproduction of cells known as cancer. But all fats may not be equally guilty. In several studies, fat from meat seems linked to an increased risk of colon cancer, but fat from dairy foods comes up clean. In the end, the link between dietary fat and cancer remains up in the nutritional air . . . so to speak.

The American Cancer Society Advisory Committee on Diet, Nutrition, and Cancer Prevention issued a set of nutrition guidelines that shows how to use food to reduce the risk of cancer. These are the American Cancer Society's recommendations:

✔ **Choose most of the foods you eat from plant sources.** Eat five or more servings of fruits and vegetables every day. Eat other foods from plant sources, such as breads, cereals, grain products, rice, pasta, or beans, several times a day.

✔ **Limit your intake of high-fat foods, particularly from animal sources.** Choose foods low in fat. Limit consumption of meats, especially high-fat meats.

✔ **Be physically active.** Achieve and maintain a healthy weight. Be at least moderately active for 30 minutes or more on most days of the week. Stay within your healthy weight range.

✔ **If you drink alcohol, drink in moderation.** Chapter 9 lays it out: Moderate consumption means no more than one drink a day for a woman, two for a man.

Four degrees of vegetarianism

Vegetarianism isn't one diet; it's four plant-based menu plans, each one distinguished by what's allowed to be on the dinner plate along with the plants.

✔ Vegetarian variation #1 is a diet for people who don't eat meat but do eat fish and poultry or just fish. (Fairness dictates that I state that many strict vegetarians don't consider people who eat fish or poultry to be vegetarians.)

✔ Vegetarian variation #2 is a diet for people who don't eat meat, fish, or poultry but do

eat other animal products, such as eggs and dairy products. Vegetarians who follow this regimen are called *ovo-lacto vegetarians* (ovo = egg; lacto = milk).

✔ Vegetarian variation #3 is a diet for people who eat absolutely no foods of animal origin. Vegetarians who eat only plant foods are called *vegans*.

✔ Vegetarian variation #4 is a diet comprising only fruit. Naturally, vegetarians who use this diet are called *fruitarians*.

DASHing to healthy blood pressure

More than 50 million Americans have high blood pressure (also referred to as *hypertension*), a major risk factor for heart disease, stroke, and heart or kidney failure.

As you can read in *High Blood Pressure For Dummies* (Wiley) by Alan L. Rubin, MD, the traditional treatment for hypertension has included drugs (some with unpleasant side effects), reduced sodium intake, weight reduction, alcohol only in moderation, and regular exercise. But data from the National Heart, Lung, and Blood Institute (NHLBI) study, "Dietary Approaches to Stop Hypertension" (2002) — DASH, for short — and a second NHLVI study, DASH Sodium (2000), offer strong evidence that the diet that protects your heart and reduces your risk of some forms of cancer may also help control blood pressure.

The DASH diet is rich in fruits and vegetables, plus lowfat dairy products with controlled sodium levels. No surprise there. But the diet is lower in fat than the ordinary lowfat diet prescribing no more than 35 percent of your total calories from fat. In line with the recommendations in the USDA/U.S. Department of Health and Human Services Dietary Guidelines for Americans 2010, DASH suggests that you aim for no more than 27 percent of your total calories from fat.

The difference does seem to make a difference. Your blood pressure is measured in two numbers that look something like this: 130/80. The first number is your *systolic pressure*, the force exerted against artery walls when your heart beats and pushes blood out into your blood vessels. The second, lower number is the *diastolic pressure*, the force exerted between beats.

When male and female volunteers with high blood pressure followed the DASH diet during clinical trials at medical centers in Boston, Massachusetts; Durham, North Carolina; Baltimore, Maryland; and Baton Rouge, Louisiana, their systolic blood pressures dropped an average 11.4 points and their diastolic pressures an average 5.5 points. And unlike medication, the diet produced no unpleasant side effects — except, of course, for that occasional dream of chocolate ice cream with real whipped cream, pound cake. . . .

Conquering the common cold

This section is not about chicken soup. That issue has been settled, and Dr. Mom was right. In the 1980s, Marvin Sackler of Mount Sinai Medical Center in Miami, Florida, published the first serious study showing that cold sufferers who got hot chicken soup felt better faster than those who got plain hot water, and dozens of studies since have said, man, he's right. Nobody really knows why chicken soup works, but who cares? It works.

So I'll move on to other foods that make you feel better when you have the sniffles — for example, sweet foods. Scientists do know why sweeteners — white sugar, brown sugar, honey, molasses — soothe a sore throat. All sugars are *demulcents,* substances that coat and soothe the irritated mucous membranes.

Lemons aren't sweet, and they have less vitamin C than orange juice, but their popularity in the form of *hot lemonade* (tea with lemon and sugar) and sour lemon drops is unmatched. Why? Because a lemon's sharp flavor cuts through to your taste buds and makes the sugary stuff more palatable. In addition, the sour taste makes saliva flow, which also soothes your throat.

Food and sex: What do these foods have in common?

Oysters, celery, onions, asparagus, mushrooms, truffles, chocolate, honey, caviar, bird's nest soup, and alcohol beverages. No, that's not a menu for the very, very picky. It's a partial list of foods long reputed to be *aphrodisiacs,* substances that rev up the libido and improve sexual performance. Take a second look, and you'll see why each is on the list.

Two (celery, asparagus) are shaped something like a male sex organ. Three (oysters, mushrooms, and truffles) are said to arouse emotion because they resemble parts of the female anatomy. (Oysters are also high in zinc, the mineral that keeps the prostate gland healthy and ensures a steady production of the male hormone testosterone. A 3-ounce serving of Pacific oysters gives you 9 milligrams of zinc, about 82 percent of the 11 milligrams a day recommended for adult men.)

Caviar (fish eggs) and bird's nest soup are symbols of fertility. Onions — and *Spanish fly* (cantharides) — contain chemicals that produce a mild burning sensation when eliminated in urine; some people, masochists to be sure, may confuse this feeling with arousal. Honey is the quintessential sweetener: The Bible's Song of Solomon compares it to the lips of the beloved. Alcohol beverages relax the inhibitions (but overindulgence reduces sexual performance, especially in men). As for chocolate, well, it's a veritable lover's cocktail, with stimulants (caffeine, theobromine), a marijuana-like compound called anandamide, and phenylethylamine, a chemical produced in the bodies of people in love.

So do these foods actually make you feel sexy? Yes and no. An aphrodisiac isn't a food that sends you in search of a lover as soon as you eat it. No, it's one that makes you feel so good that you can follow through on your natural instincts. Which is as fine a description as you're likely to get of oysters, celery, onions, asparagus, mushrooms, truffles, chocolate, honey, caviar, bird's nest soup, and wine.

Hot stuff — such as peppers, horseradish (freshly grated is definitely the most potent), and onions — contain mustard oils that irritate the membranes lining your nose and mouth and even make your eyes water. As a result, it's easier to blow your nose or cough up mucus.

Finally, there's coffee, a real boon to snifflers. When you're sick, your body piles up *cytokines,* chemicals that carry messages among immune system cells that fight infection. When cytokines pile up in brain tissue, you get sleepy, which may explain why you're so drowsy when you have a cold. True, rest can help to boost your immune system and fight off the cold, but once in a while you have to get up. Like to go to work.

The caffeine in even a single cup of regular coffee can make you more alert. Caffeine is also a mood elevator (see Chapter 24) and a *vasoconstrictor* (a chemical that helps shrink swollen, throbbing blood vessels in your head). That's why it may help relieve a headache. When I have a cold, one cup of espresso with tons of sugar can make life bearable. But nothing's perfect: Drinking coffee may intensify the side effects of OTC (over-the-counter) cold remedies containing decongestants and/or caffeine that make some people feel jittery.

Check the label warnings and directions before using coffee with your cold medicine. Vasoconstrictors reduce the diameter of certain blood vessels and may restrict proper circulation. Couldn't hurt to check with your doctor, too, if you're taking meds for a chronic condition such as high blood pressure.

Eating for a Better Body (And Brain)

Citrus fruits are rich in vitamin C, an antioxidant vitamin that seems to slow the development of cataracts. Bran cereals provide fiber that can rev up your intestinal tract, countering the natural tendency of the contractions that move food through your gut to slow a bit as you grow older (which is why older people are more likely to be constipated). Getting enough calories to maintain a healthy weight helps protect against wrinkles. And although a diet with adequate amounts of fat doesn't totally prevent dry skin, it does give you a measure of protection. That's one reason why virtually all sensible diet gurus, including the American Heart Association and the Dietary Guidelines, recommend some fat or oil every day.

And now for a word about memory. Actually, two words: Varied diet.

As long ago as 1983, a study of 250 healthy adults, ages 60 to 94, at the University of New Mexico School of Medicine showed that the people who ate a wide range of nutritious foods performed best on memory and thinking tests. According to researcher Philip J. Garry, PhD, professor of pathology at New Mexico School of Medicine, overall good food habits seemed to be more important than any one food or vitamin. Maybe people with good memory are just more likely to remember that they need a good diet.

Or maybe it's really the food. In 1997, another survey, this time at Complutense University (Madrid, Spain), showed that men and women age 60 to 90 who eat foods rich in vitamin E, vitamin C, folic acid, dietary fiber, and complex carbohydrates do better on cognitive tests. Is it the antioxidant vitamins? Does a lowfat diet protect the brain? No one knows for sure right now, but it may turn out that sticking with this same-old, same-old lowfat, high-fiber diet as you grow older may help you to remember to stick to the same-old low-fat, high-fiber diet — for years and years and years. (For more on feeding your brain at any age, see Chapter 24.)

Delivering Meds with Dinner

If an adventurous band of plant biologists have their way, the world's children — and their needle-phobic parents — will someday get their vaccine inoculations with dinner rather than from a sharp stick in the arm.

Vaccines protect by introducing a substance called an antigen into your body. The *antigen* — a live or killed microbe particle — provokes an immune response in which you make antibodies to fight the antigen. This reaction inoculates you by teaching your body how to fight a specific infectious agent, such as the flu virus. If you're exposed later on, you're ready to beat the bug.

Most modern vaccines are injected. Some, like the polio vaccine, may be delivered on a sugar cube. Others can be inhaled. But for 15 years, Charles Arntzen, founder of Arizona State University's Biodesign Institute at Arizona State University, and his fellows across the country have been working toward creating *edible vaccines* — vaccines created via genetic engineering, by inserting the antigen, a viral gene, into food.

Not just any food, mind you. Heat destroys vaccines, so to get the benefits, you'd have to eat the food raw. To date, researchers have concentrated on potatoes, tomatoes, and bananas, with the emphasis on the latter two because — let's face it — raw potatoes are no treat.

The primary target for the vaccines is diarrheal disease, such as cholera and E. coli, which kill more than 2.5 million children under the age of 5 every year. Other possibilities include the Norwalk virus that's played havoc with cruise liner vacations, hepatitis B, and HIV, the virus that causes AIDS.

In trials with cows, mice, rabbits, and mink, antigen-containing tobacco leaves, alfalfa, tomatoes, and lettuce leaves have been able to trigger immune reactions to diseases as varied as anthrax and the common cold. In a handful of FDA-approved human studies at the National Vaccine Testing Center, the University of Maryland, and Roswell Park Cancer Centre in Buffalo, New York, human volunteers who ate about 100 grams (3.5 ounces) of raw potatoes containing anti-diarrheal or hepatitis vaccines showed an immune response similar to what you might expect from an injected vaccine.

Most researchers expect edible vaccines for animals to show up before edible vaccines for human beings. When the human versions do arrive, the plant scientists say they'll be cheap, administered without a needle and without a doctor.

Just don't expect to toss some seeds in the window box and grow your own. For one thing, fresh food has a relatively short shelf life. You can't stick your vaccine-laden banana in the fridge and use it sometime in the next six months. Second, unless the food is grown in controlled conditions, you can't be sure it has the correct amount of protective antigen. Finally, nobody wants these genetically modified foods to somehow slip into the general food supply.

In the end, the plant guys say, the banana, tomato, potato, or other vaccine-toting food will probably be sliced and diced, frozen, or ground to powder and pressed into chips or tucked into a pill to make a stable med that can be produced with basic agricultural and food-processing technologies available virtually anywhere around the globe.

No needles, no doctors, no fuss. Now that's a med any mother could love.

The Last Word on Food versus Medicine

Sometimes, a person with a life-threatening illness is frightened by the side effects or the lack of certainty in standard medical treatment. In desperation, she may turn down medicine and turn to diet therapy. Alas, this decision may be hazardous to her already-compromised health.

No reputable doctor denies the benefits of a healthful diet for any patient at any stage of any illness. Food not only sustains the body but also can lift the spirit. But although food and diet may enhance the effects of many common drugs, no one has found them to be an adequate, effective substitute for (among other medicines).

- ✔ Antibiotics and other drugs used to fight infections
- ✔ Vaccines or immunizations used to prevent communicable diseases
- ✔ Anticancer drugs

If your doctor suggests altering your diet to make your treatment more effective, your brain will tell you, *Hey, that makes sense.* But if someone suggests chucking your doctor and tossing away your medicine in favor of food therapy alone, heed the natural warning in your head. You know there's no free lunch and — as yet — no truly magical food, either.

The history of food and medicine

Common wisdom to the contrary, doctors do have a sense of humor. Witness this "history of medicine" attributed to that famous author Anonymous and currently making the rounds of medical meetings and blogs:

2000 B.C. "Here, eat this root."

A.D. 1000 "That root is heathen. Here, say this prayer."

A.D. 1850 "That prayer is superstition. Here, drink this potion."

A.D. 1940 "That potion is snake oil. Here, swallow this pill."

A.D. 1985 "That pill is ineffective. Here, take this antibiotic."

A.D. 2000 "That antibiotic doesn't work. Here, eat this root."

Part VI
The Part of Tens

The 5th Wave   By Rich Tennant

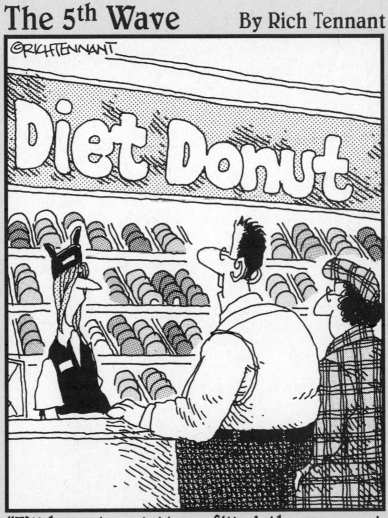

"I'll have two lettuce filled, three carrot glazed, five celery frosted..."

In this part . . .

1f you've ever read a *For Dummies* book, you know what to expect here — nifty lists of useful factoids that make great conversation starters and help you wind your way through the subject at hand.

In this book, that means ten great nutrition Web sites, ten superstar foods, ten terrific foods starting with the letter *P* (really), and ten easy ways to cut the calories without eliminating tasty food. On a scale of 1 to 10, that adds up to an easy 10.

Chapter 27

Ten or So Nutrition Web Sites

*T*he current and one archived nutrition-oriented Web sites listed in this chapter give you accurate, balanced information: nutritional guidelines, medical news, interactive sites, directories, and more. And these sites are only a start. Had Wiley Publishing called this part of the book The Part of Hundreds rather than The Part of Tens, it would have been a cinch to include many more.

But there is no reason a curious reader cannot find additional sites. Type "nutrition information" into the search bar and up come McDonald's, a bunch of university sites, and government sites here and abroad. Check carefully to assure yourself that the site is reliable (the suffixes gov and edu are a good sign) and away you go.

U.S. Department of Agriculture Nutrient Database

```
www.nal.usda.gov/fnic/foodcomp/search
```

The USDA Nutrient Database is the ultimate food info chart, with nutrient data for more than 5,000 foods in several serving sizes and different preparations. Each entry is a snapshot of a specific food serving (for example, a raw apple with skin) that lists the amount of

✔ **Water** (by weight)

✔ **Energy** (calories)

✔ **Protein**

✔ **Total fat**

✔ **Carbohydrates**

✔ **Dietary fiber**

✔ **Sugars**

✔ **Minerals:** Calcium, iron, magnesium, phosphorus, potassium, sodium, zinc, copper, and selenium

✔ **Vitamins:** Vitamin C, thiamin (vitamin B1), riboflavin (vitamin B2), niacin, vitamin B6, folate, choline, vitamin B12 (naturally occurring or, added), vitamin A (total), vitamin A as retinol, alpha carotene, beta carotene, cryptoxanthin, lyciopene, lutein, luteine + zeaxanthin, vitamin E (naturally occurring), vitamin E (added), vitamin D, and vitamin K

✔ **Lipids (fatty acids):** Total saturated, monounsaturated, and polyunsaturated fatty acids, plus cholesterol

✔ **Amino acids**

✔ **Other:** alcohol, caffeine, theobromine (the stimulant found primarily in tea)

When you open this site, the first page that comes up is headlined Search the USDA National Nutrient Database for Standard Reference. To find the food you're looking for, type its name — "apple," for example — into the empty box below and then click Submit. You then see a list of possibilities, such as "Babyfood, juice, apple and grape" or "Babyfood, dinner, apples and chicken, strained." Ignore the fancy stuff and scroll down to something basic, such as "Apples, raw, with skin." Click the circle next to that entry and click Submit, and a new screen lists various forms of raw apple, such as "100 grams" or "1 cup, quartered or chopped" or "1 large (3-¼" dia) (approx 2 per lb)." Choose the box in front of the serving you prefer, click the button marked Submit, and there you are — calories and nutrients for one large apple!

Click the button marked Nutrient Lists from the main page to access a list of foods showing the content of a single nutrient, such as protein, calories, vitamin C, calcium, or beta-carotene. Then follow directions to get the list you want, with the foods arranged either in alphabetical order or by the amount of the nutrient in the food.

Note: The lists are displayed as PDF (portable document format) files; to read them, you need Adobe Acrobat Reader, available free at `http://get.adobe.com/reader/?promoid=BUIGO`.

USDA Food and Nutrition Information Center (FNIC)

www.nal.usda.gov/fnic

Have you worked your way through every single one of the several thousand listings on the USDA Nutrient Database in the previous section? Then come on over to FNIC, which is part of the USDA National Agricultural Library.

To access its info, slide your mouse over to the box on the left side of the home page and pick a subject. The choices are Dietary Guidance; Lifestyle Nutrition; Diet and Disease; Food Composition; Weight and Obesity; Food Safety; Food Labeling; Dietary Supplements; Nutrition Assistance Programs; Surveys, Reports and Research; and Professional and Career Resources.

My particular favorite is Surveys, Reports and Research. All categories are updated frequently. As a result, this one is a superlative guide to the latest food and nutrition news, including legislation.

U.S. Food and Drug Administration

www.fda.gov

Entering the FDA Web site is like opening the door to the world's biggest nutritional-information toy store. So much stuff is on the (virtual) shelves that you hardly know which item to grab first. Luckily, in this store, all the toys are free, and plenty of links to other helpful information mean you can linger here happily for days. Weeks. Years. Maybe forever.

The FDA's charter includes drugs as well as food, so on the left of the home page, you can click links to information on medicines for people and pets, poisons and side effects, medical devices (think pacemakers), and products that give off radiation. The link titled How to Comment on Proposed Regulations makes it possible for you to add your two cents, maybe more, regarding new rules proposed by the FDA, such as the New Final Rule to Ensure Egg Safety, Reduce Salmonella Illnesses that went into effect as this page was being typed.

Of course, for people who want to know everything about food, the main event on the left side of the page is the button marked Food. Click the Food link, and you move to the main page of the food section with links to Biotechnology, Dietary Supplements, Food Defense & Emergency Response, Food Ingredients & Packaging, Food Safety, Guidance, Compliance & Regulatory Information, International Activities, Labeling & Nutrition, News & Events, Resources for You, and Science & Research.

My particular favorite here is Resources for You because the day I tried it, clicking the link took me to "The new Food Safety Alerts & Tips Widget." What's a *widget?* A thingee that lets a computer user "interface with the application and operating system." For example, the ubiquitous and universally annoying Microsoft Office Assistant is a widget.

American Dietetic Association

www.eatright.org

This site features nutrition recommendations, tips, guidelines, research, policy, and stats from the world's largest membership association of nutrition professionals, primarily registered dietitians. (For a quick rundown on who's who in nutrition science, see Chapter 1.)

The ADA home page features links to categories (such as Professional Development) that are clearly meant to appeal to association members. But the site also has tidbits for consumers, such as daily nutrition tips, a monthly feature, and nutrition position papers.

Click For the Public to access a page with links to subjects of general concern such as childhood obesity, food safety, sports nutrition, and — a real bonus — sources in languages other than English.

In other words, if you can bend your brain around the much-too-adorable net address ("eatright"? Give me a break!), this site, written and reviewed by nutrition professionals, is a true treasure trove.

The American Heart Association

www.americanheart.org

The indisputable link between diet and heart disease risk, not to mention the AHA site's user-friendly approach, makes this site a must-stop on your nutritional tour of the Web.

Starting at the home page, click Getting Healthy at the top. When the page changes, slide your mouse to Nutrition Center. Up pops a list of subjects, such as a dictionary of nutrition, a guide to healthy restaurant choices, nutrition quizzes, and so on. You can click Fats and Oils for the absolute expert's guide to fatty ingredients or click Physical Activity for the serious or beginner athlete's guide to exercising your heart muscle.

All in all, a thoroughly valuable series of clicks.

The American Cancer Society

www.cancer.org

Until now, the American Cancer Society was barely a blip on the screen of nutrition sources. Today, with a growing number of well-designed studies to demonstrate that some foods and diet regimens may reduce your risk of certain types of cancer while others put you in harm's way, the ACS Web site offers solid reporting on this area of nutritional research.

True, most of the nutrition news you find here is available elsewhere, but this site's defined focus provides easy access to other cancer-related topics.

For example, when you click the Stay Healthy button at the top of the ACS home page, that brings up a page with three broad choices:

- ✔ Eat Healthy
- ✔ Get Active, Eat Healthy
- ✔ Find Healthy Recipes

Each offers consumer-friendly information and advice directly linked to specific aspects of cancer prevention or cancer treatment, such as the article "Diet and Physical Activity: What's the Cancer Connection?"

The Food Allergy and Anaphylaxis Network

www.foodallergy.org

The Food Allergy and Anaphylaxis Network (FAAN) is a nonprofit membership organization (individual membership fee: $50/year or $500/lifetime) whose participants include families, doctors, dietitians, nurses, support groups, and food manufacturers in the United States, Canada, and Europe. The group provides education about food allergies in addition to support and coping strategies for people who are allergic to specific foods.

From FAAN's home page, you can link to updates, daily tips, newsletter excerpts, and all the usual service-oriented goodies. The site's best feature is a no-charge e-mail alert system. Click the link under Special Allergy Alerts, fill out the form, and submit it to the site. You're now connected to an early warning system with allergy-linked news and information about recalls of troublesome products, such as bags of cashews that may mistakenly contain peanuts.

This no-nonsense, highly accessible site is required reading for people with food allergies. Others, such as families and friends, can also benefit from its solid information and support services.

International Food Information Council (IFIC)

www.ific.org

The International Food Information Council (IFIC), created in 1985, is a nonprofit organization dedicated to improving the relationship between the nutrition community — scientists, food manufacturers, health professionals, government officials — and the news media. Although the council's membership includes corporations that make and sell food products, IFIC plays no role in marketing products or promoting its members. Its aim is to make sure that consumers get accurate information about diet and health.

The home page has the requisite For Consumers link, but the link to Hot Topics and Newsletter are well worth investigating. The site also offers articles on basic nutrition topics, such as functional foods, oral health, dietary fats and fat substitutes, and additional resources. The writing is accessible, the information impeccable.

IFIC is a trade group, so purists may complain about some IFIC positions, such as its endorsement of some food additives, but the site's intelligent approach to complex and emotional issues allows you to make up your own mind.

Mayo Clinic

www.mayoclinic.com

When you open the home page, type **nutrition** into the search box. The day I reviewed the site for this new edition of *Nutrition For Dummies,* that search pulled up 28 pages with 271 entries ranging from "Nutrition and healthy eating" to "Sea salt vs. table salt: Which is healthier?"

Of course, nutrition information isn't all this award-winning site has to offer. In fact, the virtue of a site created by one of America's premier medical centers is that it's packed with, well, medical links, many nutrition-related.

For example, when you're done with nutrients, return to the home page and use the A-B-C box to look up any one of hundreds of diseases and medical conditions. Or check out your symptoms or scroll through a list of medical tests using the same A-B-C buttons.

Is it any wonder that this site picks up awards every year or so?

American Council on Science and Health (ACSH) and the Center for Science in the Public Interest (CSPI)

```
www.acsh.org
```

```
www.cspinet.org
```

The American Council on Science and Health and the Center for Science in the Public Interest are two nonprofit consumer-friendly organizations that usually sit on opposite sides of any nutritional issue. ACSH is cool; CSPI is a hot-button advocate.

For example, CSPI believes many additives are hazardous to your health; ACSH says some additives are useful in some foods for some people. This kind of disagreement often means that if you punch up the same search word or phrase on both sites, you'll be able to nail down the pros and cons of a particular issue.

Both sites feature news releases, position papers, online membership enrollment, order forms for publications, and links to other sites.

Which site you prefer is pretty much a matter of personality, but you really can't go wrong with either one.

WebMD

```
www.webmd.com/default.htm
```

The home page of the Net's all-purpose medical information site has a button for Healthy Eating and Diet.

Clicking that button opens a page with lists of subjects too numerous to type in one simple entry here. However, if you've ever planned, are planning now, or plan in the future to lose weight, it would be folly not to ask you to scroll down the page to a box on the right side labeled Diets A–Z, which really is

A (Atkins) to Z (The Zone) and pretty much every other weight loss scheme (okay, regimen) in-between.

As on all WebMD-related sites (Medscape.com, eMedicine.com, theHeart. org), the material is current, accessible, and sound.

The Archive

The Tufts University Nutrition Navigator was the mother of all Internet nutrition guides. The site, developed by the Tufts University Gerald J. and Dorothy R. Friedman School of Nutrition Science and Policy, evaluated several hundred other nutrition Web sites on a 25-point scale measuring content and reliability on a scale ranging from Among the Best (22–25 points) down to Not Recommended (below 12 points). The site categories included those devoted to women, men, family, older adults, general nutrition, health professionals, educators, journalists, weight management, special dietary needs, and the always popular hot topics.

The site should be included in this list, but when I went to verify the details for this book,

this message popped up: "This web site is not currently conducting new review of nutrition web sites. However, the reviews and ratings contained on these pages still remain of value when taken in the context in which they were originally written."

The Tufts people say that the Friedman School is working to create a "virtual Community of Practice" to serve the same broad purpose as the Navigator in providing reliable information. Click the site (`http://navigator.tufts.edu`) to add your name to their e-mail list.

In a perfect world, you might one day discover *You've Got Mail* from a new navigator.

Chapter 28

Ten or So Superstar Foods

*E*ver since Eve pulled that apple (really a pomegranate) off the tree of knowledge in the Garden of Eden, people have been attributing special powers to one food or another.

This chapter is by no means the complete A+ list. For example, I don't include chicken soup, because what more can anyone say about this universal panacea? How about this: These ten or so foods are super good enough.

Alcohol

Moderate alcohol consumption relaxes muscles and mood, expands blood vessels to lower blood pressure temporarily, and lowers the risk of heart disease, either by reducing the stickiness of *blood platelets* (small particles that can clump together to form a blood clot), by relaxing blood vessels (making them temporarily larger), or by increasing the amount of HDLs ("good cholesterol") in blood. Although some forms of alcohol, such as red wines, have gotten more press attention with regard to these effects, the fact is that controlled studies show similar effects with all forms of alcohol beverages — wine, beer, and spirits.

Common wisdom to the contrary, alcohol sometimes may also be beneficial to the brain. Yes, drinking can make you fuzzy, which is why you should never drink and drive. However, recent studies suggest that red wine may reduce the adverse effects after a stroke, and a report from the Institute of Preventive Medicine at Kommunehospitalet in Copenhagen, Denmark, and

Johns Hopkins University in Maryland shows that regular consumption of moderate amounts of wine may keep minds sharp into older age. (Check it out in Chapter 10.) So, the next time you lift a (moderate) glass and toast "To your health," consider yourself right on the money.

Beans

All beans are rich in soluble dietary fiber, the *gums* and *pectins* that mop up fats and cholesterol to prevent their being absorbed by your body. (Oats, which also are rich in gums, particularly gums called *beta glucans,* produce the same effect.)

Beans are also valuable for people with diabetes. Because they're digested very slowly, eating beans produces only a gradual increase in the level of sugar circulating in your blood. As a result, metabolizing beans requires less insulin than eating other types of high-carb foods, such as pasta and potatoes (see Chapter 9). In one now-classic study at the University of Kentucky, a diet rich in beans made it possible for people with Type 1 diabetes (their bodies produce virtually no insulin) to reduce their daily insulin intake by nearly 40 percent. Patients with Type 2 diabetes (their bodies produce some insulin) were able to reduce insulin intake by 98 percent.

Just about the only drawback to a diet rich in beans is gas resulting from the natural human inability to digest some dietary fiber and complex sugars such as *raffinose* and *stachyose,* which sit in your gut as fodder for the resident friendly bacteria that digest the carbs and then release carbon dioxide and methane, a smelly gas.

 One way to reduce intestinal gas production is to reduce the complex sugar content of the beans before you eat them. Here's how: Bring a pot of water to a boil. Turn off the heat. Add the beans. Let them soak for several hours. The sugars leach out into the water, which means you can discard the sugars by draining the beans and adding fresh water to cook in. If that doesn't do the job, try two heat-and-soak sessions before cooking.

Berries

Berries are top of the list among foods rich in antioxidants, the naturally occurring compounds that inactivate *free radicals,* particles that would otherwise damage cells. In addition, eating berries may step up the activity of cells in the liver that reduce the production of cholesterol and other artery-clogging fats. Nobody knows for sure exactly how many berries you have to eat to lower your cholesterol, but some studies suggest that ounce for ounce, blueberries have one of the highest antioxidant contents in the vegetable and fruit world. As a result, several studies show that eating berries may reduce the risk of heart attack by preventing the small particles known as platelets from clumping together into blood clots.

Even better, eating blueberries (the designated star of the group) may improve memory. The first evidence came from animal studies in 2008; then, in 2010, a report in the *Journal of Agricultural and Food Chemistry* reported that volunteers in their 70s with early memory problems who drank 2 to 2.5 cups of blueberry juice a day every day for two months showed "significant" improvement on memory and learning tests. The control group — people who did not get the juice — showed no such change. (More on food and the brain in Chapter 24.)

Bison

Bison is back. The really big *bovid ruminant* (translation: an animal related to a cow) is no longer an endangered species. In fact, according to the 2,500-member National Bison Association, the bison herd, once hunted almost to extinction, is currently up to 500,000 animals, most on private ranches.

The Association estimates that Americans now consume up to 1 million pounds of bison each month. And no wonder: Ounce for ounce, bison — water buffalo, an African animal whose milk is also nutritionally valuable — has less fat, less sat fat, less cholesterol, fewer calories, and more protein than beef. It's pretty tasty, too, with a rich, meaty flavor that survives broiling and grilling but may, alas, turn dry when roasted — which is why most Americans get their bison as a broiled burger.

But here's a caution: Never say "buffalo" when you mean "bison." The scientific name for American bison is *Bison bison*. The word *buffalo* comes from French explorers who called bison "boeuf" (meaning beef). English changed that to "buff." Common usage smoothed that out to "buffle" and eventually "buffalo." Actual buffalo are native to Asia and Africa. Which kind of makes you wonder why the National *Bison* Association named 2010 The Year of the *Buffalo*.

Breast Milk

Human breast milk is more nutritious than cow's milk for human babies. It has a higher percentage of easily digested, high-energy fats and carbohydrates. Its proteins stimulate an infant's immune system, encouraging his or her white blood cells to produce plenty of infection-fighting antibodies, including those that go after viruses linked to infant diarrhea, which accounts for 23 percent of all deaths among children younger than 5. And get this: In

2004, a report in the British Medical Journal *Lancet* said that feeding a baby breast milk rather than formula for the first month of life may lower the child's cholesterol levels later in life, reduce the child's eventual risk of high blood pressure, and keep a person slimmer as he or she grows older.

And if that were not enough, in the spring of 2010, a researcher at the University of California San Diego reported that *lauric acid,* an ingredient in human breast milk (and coconut oil) may be a promising topical treatment for acne treatment.

All in all, a pretty good way to start off in life and sail through adolescence, don't-cha think?

Chocolate

Westerners have been fools for chocolate ever since the Spanish conquistadors discovered it at Montezuma's Mexican court. And why not? The cocoa bean is a good source of energy, fiber, protein, carbohydrates, B vitamins, and minerals (1 ounce of dark sweet chocolate has 12 percent of the iron and 33 percent of the magnesium a healthy woman needs each day).

Chocolate is heart healthy. True, chocolate's fat, cocoa butter, is 59 percent saturated fatty acids, primarily stearic acid. But unlike other saturated fats, stearic acid neither increases LDLs ("bad cholesterol") nor lowers HDLs ("good cholesterol"). In addition, stearic acid makes blood platelets less likely to clump together into a blood clot, thus lowering the risk of heart attack or stroke. And, like other beans, cocoa beans contain gums and pectins that sop up fats before they reach your bloodstream (see "Beans," earlier in this chapter). Finally, a study published in the *Proceedings of the National Academy of Sciences* in January 2006 credits the cocoa compound (–)epicatechin (translation: *minus epicatechin*) with the ability to help blood vessels relax — lowering blood pressure and once again reducing the risk of heart attack.

Chocolate is also rich in antioxidants, the naturally occurring compounds that inactivate free radicals (small particles that can damage cells). In 2007, when the U.S. Department of Agriculture created a scale to rank the antioxidant content of several hundred foods, red beans came in at #50 but unsweetened cocoa powder was #10; unsweetened baking chocolate, #16; and dark chocolate candy, #31.

Does all this mean chocolate is a bona fide component of a healthful diet? Yes. Especially because (see Chapter 24) it's a veritable happiness cocktail containing *caffeine* (a mood elevator and central nervous system stimulant), *theobromine* (a muscle stimulant), *phenylethylamine* (another mood elevator), and *anandamide,* a chemical that stimulates the same areas of the brain that marijuana does, although you'd have to consume 25 pounds or more unsweetened chocolate at one sitting to get even the smallest marijuana-like effect.

Coffee

For years, there was nothing but bad news about coffee. Pancreatic cancer. Cystic breasts. High cholesterol. Heart disease. Stroke. Birth defects. Heartburn and reflux. But more recent research shows no link at all between drinking coffee and an increased risk of any of these conditions. True, coffee may upset your stomach and keep you up at night, but as *Heartburn & Reflux For Dummies* (written by me and published by Wiley) explains, for most people, these effects are almost always linked to excess consumption, an amount that varies from person to person.

In moderation, regular coffee, like alcohol, qualifies for anybody's list of super foods. Its most active ingredient, caffeine, elevates your mood and increases your ability to concentrate; may improve your athletic performance (although for NCAA athletes, urine concentrations greater than 15ug/ml is illegal); can help shrink the swollen, throbbing blood vessels that make your head ache; and boosts the effect of painkillers, which is why caffeine is often included in over-the-counter analgesic (pain-relieving) products.

Two studies released 12 days apart in the spring of 2010 have even better news about java. The first, published in the *Journal of Agriculture and Food Chemistry,* suggests that regular coffee consumption may reduce the risk of Type 2 diabetes, at least in laboratory mice. The second, published in the journal *Cancer Epidemiology, Biomarkers & Prevention,* posits the possibility that drinking coffee may reduce the risk of human cancers of the head and neck.

Obviously, there is more to come.

Nuts

Pass up the pretzels. Skip the chips. At snack time, reach for the almonds. Although nuts are technically a high-fat food, multiple studies, including several at California's Loma Linda University, say that adding moderate amounts of nuts to a cholesterol-lowering diet or substituting nuts for other high-fat foods, such as meats, may cut normal to moderately high levels of total cholesterol and LDLs ("bad cholesterol") by as much as 12 percent.

These guys should know. A while back, they made headlines with a walnut study in which volunteers were given one of two diets, both based on National Cholesterol Education Program (NCEP) recommendations. People on Diet #1 got 20 percent of their calories from fats in oils and fatty foods, such as meat. Folks on Diet #2 got 20 percent of their calories from high-fat nuts instead of meat, but both controlled-fat diets appeared to lower cholesterol levels.

The take-home message here is that although nuts are high in fat, their fats are polyunsaturated fatty acids and monounsaturated cholesterol busters (more about them in Chapter 7). And nuts also provide other heart-healthy nutrients such as arginine (an amino acid your body uses to make a clot-blocking compound called nitric oxide) and dietary fiber.

So feel free to go (sensibly) nuts for nuts.

White Tea

Black and green? So 20th century. The hot new color in tea is white. The leaves for all three teas come from one plant, *Camellia sinensis.* But those leaves meant for black and green teas are rolled and fermented before drying, while those destined for white teas — which actually brew up pale yellow-red — aren't. Nutritionally, this small change makes a big difference.

Flavonoids are natural chemicals credited with tea's ability to lower cholesterol, reduce the risk of some kinds of cancer, and protect your teeth from cavity-causing bacteria. Fresh tea leaves are rich in flavonoids called *catechins,* but processing the leaves to make black and green teas releases enzymes that enable individual catechins to hook up with others, forming new flavor and coloring agents called *polyphenols* (poly = many) that give flavor and color to black and green teas. Because white tea leaves are neither rolled nor fermented, fewer of their catechins marry into polyphenols. According to researchers at the Linus Pauling Institute (LPI) at Oregon State University, the plain catechin content of white tea is three times that of green tea. Black tea comes in a distant third.

Why should you care about this? Because all those catechins seem to be good for living bodies. For example, when LPI researchers tested white tea's ability to inhibit cell mutations in bacteria and slow down cell changes leading to colon cancer in rats, the white tea beat green tea, the former health champ. And when scientists at University Hospitals of Cleveland and Case Western Reserve University applied creams containing white-tea extract to human skin (on volunteers) and exposed the volunteers to artificial sunlight, the creamed skin developed fewer pre-cancerous changes. To be fair, green tea preparations were also protective, but white tea has less caffeine than either green or black tea, which makes it the perfect brew for a recovering caffeine fiend.

Whole Grains

Are you a man who plans to live forever? Then a team of nutrition scientists at Harvard/Brigham and Women's Hospital in Boston have three words for you: whole grain cereal. When the investigators took a look at the health stats for a one-year period in the lives of the 86,190 male doctors in the long-running Physicians' Health Study, they found 3,114 deaths among the study volunteers, including 1,381 deaths from heart attack and stroke. Then they looked a little closer and discovered that eating habits count. Men who ate at least one serving of whole grain cereal a day were 27 percent less likely to die than were men who ate refined grain products. The whole-grain group was also as much as 28 percent less likely to succumb to a heart attack, regardless of how much they weighed, whether they smoked or drank alcohol or took vitamins pills or had a history of high blood pressure and high cholesterol.

Nobody yet knows exactly why this should be so. But they do know that whole grains are a treasure trove of dietary fiber, vitamins, minerals, and other phytochemicals (plant compounds such as antioxidants) that protect by lowering blood pressure and cholesterol while improving the body's ability to process nutrients, particularly carbohydrates.

The question is, how much cereal must you eat to benefit? The studies say more is better, but one serving a day is better than none at all. To find the right cereal, check the Nutrition Facts label. If whole grain is the first ingredient and each serving has at least 2 grams dietary fiber, you've found breakfast. Hate cereal? Whole-grain bread is an acceptable alternative. And, yes, whole grains are an equal opportunity dish. Earlier studies suggest that women, too, may come out ahead by adding whole grain to their daily diets.

Yogurt

Yogurt is milk with added friendly bacteria that digest milk sugar (lactose) to produce lactic acid, a natural preservative that gives the flavor of yogurt its pleasant bite. Yogurt is definitely magical for people who are *lactase deficient* (meaning they don't produce enough lactase to digest milk sugar, so they get gassy whenever they drink milk).

But there's no evidence to show that yogurt is a longevity tonic, a claim traced back to Ilya Ilyich Metchnikoff, a Russian Nobel Prize winner (1908; Physiology/Medicine), who believed that people die prematurely entirely because of the action of "putrefying bacteria" in the intestines. Searching for a way to disarm the putrefiers, Metchnikoff ended up in Bulgaria, a place where a significant percentage of the population lived into their late 80s.

Historians may argue that the only way to live that long in Bulgaria was to avoid Bulgarian politics, but Metchnikoff credited the organisms used to make Bulgarian cultured milk. He was wrong. The bugs, christened *L. bulgaricus,* make nice yogurt but don't take up residence in the human gut. This hardly mattered to Metchnikoff, who died in Paris in 1916, at the relatively young age of 71. His faith in yogurt, however, continues to cycle in and out of fashion.

Chapter 29

Ten Terrific Foods Starting with the Letter P

*I*f your first thought on seeing the title of this chapter was "It's a joke?" then think again. Count the listings in your favorite food book, and you're likely to discover that more foods have names beginning with *P* than with any other letter of the alphabet. Choosing ten nutritious ones is a cinch.

Note for the curious: As is the case all through this book, the nutrient numbers in this chapter come from the *USDA National Nutrient Database for Standard Reference.* The Web site (see Chapter 27) is online at www.nal.usda.gov/fnic/foodcomp/search.

Papaya

The papaya, also known as the *paw-paw,* is a pear-shaped melon with versatile pale yellow flesh that you can serve cooked when unripe or enjoy straight when ripe (look for an orange-y gold rind). Either way, one small papaya provides about half an adult's daily value of vitamin A, more than a day's worth of vitamin C, and about 10 percent of the daily dietary fiber allotment.

In 2010, the *Journal of Ethnopharmacology,* a publication dedicated to "people's use of plants, fungi, animals, microorganisms, and minerals and their biological and pharmacological effects," carried a report from researchers at the University of Florida and the University of Tokyo saying that adding extract of dried papaya leaves to breast, cervical, liver, lung, and pancreatic tumors grown in a laboratory setting seemed to step up the production of a molecule that interferes with cancer cell growth without harming normal cells. Which component in the extract does the heavy lifting is still unknown.

While waiting for the next study, smart cooks should know that the leaves of the papaya plant are also useful in the kitchen. The leaves are packed with *papain,* the *proteolytic* (protein-breaking) enzyme found in commercial meat tenderizers. In Central America, where the papaya was born, wrapping meat in papaya leaves is the standard tenderizing technique. But papain can irritate the skin, so handle the leaves with care. Or, given the scarcity of papaya leaves in modern food markets, just pick up the store-bought product.

Parsley

Parsley is a member of the carrot family. Curley leaf or flat, this herb is unlikely to be a major part of anyone's daily diet, but as Spencer Tracey said of Katherine Hepburn in the 1930 movie *Pat and Mike* (ask your grandmother), "Not much meat on her, but what there is, is cherce," Brooklyn-ese for "choice."

For example, ½ cup of fresh chopped parsley tossed in a salad adds 1,500 IU/450 mcg vitamin A (more than 30 percent of the current RDI for an adult), 40 mg vitamin C (more than 40 percent of the adult RDI), and 1.9 mg iron (more than 20 percent of the adult RDI).

Pear

The pear is a botanical cousin of the apple, a late-summer early-fall fruit that grows most plentifully in the American northwest. (Washington State is the leading producer of both apples and pears.)

Although the apple is more popular, the pear is a better bet, nutritionally speaking. True, a 5-ounce fresh pear has 9 more calories than a 5-ounce apple, but the pear has 25 percent more protein than the apple, 30 percent more dietary fiber, including soluble pectin in the flesh and the insoluble fibers hemicellulose in the peel and lignan in those tiny gritty particles that crunch when you chew the pear. The pear also has 40 percent more iron and 50 percent more *lutein* (a naturally occurring plant chemical that protects vision).

Pears resent rough handling. Bruising or slicing one releases *polyphenoloxidase,* an enzyme that hastens the oxidation of *phenols* (alcohols) in the fruit, producing clumps of flesh-darkening brownish compounds. You can slow this natural reaction by dipping sliced pears in a protective acidic antioxidant solution, such as lemon juice or vinegar and water. (Yes, this trick also works for apples, bananas, potatoes, and some other fruits and veggies.)

Unfortunately, not every part of the pear is people-friendly. Like peach pits, apricot pits, and apple seeds, pear seeds contain *amygdalin,* a cyanide/sugar compound that breaks down into hydrogen cyanide in the stomach. An occasional seed isn't necessarily hazardous for an adult, but swallowing only a few may be lethal for a child.

Peas

Like other legumes (beans and peanuts), peas are high in dietary fiber (4.4 grams per half cup) and protein rich (4.29 grams). One-half cup peas has 477 IU vitamin A (16 percent of the RDA for a man, 21 percent for a woman), 11.36 mg vitamin C (19 percent of the RDA), and 1.24 iron (8 percent of the RDA for a woman of child-bearing age).

They taste good, too. Peas start out high in sugar, but within hours after picking, nearly half the sugar turns to starch. The fresher you get them, the sweeter they will taste. You can pop them raw, straight from the pod into your mouth or your salad. If you cook them, better make it quick. Chlorophyll, the pigment that makes green peas green, is sensitive to acids. When green vegetables, including peas, are heated, the chlorophyll reacts with acids in the cooking water or in the pea itself, forming a brownish pigment called *pheophytin* that turns peas olive drab. Swift cooking avoids this curse of steamed table cuisine.

Despite their virtues, peas are not perfect. Legumes rank among the foods most likely to trigger allergic reactions. Some nutrition guides warn that dried peas may interact with the antidepressant drugs known as MAO (mono amineoxidase) inhibitors and send your blood pressure soaring. *Purines,* byproducts of protein metabolism, may worsen the pain of *gout* (a form of arthritis). Some nutritionists think that dried peas may have enough protein to produce this effect.

Pick a peck of perfect peas

Not all peas are the same. For example, *fresh peas* are garden peas, straight from the pod. *Petits pois* is French for "small peas," peas that are mature but not yet full size. *Dried peas* are whole peas minus the natural moisture, which means they must be soaked before cooking. *Split peas* are dried peas that have been boiled, skinned, and split in half; these dried peas can be cooked without soaking. Because dried peas are minus the natural water, you get more pea solids per ounce and thus more nutrients — including calories, of course. *Pea pods* are very early pods with only a hint of peas inside; the most tender are called *snow peas; sugar peas* are a variety of snow peas. And here's a bonus: When you eat the pods with the peas, you add dietary fiber to your diet.

Plantain

The *plantain* is a kind of banana, but unlike the peel-and-eat fruit, the plantain is classified botanically as a vegetable. Unlike the banana, the plantain doesn't convert its starches to sugars as it ripens, so you have to cook the plantains before serving to make the starch granules in them swell and break open so that the flesh softens. (The "fried bananas" so popular in Latin American cuisine are usually fried plantains.)

The upside, though, is that ounce for ounce, the plantain has more than ten times as much vitamin A as a banana, twice the vitamin C, and one-third more potassium.

The even better upside is that plantains, like bananas, are rich in serotonin, dopamine, and other naturally occurring *neurotransmitters* (chemicals that make it possible for brain cells to communicate) that act as mood elevators. And if the latest chocolate research is right, you might increase the Bliss Potential by dipping those plantains in melted dark chocolate (see Chapter 28).

Pork

Ounce for ounce, pork has fewer calories and less total fat, sat fat, and cholesterol than lamb and beef. And as you read this book, a team of Canadian researchers at the Lacombe Research Centre in Alberta, the University of Alberta, and the Prairie Swine Centre in Saskatoon, Saskatchewan, is charging ahead with its attempts to pack pork with heart-healthy omega-3 fatty acids. The scientists are feeding their test animals omega-3-rich flaxseed and canola oil to discover just how much they can enrich the pork while keeping it stable in storage and tasty on the plate.

Of course, some folks say might say, why bother? If your goal is to consume omega-3s, why not just eat fish and seafood, the primary source of these good fats? But science marches on. Sooner or later, an omega-3 pork chop is sure to hit your table. Until then, Table 29-1 lists the comparable fat stats on pork, lamb, and beef.

Table 29-1	Fat Content (100 g./3.5 oz. Roasted Loin)		
	Pork	*Lamb*	*Beef*
Calories	142	217	257
Total fat (g)	4.9	11.4	15.8
Saturated fat (g)	1.7	4.6	6.2
Cholesterol (mg)	53	90	83

Potato

The humble potato is a filling food with indisputable nutrition virtues. One 7-ounce oven-baked potato, skin included, dishes up 220 calories, mostly starchy carbs, plus 4 g dietary fiber, 5 g protein, and practically no fat. True, the proteins are "incomplete," with limited amounts of some essential amino acids. But you can remedy that by serving potatoes the traditional way, boiled, with a little milk poured on. Or you could melt some (lowfat) cheese into a baked potato. (See Chapter 7 for more on the nature of proteins.)

Potatoes, which have lots of vitamin C, were once eaten raw to prevent *scurvy*, the vitamin C deficiency disease. You should know that the fresher the potato, the higher the C. After three months' storage in a cold place, a potato loses about one-third of its vitamin C; after six months, about two-thirds. Long storage also turns the potato's starches to sugar, so it tastes sweeter and less potato-like. But here's a fabulous factoid: The conversion of starch to sugar is temperature-related; if the potatoes are stored back at 70 to 75 degrees Fahrenheit, the sugars revert to starch. Amazing.

The devastating mid-18th century Irish potato famine was caused by *Phytophthora infestans,* a fungus that rotted the crops, but potatoes can be pretty mean critters on their own. The potato is a member of the nightshade family that produces a nerve poison called *solanine* (hence the potato's scientific name, *solanum tuberosum*), which makes it hard for your cells to transmit messages back and forth. Solanine, found in the green parts of the plant (leaves, stem, green spots on the skin), doesn't dissolve in water and is unaffected by heat. Any solanine present in a raw potato will still be there after you cook it. Yes, an adult might have to eat about 3 pounds of potatoes or 2.4 pounds of potato skins at one sitting to develop solanine poisoning, but better safe than sorry: Toss any potato with sprouts or green spots.

Prawns

American and Britons both speak English, but sometimes the same word means one thing in the United States and another in the U.K. Case in point: Prawns. In the States, a prawn is a very big shrimp; in the Kingdom, it's any shrimp at all.

For a few years, prawns, like lobsters, crabs, oysters, clams, and mussels, were banned from a healthy diet due to a high cholesterol content. But as nutrition scientists zeroed in on the role played by various kinds of fatty acids, particularly the nefarious saturated fat (for more on that, check out Chapter 8), foods low in sat fats were welcomed back onto the menu.

True, a 100 g/3.5 oz. serving of prawns has about 195 mg cholesterol versus about 82 mg for a similar serving of 90 percent lean hamburger. But the burger has 4.2 g sat fat, 23 percent of the total recommended daily allowance, and 14 times the 0.3 g sat fat in the prawns. In addition, like other fish and seafood, prawns are a good source of heart-healthy omega-3 fatty acids, plus minerals such as magnesium and zinc, all wrapped in a diet-pleasing 99 calories per serving.

Prunes

If you call a prune a dried plum, do you love it more? In 2000, The California Prune Board, voting "Yes," convinced the Food and Drug Administration to approve renaming the fruit, which is why cartons of prunes are now labeled "dried plums."

Of course, no matter what you call it, the prune is a food jam-packed with antioxidants, vitamin A, *nonheme iron* (the form of iron found in plants), and fiber. Lots of fiber: Ounce for ounce, the fruit has more dietary fiber than dry beans.

But who's kidding whom? The prune's true nutritional claim to fame is still its reliable ability to relieve constipation. Prunes contain *dihydrophenylisatin,* a naturally occurring chemical relative of *biscodyl,* the active ingredient in many over-the-counter laxatives. The dihydrophenylisatin is a stimulant that triggers intestinal contractions to move food along.

As a result, if you eat too many prunes, you may experience diarrhea. But you'd expect that. What may take you by surprise is an allergic reaction to sulfites used to prevent the flesh of dried fruit, including prunes, from darkening. To reduce the risk of serious side effects, including potentially lethal *anaphylaxis* (a whole body reaction that can include respiratory problems), all dried fruit containing sulfites carries a prominent warning on the label. For more about food allergies, see Chapter 23.

Pumpkin

The pumpkin, a New World original now grown on every continent except Antarctica, is a member of the squash family with nary a smidgen of waste. Boiled pumpkin flowers and leaves are green veggies. Dried or roasted pumpkin seeds are high-protein, high-fiber snacks. Pumpkin meat is an extraordinarily good source of vitamins A and C. In fact, just about the only unappetizing thing named pumpkin is the pumpkinseed, a fish not a plant, and a bone-y, though delicious, one to boot.

The most nutritious pumpkins are the golden cylindrical varieties, such as the Dickenson pumpkins grown and processed by Libby, the leading marketer of canned pumpkin. In fact, canned pumpkin is one time when processed beats natural hands down: Ounce for ounce, plain canned pumpkin has up to 20 times as much vitamin A, and up to 2.5 times as much calcium as boiled fresh pumpkin.

With all this goodness, is it any wonder that farmers around the world compete to see who can bring in the biggest pumpkin of them all? The current record-holder is a 1,725-pound giant crowned at the Ohio Valley Giant Pumpkin Growers (OVGPG) Giant Pumpkin Weigh-Off on Saturday, October 3, 2009. You can access a list of the world's biggest pumpkins at www.back yardgardener.com.

Bet you can't look without saying, "Wow."

Chapter 30

Ten Easy Ways to Cut Calories

In This Chapter

▶ Lowering the fat content of a dish

▶ Cutting back instead of cutting out

▶ Switching to healthful alternatives

▶ Noting a special tip for chopped meat

*L*osing weight is simple math. If you cut 3,500 calories out of your diet in the course of a week without reducing your daily activity, you can say goodbye to a whole pound of fat.

Yes, reading that sentence is easier than actually doing it, but two tricks make the job easier. First, cut calories in small increments — 50 here, 100 there — rather than in one big lump. Second, instead of giving up foods you really love (and then feeling deprived), switch to lowfat versions.

This chapter tells you how to make ten little changes, sometimes with brand-name products included so that you can compare different versions of a food — and sometimes different versions from the exact same company.

Switch to Lowfat or No-Fat Dairy Products

Milk and milk products are the best source for the calcium that keeps bones strong. But these same products may also be high in cholesterol, saturated fat, and calories. Reduce all three by choosing a low- or no-fat milk product.

For example, a cup of whole milk has 150 calories, but a cup of skim milk has only 85. One slice of regular Kraft American cheese has 60 calories, but one slice of Kraft Free American cheese has only 30. A sandwich made with three slices of cheese is 90 calories lighter if the cheese is "free." And not to worry about a smoothly melted, lowfat, grilled cheese sandwich. Over the years, the tech guys at the food companies have found some mysterious way to make the substitute melt just as pleasantly as the "real" cheese.

Use Sugar Substitutes

Coffee and tea have no calories, but every teaspoon of sugar you stir into your cup has 15 big ones. Multiply that by four (1 teaspoon each in four cups of coffee), and your naturally no-cal beverage can add 60 calories a day to your diet.

Sixty calories a day times seven days a week equals 420 calories, about as many as you get from four or five medium slices of unbuttered toast or five medium apples. So is this a good time to mention that one packet of sugar substitute has absolutely zero calories? Yes.

Serve Stew Instead of Steak

No matter how you slice it, red meat is red meat — cholesterol, saturated fats, and all. But if you stew your beef or lamb or pork rather than broiling or roasting it, you can skim off a lot of high-calorie fat. Just make the stew and then stick it in the fridge for a couple of hours until a layer of fat hardens on top. Spoon it off: Every tablespoon of pure fat subtracts 100 calories from dinner. And, yes, you can also cut off all visible fat before preparing the meat. Same 100 calories per tablespoon of fat.

Choose Lowfat Desserts

Who says you have to suffer to cut calories? One-half cup of Häagen-Dazs chocolate ice cream has 270 calories. One-half cup of Häagen-Dazs lowfat chocolate sorbet has 130 calories. Switching from the first to the second is no sacrifice in satisfaction.

Peel the Poultry

Most of the fat in poultry is in or just under the skin. A fried chicken breast with skin has 217 calories; without the skin, it has only 160. Half a roasted duck (with skin) has a whopping 1,287 calories; without skin, it's only 444. Even if you have a fried chicken breast every night for a week, you can save 399 calories by taking the skin off before cooking the bird. Share seven skin-less half-ducks with a friend, and you each save 2,950 calories a week by removing the skin. That's practically a pound right there.

Don't Oil the Salad

True, salad can be a lowfat, low-calorie meal. Throw in some breast of chicken and a couple of no-fat croutons or cheese cubes, and it's still mostly crunch.

But the dressing can do you in. For example, 2 tablespoons of Wishbone Italian Dressing contain 80 calories; 1 tablespoon of Hellmann's regular "real mayonnaise" has 90 calories. What to do? Switch.

Two tablespoons of Wishbone Fat Free Italian dressing add just 16 calories. One tablespoon of Hellmann's Light has only 45, half the calories of the regular. Have salad once a day for a week, and you can save 448 calories with fat-free rather than regular salad dressing or save 315 calories with light mayonnaise rather than regular.

Don't oil your pots and pans, either. Bake with parchment paper instead of greasing the pan or spraying with cooking spray. Sauté with natural juices in nonstick pans. Every tablespoon of fat you don't use means approximately 100 fewer calories in the dish.

Make One-Slice Sandwiches

Depending on the brand, one slice of bread in your daily luncheon sandwich may have anywhere from 65 to 120 calories. Do like the Scandinavians do: Eliminate one slice and serve your sandwich open-face. This strategy can cut up to 840 calories from your weekly total. And making that one bread slice whole wheat adds dietary fiber to your menu.

Eliminate the High-Fat Ingredient

A bacon, lettuce, and tomato sandwich usually comes with three strips of bacon, each one worth 100 calories. Leave off one strip and save 100 calories. Leave off two, save 200 calories. Leave off three, save 300 calories — and enjoy your lettuce and tomato sandwich with lowfat mayonnaise.

Here are some other ways to eliminate fat calories:

- Make spaghetti sauce without olive oil (100 calories a tablespoon)
- Make split pea soup without ham (55 to 90 calories an ounce)
- Make cream sauces with skim milk instead of cream (470 calories per cup for the cream; 85 to 90 calories for the skim milk)

Season the Veggies Instead of Drowning Them in Butter

Season your vegetables with herbs instead of greasing them, and you save 100 calories for every unused tablespoon of butter, margarine, or oil. Think dill on the potatoes, chives on the corn, oregano on the green beans — whatever catches your imagination.

Wash the Chopped Meat

Fill a teapot. Turn on the burner. While the water is coming to a boil, put the chopped meat in a frying pan and cook it until it browns. Pour off the fat, turn the meat into a strainer, and pour a cup of hot water over it. Repeat two times. Every tablespoon of fat that melts or drains from the meat saves you 100 calories, plus cholesterol and saturated fat. Use the defatted meat in spaghetti sauce. (Check out Figure 30-1 for the visual presentation!)

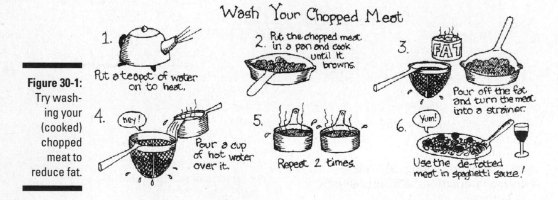

Figure 30-1: Try washing your (cooked) chopped meat to reduce fat.

Wash Your Chopped Meat

1. Put a teapot of water on to heat.

2. Put the chopped meat in a pan and cook until it browns.

3. Pour off the fat and turn the meat into a strainer.

4. hey! Pour a cup of hot water over it.

5. Repeat 2 times.

6. Yum! Use the de-fatted meat in spaghetti sauce!

Index